Explorations Between Psychoanalysis and Neuroscience

Explorations Between Psychoanalysis and Neuroscience brings together the life's work of David Olds, pioneering psychoanalyst, psychiatrist, philosopher, and key figure in neuropsychoanalysis.

Throughout the chapters, the reader is taken on a journey through Olds' theories on psychoanalysis and neuroscience as he develops new ways of examining the brain and human thought. Olds instills in the reader the importance of taking an interdisciplinary approach to psychoanalysis, psychiatry and working with patients. He expands upon his philosophical background and integrates evolutionary biology, neurobiology, cognitive science, and semiotics to show the importance of dual aspect monism in neuropsychoanalysis. The theories developed by Olds and presented in this volume will help analysts working with patients facing issues with memory, affect, consciousness, cognition, and trauma, among other difficulties.

This book will be essential reading to psychoanalysts and psychiatrists, as well as anybody interested in neuropsychoanalysis and the importance of an interdisciplinary approach to analytic thinking and practice.

David D. Olds, MD is a Clinical Professor of Psychiatry in the Columbia University Department of Psychiatry and a senior Training Psychoanalyst at the Columbia Psychoanalytic Center, USA. He has been leading and teaching courses in integrating the brain-mind relationship since the 1980s.

The Routledge Neuropsychoanalysis Series
Series editor: Mark Solms

The attempt to integrate the findings and methods of psychoanalysis with those of the neurological sciences can be said to have begun in 1895, with Freud's Project for a Scientific Psychology. Ongoing, sporadic efforts continued throughout the 20th century. However, the field really took off when the journal Neuropsychoanalysis was founded in 1999 and the International Neuropsychoanalysis Society was established in 2000. Ever since, a themed annual congress has been held in different cities around the world. Today, it is fair to say that these efforts have generated the most rapidly growing and influential body of knowledge and clinical practice in the broader field of psychoanalysis.

The establishment of this book series in 2023 marked another important milestone in the development of the field. Under the editorship of Mark Solms, the co-chair of the International Neuropsychoanalysis Society, it publishes books by leading proponents – and critics – of neuropsychoanalysis. The books in this series focus not only on the scientific findings of neuropsychoanalysis and on its theoretical yield, but also on its history, its philosophical implications and its clinical practice, as well as its ramifications for neighbouring disciplines and for the mental and neurological sciences as a whole.

The Spirit of the Drive in Neuropsychoanalysis
Mark Kinet

The Unconscious in Neuroscience and Psychoanalysis
On Lacan and Freud
Marco Máximo Balzarini

Explorations Between Psychoanalysis and Neuroscience
At the Edge of Mind and Brain
David D. Olds

Explorations Between Psychoanalysis and Neuroscience

At the Edge of Mind and Brain

David D. Olds

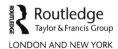

Routledge
Taylor & Francis Group

LONDON AND NEW YORK

First published 2024
by Routledge
4 Park Square, Milton Park, Abingdon, Oxon OX14 4RN

and by Routledge
605 Third Avenue, New York, NY 10158

Routledge is an imprint of the Taylor & Francis Group, an informa business

Designed cover image: © Ellen Rees

British Library Cataloguing in Publication Data
A catalogue record for this book is available from the British Library

Library of Congress Cataloging-in-Publication Data
A catalog record has been requested for this book

ISBN: 978-1-032-50766-8 (hbk)
ISBN: 978-1-032-47388-8 (pbk)
ISBN: 978-1-003-39955-1 (ebk)

DOI: 10.4324/9781003399551

Typeset in Times New Roman
by Taylor & Francis Books

Contents

Figures

To Ellen.

A loving, inspiring, and profound companion.

Acknowledgments

My wife, Ellen Rees, contributed to every step of the book's creation. Great editing help, along the way, for my writing, came from the editorial wisdom of John Kerr. Bonnie Litowitz helped me learn and write about semiotics and has helped very much in organizing this book. A major engagement in my years at Columbia was the activity spent with the development of the inter-disciplinary course for candidates. This course expanded pretty rapidly over the years, encouraged by our Curriculum Chair, Betsy Auchincloss, who saw the importance of the whole endeavor. The atmosphere at Columbia has been very congenial to this thinking and writing. A good number of eager and intelligent faculty have taken part in the teaching. The development of the course took place in parallel with the growth of the Neuropsychoanalytic movement, and our faculty learned much from the leaders of that group, most notably Mark Solms, who founded the organization, nurtured it with his lectures and his writing and is now the editor of this book series. I became a member of the group and later a co-editor of the journal *Neuropsychoanalysis*, admiring the very skilled and creative leadership of Maggie Zellner. And, for the book, thanks are due to the editors from Routledge, Zoe Meyer, Priya Sharma, Reanna Young, and Driss Fatih, who led me through this unfamiliar space.

Introduction

It has taken me many years to assemble this book. Its over-arching, if complex goal, has been to make an early attempt to translate between, psychoanalytic theory, and the scientific endeavors that can be seen as the neighbors of psychoanalysis. As a resident in psychiatry, I was fascinated by the multidisciplinary research being done and presented to our young minds. But I had little talent for the slow, rigorous, and sometimes frustrating process that attended the researcher's medium. With a major in philosophy, I had become more comfortable with the armchair speculations that I had learned to enjoy. I took pleasure in my slow and haphazard musing, and I had an unexpected encouragement from countless hours, as officer of the deck, during my three years in the navy on an icebreaker and later a tanker on long sea voyages. There is something meditative, standing quietly on the ship's bridge, with a 360-degree view of the horizon. Even now I am calmed by the uninterrupted contemplation of that vision.

This book may be an extension of that phenomenon. It draws together some of the vast world of living creatures and their varied and seemingly miraculous interactions within their lives, and the several-layered behavioral schemas that they use to maintain their existence. The book describes the history of my engagement in those layers, as our sciences have portrayed the results, now still in their early stages. I hope to present the complex picture to the reader seeking knowledge.

My medical and psychiatric training took place at Columbia. After residency, in the 1970s, I began psychoanalytic training at the Columbia Psychoanalytic Center, at a time when the neural sciences were beginning their emergent multidirectional involvement with the mental-theory world. I always felt some conflict as I approached simultaneously several different neighboring areas. In the midcentury there was lots of opposition from the more doctrinaire psychoanalysts, who saw these explorations as a kind of acting out of one's hostile transference to Freud. There was also a concern about the flirtation with reductionism, which has always had its risks in the area of mechanizing the mind. There did develop in the world of philosophy a region of attempted integration, and considerable progress was made—for

DOI: 10.4324/9781003399551-1

instance, by Crick, Dennett, Damasio, and Freeman, to mention a few of a pretty long list. These varied works range from a strict monism, in which the only mental reality is the brain and its neurons, to an acceptance of various levels of dualism.

A pair of parallel tracks developed as the neural sciences progressed to learn more and more about the brain, while psychoanalysis made its own progression through a different series of theories, developing intact—and often intensely disagreeing—conceptions of the psyche and the clinical mind. Included here would be ego psychology, Kleinian, Kohutian, object relations, and interpersonal models. To me this was an exciting discourse, which is more and more full of surprises and interesting interactions between the empirical discoveries of neuroscience and the syntheses of analysts' personalities and clinical observations that mediated clinical practice. And both traditions marched, accompanying each other in often varying directions. And, I have found the mutual feedback and controversy to be one of the more fascinating phenomena of the century.

This mélange of activities fascinated me, given the broad range of psychological phenomena that needed to be integrated in order to understand the human. Psychoanalysis became central to my interests, but I kept looking into the other scientific disciplines, that were then still in their youth.

In this book, the essays follow an order similar to that of my looking into the neighboring disciplines, although in some cases a topic gets several treatments enabled by my advancing studies and my gradually increasing knowledge. And as usual in this approach to current science, some theories and conclusions become outdated, and have to be corrected as new theory emerges. Not surprisingly, some of my interests proceeded in parallel, so it makes sense here to cluster together those on similar topics.

The first chapters bring in efforts to combine mind and brain, developing a "behavioral schema," which looked at four modes of treatment—behavioral, biological, internalizing, and cognitive, all operating and contributing to the complicated behavior of a person.

In the 1990s I encountered the work of the explorers of semiotics and began to see that as a good way of engaging with the mind-brain dilemma. Important to me was the work of Bonnie Litowitz, and her paper in the book (Litowitz, 1991). This led to three papers in which I explored this issue and came, in the third paper, to a semiotic model of affect.

At about the same time I began to be curious about the complexity models that were then emerging. This led to the connectionism paper and its attempt to organize the multiple themes in brain science. In this process I encountered work on dynamic systems and their attention to theories about the mind—the work of Freeman, Galatzer-Levy, Piers, and others, and used that model in thinking of mental function. Drawing on the work of Edward Thorndike in the 1920s, a related model, connectionism, was being used interestingly in understanding how neural networks could be seen as basic to brain function.

While analysts were most interested in the unconscious, brought forward in Freudian models of mind, I found consciousness itself quite interesting and wrote several papers on the subject, one written with the prominent explorer in this area, Regina Pally, in 1998. I also wrote one in which I tried to explore a semiotic model of consciousness. This led to the paper on a semiotic model related to psychoanalysis, and to a very interesting on-line debate on the subject, which went on for some months.

Subsequently, I grew more interested in taking a psychoanalytic concept and seeing how far we could go with using other sciences to understand it. That led to the paper on Identification, which was my most complete attempt to do that.

In the 1990s I began hearing about a series of lectures by the South African psychologist, Mark Solms, at the New York Psychoanalytic Institute, and started attending them regularly. Solms was travelling from England once a month and giving very articulate and up-to-date thinking about the mind-brain interface. These lectures were attended by a stable group, mostly psychoanalysts. During this time Solms named the endeavor, *Neuropsychoanalysis*. That name held, and the discipline has spread mostly in North and South America, and Europe. In the year 2000 the first annual congress of the Neuropsychoanalysis Society was held in London. Among the speakers were Oliver Sacks, Jaak Panksepp, and Solms. There has been an annual congress since then, last year in San Juan, and this year in Tel Aviv.

After attending the lectures by Solms, I soon became an enthusiastic member of the group, and I have used it as background support in writing the later essays in this book. Currently, I am one of the editors of their journal, entitled unsurprisingly, *Neuropsychoanalysis.*

In the current model, we have a conscious brain being in continuous output, influenced by both conscious and unconscious brain activities, including the affect system, as well as the perceptual and memory systems. As time goes on, we are finding more detail about how the brain works to produce the mental. One thing that becomes clear, is that much mental direction emerges not only from one brain but from two or more interacting brains. This fact has brought increasing prominence to dynamic systems theories, which conceptually can handle the resulting complexity, and the not always predictable behavior of participants. And it has also provided encouragement to the interpersonal psychoanalytic schools developing at that time.

The model that neuropsychoanalysis makes use of is one we call *dual aspect monism*. This point of view depends upon the concept that the *aspect from which we look* toward the brain/mind determines our understanding of mental phenomena, each viewpoint dealing with *one and the same brain*. The two aspects from which we consider the brain/mind, are 1) the brain, which we view from hearing and seeing what a person thinks and knows, and possibly including the use of neuro-imaging methods; and 2) the mind, which we view from the aspects of introspection and empathy.

One point that some have noted is that much of the book is devoted to semiotic theory and understanding. And, I have come to understand that there is important interaction between the dual aspect concept and semiotics. Both ideas have a dual aspect, which in the case of semiotics is the idea of Saint Augustine that "a sign *stands for* something that is other than itself." This is another kind of dualistic notion that includes two entities bound by the 'standing for' relationship. This is of course most clear in language – where *words stand for* things – but also in other kinds of coding, and in the connections in the biological hierarchy of organic life. An example would be that of neural patterns which stand for mental phenomena.

This brings in the "aspect" from which one is thinking. And, it leads us to the recently appreciated affect systems of Jaak Panksepp, which have been further elucidated by Solms (2021) and by Doug Watt (forthcoming, 2023). A prominent example is the complexity of bodily, physiological and mood changes that add up to an awareness of depression. Scientists are mapping out the multiple biological changes that indicate the altered mood at the same time that the person consciously experiences the inner aspect of depression.

We see here that we have two slightly different versions of dualism. In dual aspect monism we make use of the aspect or viewpoint from which we are observing a phenomenon, and we emphasize that we are observing the same brain from these two viewpoints. The other version, semiotics, takes two points of view while maintaining that one stands for the other. The first focuses on the two viewpoints from the subjective self, the second pairs the two phenomena as *one stands for the other*, this being less subjective and more implying that there is a natural standing-for in the world "out there." Notable in this development is that neuropsychoanalysis and semiotics are, in this book, introduced to each other.

In the semiotics discussion, I refer to a *system* that makes use of signs so that they perform their communicative functions. By that system I decide that one thing signifies, or represents, another, because of similarities in their make-up from an objective point of view. The system is one that takes characteristics of one thing and says that they equate to those of the other in some essential way, allowing one to *stand for* the other. On the other hand, with the dual aspect model, we attribute similarity or signifying to the objects as looked at from *two points of view* by my sensory system. It is curious that the *neuropsychoanalytic* approach will lead one to think about *aspect* (a property of the viewer), and the *semiotic* model will focus on the *standing-for* (a property of the object). Another point about the semiotic model is that if we go back to molecules and how they stand for things, we note that the standing for is a product of what the sign *is*, as in its shape, it size, the order of its parts, even its distance from the viewer. Very important is that at the beginning of life on our planet we have molecules constituting DNA and

RNA, which, by simply having the order of nucleotides, leads to an order of RNA, which leads to a certain protein, which begins the process of construction of living organisms. (For more detail about this, see Deacon, 2021.)

In any discussion, the question often comes up: why do we need to study what is being learned in these neighboring sciences? The question implies both the idea that biological knowledge interferes with psychoanalytic thinking and technique, along with the notion that it is a foreign and irrelevant body of knowledge, wasting the time of the analyst learning the discipline. We may also at times be concerned that this attention can lead to a distracting intellectualism, and can cause a distancing from affect and from clinical engagement. However, as I discuss in several chapters, a range of biological knowledge can be important to clinical skill; it is also extremely interesting. Many people working in this interdisciplinary area are comfortable with the idea that a broader spectrum of knowledge can enrich technique. An understanding of the human being from the point of view of a multilayered hierarchy equips the practitioner to work in a more nuanced way, bringing in concepts that handle the complexity of the human mind, and the human social milieu, more effectively and more creatively.

One thing about the book is that it is a version of the history of the evolution of our thinking over the past 50 years. It shows many of the steps along the way, and some of the wrong turns.

During the 1980s I began developing a course at the Columbia Psychoanalytic Center, which attempted to take what we were learning, and to offer it to psychoanalytic students. Along the way Ellen Rees joined me as co-chair of the course, and years later, she and I wrote the paper, which is the most recent chapter of this book. That chapter recounts the history of the course and some of the experiences that characterized it. The course started out with four sessions, and worked its way up to 26 sessions for fourth year students. The written account about the course has been well received, and it has proven useful to other institutes that want to put together such a course.

As you will see, the chapters in the book are copies of my published papers in the literature. The book is a collection of chapters, many of which take you in different directions. But they do follow the history for our thinking, and they should provide a basis for understanding the fascinating conglomeration that leads to the cutting edge of neuropsychoanalytic models that we have today, and in the near future.

January 2024

References

Deacon, T. W. (2021) How Did Molecules Become Signs? *Biosemiotics*, 16 (3): 1–13.
Litowitz, B. (1991) Elements of semiotic theory relevant to psychoanalysis. In *Semiotic Perspectives On Clinical Theory and Practice: Medicine, Neuropsychiatry*

and Psychoanalysis, ed. B. Litowitz & P. S. Epstein, pp. 81–108. DeGroyter/
Mouton.

Panksepp, J. (1998) *Affective Neuroscience: The Foundations of Human and Animal
Emotions*. New York: Oxford University Press.

Solms, M. (2021) *The Hidden Spring: A Journey to the Source of Consciousness*. New
York: Norton.

Watt, D. (forthcoming) The Separation Distress Hypothesis of Depression – An
Update and Systematic Review. *Neuropsychoanalysis*.

Chapter I

Stagnation in Psychotherapy and the Development of Active Technique[1]

Introduction

Active Technique in Psychoanalysis

Ferenczi (1920) described active technique as an extension of Freud's basic theory to include methods for forcefully overcoming resistance. In his view, Freud's basic technique, involving attention to free associations and formulation of interpretations, was useful most of the time. In some cases, however, he saw a static situation developing; "the patient makes himself at home," and the pathology is maintained by the comfortable, passive procedures of the analysis. In such cases he recommended active methods, both to get the analysis moving and to increase the depth of the understanding.

Ferenczi viewed symptoms and habits as displacements of libido from normal genital pathways of discharge by regression to urethral and anal pathways as well as to other somatic automatisms. In theory, his technique involved prohibitions and injunctions which would block the pathological forms of discharge and create tension and conflict, leading to new associations and revelations at the psychic level. The practical principle was to "go against the grain" of the behavior. If a patient defecated with compulsive regularity, he would be instructed to retain his feces. If a patient was sexually active, the doctor would enjoin abstinence. According to the libido-economic theory these manipulations would lead to a buildup of pressure which would overcome psychic resistance.

A good example of his style is seen in the case of "a young Croatian woman, a musician, who suffered from a host of phobias and obsessional states...." Her conflicts over exhibition gave rise to severe stage fright and fears of being observed because of her "too voluminous breasts..." (p. 202). Her analysis began to stagnate despite her increasing intellectual insight. At one point she mentioned a song which she was too ashamed to sing. The doctor asked her to sing the song and eventually she was able to do so, even with appropriate provocative gestures. As a result, she became conscious of

DOI: 10.4324/9781003399551-2

her exhibitionistic yearnings and conflict over them, and even of genital arousal during uninhibited performances. The next step was to prohibit the newly available activities.

> "Then, when the satisfaction of the newly pleasurable activity was denied her, the psychic impulse once aroused found the way to the repressed material, to infantile reminiscences. As a result, we were then able to take cognizance of reminiscences and constructions of infantile genital play, the chief source of her exaggerated sense of shame."
>
> (p. 205)

Ferenczi's work emerged from the welter of experimentation done by the pioneer psychoanalysts in the first two decades of the century. He could well claim Freud as an authority for Freud himself had used active techniques. In the treatment of the "Wolf Man," Freud used two measures: one was the promise of a complete cure, the other was the threat of termination as an aid to overcoming the patient's resistance (Freud, 1918). The most enduring of Freud's active devices was the injunction to the phobic patient to enter the feared situation (Freud, 1919). Interestingly, it can be said that the classical technique, involving the recumbent position, the basic rule of free association, and the strictures against acting out, is an active measure with quite specific instructions to the patient. Freud established these technical procedures, in the spirit which Ferenczi followed, to establish a state of frustration combined with freedom. The method of blocking the normal flow of libido and restricting motor activity at the same time as allowing complete freedom of speech produced a technique designed to force repressed impulses, memories, and fantasies to the surface in words.

By 1914 Freud had become more interested in the transference and in a technique which would allow a new version of the infantile neurosis—the transference neurosis—to flower in relation to the analyst (Freud, 1914). This delicate process required of the analyst a more abstinent and neutral style. The mainstream of psychoanalysis grew hostile to the practice of active techniques beyond the standard instructions. Glover (1955) discussed Ferenczi's technique at length, finally rejecting it because of the disruption caused by the actualization of the transference when the analyst enacts the role of superego or permissive ego. He himself, however, would occasionally resort to progressively firm interdictions in cases of repetitive acting out. Eissler (1954) clarified the limits of psychoanalysis and discussed the uses of modifications of basic technique, which he called "parameters," in the treatment of more seriously disturbed patients.

By the 1950s a consensus had developed that most active techniques are inappropriate in the psychoanalysis of relatively healthy patients. It also became clear that psychoanalytic psychotherapy is not just dilute analysis, but a legitimate discipline in itself. Several writers tried to differentiate between the two techniques and clarify the properties of each. Gill (1954) produced a definition of psychoanalysis which remains central to any discussion of the topic: "Psychoanalysis is that technique which, employed by a neutral analyst, results in the development of a regressive transference neurosis and the ultimate resolution of this neurosis by the technique of interpretation alone" (p. 775). Departures from this ideal technique—usually involving modifications of the neutral stance, of the exclusive use of interpretation, and of the systematic analysis of the transference neurosis—characterize psychoanalytic psychotherapy. Gill made another important distinction between the two basic uses of psychotherapy. It is used 1) for patients whose ego structure will not tolerate the demands of analysis; and 2) for patients with relatively healthy ego structures, who for practical or motivational reasons cannot or will not undergo psychoanalysis. These distinctions remain relevant to the present day as Kernberg (1980) has recently pointed out. The latter group, relatively healthy but well-defended patients in once or twice-weekly psychotherapy, are the cases most relevant to my discussion. In such therapy a transference neurosis usually does not develop fully, and the therapist may and sometimes should be more active.

Bibring (1954) described five basic techniques which characterize any therapy: suggestion, abreaction, manipulation, clarification, and interpretation. Analysis relies mostly, but not exclusively, on the last two; psychotherapy makes more use of the first three. In practice, dynamically oriented therapists strive toward a position of neutrality. Departures from this stance tend to be unsystematic—an expression of approval or disapproval, an encouraging remark, or sometimes a directive exhortation. Behavioral therapists, on the other hand, have developed more systematic directive approaches. Of particular interest are a number of attempts to combine these approaches with dynamically oriented therapy.

Psychodynamic Behavior Therapy

Feather and Rhoads (1972), in their paper "Psychodynamic Behavior Therapy," described a major advance in the technique of behavioral treatment. They treated symptom disorders—inhibitions, compulsions, and phobias—using a behavioral technique enhanced by psychodynamic information. Instead of desensitizing a patient to cue stimuli, they worked to discover the fear underlying the symptom, and then desensitized the patient to that fear. For example, a man with a phobia involving groups of people in enclosed spaces (airplanes, theaters, or parties) was discovered to have a generic fear that in these situations he would go berserk and act outrageously—hit people, spill things, defecate, and urinate. The traditional method would be to have the patient relax while having fantasies of the individual situations (crowded theaters, airplanes, and so forth). Instead, the authors used their combined approach to desensitize the patient to the dynamic fear of his own aggression, encouraging him to relax and imagine going berserk in such places.

As the authors make clear, this method is not an analytic technique but a behavior therapy rendered more effective by paying attention to the preconscious fantasy underlying the phobia. They point to the synergy between desensitization and insight. The insight in this method involves 1) discovery of the repressed fear; 2) discovery that imagining the act is quite different from doing it; and 3) discovery of the workings of repression, which leads to a more generalized understanding of oneself. The desensitization helps to convince the patient that the fantasy is accepted, and will not be punished by the therapist, and leads to a step-by-step exposure to the feared situation *in vivo*.

Birk and Brinkley-Birk (1974), working in the same vein, described combined therapies, developing an integrated theoretical model showing how the two techniques aid each other. In their system both behavioral and interpretive interventions lead to insight, which in turn stabilizes the behavioral change.

Two-Therapist Technique

There are recent reports of psychotherapists augmenting basically analytic therapy by referring patients for concurrent behavior therapy. One project is that of Segraves and Smith (1976) in which three patients were treated in this manner. One, a woman undergoing twice-weekly therapy for aid in dealing with chronically unsatisfactory relationships with men, also suffered from a fear of birds. After seven months in psychotherapy there was apparently little progress. However, she did express an interest in treatment for the phobia and was referred to a behaviorist who treated her with 11 weekly sessions of systematic desensitization, leading up to her touching a live duck in the behaviorist's office. Just prior to touching the duck she stopped and commented, "You know, it's funny, I want to touch the duck but somehow feel it's wrong. It reminds me of dating in high school when I desired intercourse but always said 'No'." That night she dreamed that her uncle was ripping open the bloody throat of the bird.

Subsequently her psychotherapy began to move ahead. She had sexual dreams and recovered memories of childhood seductions by older men, including petting by her father. According to the authors, therapy continued for another year and a half with considerable improvement in her relationships with men, her self-esteem, and general adaptation.

Toward a Cohesive Active Technique

Is it feasible to combine these two techniques in a treatment by one therapist? Using my clinical experience, I would like to discuss such a possibility. The results suggest that the alliance between the two modes enhances the process in certain situations and does not undermine the psychotherapy. The method is similar to that of Segraves and Smith, basically analytic with the occasional imposition of an active technique, but everything is conducted by one therapist. It is not truly a combined technique as is psychodynamic behavior therapy, which mixes both forms of therapy throughout a relatively brief treatment.

The situation to be considered is this: a treatment is needed for a patient with character pathology combined with symptoms or inhibitions, a patient who may be inappropriate or unmotivated for psychoanalysis. The patient begins once or twice weekly analytically oriented psychotherapy, which in most cases proceeds to a successful conclusion using the standard techniques of clarification and interpretation, plus some use of the positive transference to prod, encourage, or dissuade. In other cases, the therapy may develop smoothly for a while and then begins to stagnate and becomes repetitive, or the patient may persist in a chronic complaint or repeated acting out, unresponsive to interpretation and confrontation. At this point the therapist employs specific active techniques, which will function to break the impasse, change the symptomatic condition, and, most important, enhance the uncovering process.

Active Techniques

Possible interventions for this purpose come from the repertoires of the behavioral and cognitive therapies. Taking into account that the available techniques are too numerous and varied for one therapist to learn—and that some, such as those using aversive shock or cinematic equipment, are not easily integrated into an analytically oriented practice—I believe that the following techniques are most useful.

Fantasy rehearsal and visualization techniques. Fantasies may be used in a formal systematic desensitization (Wolpe and Lazarus, 1968), or in a less structured technique, in which the patient is asked to visualize a scene and follow it through to its consequences. The latter method is similar to Ferenczi's (1924) use of "forced fantasies."

Record keeping. Records may be kept of a symptomatic phenomenon. Best known are the weight watcher's eating record, the insomniac's sleep log, and the headache sufferer's pain chart. A variation is the diary, which the patient can use to record phenomena the therapist wishes to call to attention or to encourage. Such a journal can be used to record sexual fantasies in a patient with sexual dysfunction, assertive behavior in a patient with problems in assertion, or anxious thoughts and associations in patients with phobias or chronic anxiety.

Contracts and financial incentives. Agreements specifying rewards or punishments are particularly useful in problems with time such as procrastination, lateness, and the inability to finish work.

Paradoxical intention. With this maneuver, described by Frankl (1960), and later elaborated by Haley (1963), the therapist directs the patient to perform the symptom, changing the patient's relationship to the symptom from helplessness to control. The therapist can make this device most useful if he or she encourages the patient to attend to associations when performing the symptom.

Effects of Active Techniques

The effects are often dramatic and convincing, sometimes unexpected. The following are the most common.

New associations. The most frequent response is new associations which may uncover historical data, recollections from childhood related to or similar to the intervention.

Response to the intervention. The patient may respond to the therapist's request in a number of illuminating ways—by compliance, active resistance, passive resistance, compliance followed by resistance, and so on. There may also be accompanying affective responses such as anger, anxiety, relief, or pleasure. There may appear to be no response at all, in which case the therapist must remain alert for subtle or delayed effects.

Elucidation of patterns. Especially with directed fantasies and record keeping, the fine anatomy of the problem may be revealed more clearly than would be the case in months of nondirective therapy. The picture that emerges helps to break the problem into small units to be dealt with separately.

Symptom substitution. Although this is denied by some behaviorists, symptom substitution does occasionally occur. Because behavioral techniques are so powerful, they may induce a patient to give up a symptom prematurely. In active technique, instead of viewing such a result as a failure, the therapist can see it as a step in the process, often an illuminating one. For instance, in the treatment of sexual problems sometimes an erectile dysfunction is replaced temporarily by premature ejaculation or by sudden loss of sexual drive. When this happens it often leads the patient to understand the symptom in a new light and to see it in terms of unconscious motivation.

Social response. Any new behavior will lead to new responses from the environment, which becomes important to the treatment. Thus, a new assertiveness may provoke anger or respect from the patient's associates, quickly leading to possibilities for a change in self-image; this breaks a recurrent cycle in which passivity depresses self-esteem, which, in turn, increases the tendency to passivity. Again, the new experience may lead to new associations and memories as well as to new integration of previously uncovered material.

Example I

A graduate student in her 20s came for therapy, complaining of diffuse problems involving self-esteem, work, and her relationship with her parents.

Psychoanalysis would have been appropriate for her, but she was unable to commit herself to it.

A twice-weekly therapy proceeded in which I took the role of helpful listener to her complaining. She asked for my suggestions but would then find them useless or impossible to follow. She derived some benefit from interpretations, especially those involving her need to complain in a way similar to that of her alcoholic mother. Much time was spent on her lack of assertiveness, both in making demands of people and in resisting her parents' demands of her.

In the second year of therapy, we seemed to have reached a plateau of despondency. She complained continually and tearfully about her passivity and inability to serve her own needs. Using a paradoxical intention technique, I instructed her to spend the next few days behaving exclusively in passive ways; whenever a choice arose between activity and passivity, she should choose the latter. Muttering that she'd never get anything done if she behaved that way, she left.

In the next session she seemed to have solved a number of the problems which had been worrying her—editing a manuscript, getting her committee to read it, and so forth. Then, she confessed that she had not been able to follow my instructions to the letter. She had in fact gone to the appropriate faculty member and found some simple practical solutions to her administrative problems.

This success was of less importance than the discussion which followed. We had to consider the complexities of her "passivity." Although she was active in finding a solution, and in disobeying my injunction, she was passive in submitting to the school's dissertation requirements. If she had been passive in regard to the practical matters she would have been in active rebellion against her committee. We came to see that the problem was not simply a lack of assertion. The trouble originated in her own projection of anger onto her professors. Assuming that a request for help would be met with refusal, she would delay "passively" until it was too late and then make the request in a sullen, hostile way, likely to invite rejection, perpetuate her role as victim, and allow her righteous anger at others. Understanding this pattern and relating it to her interactions with her mother were important steps toward clarification and insight.

Example 2

A young man with an aloof, narcissistic life style entered therapy suffering from severe work inhibitions. We proceeded in a therapy with an analytic orientation dealing with numerous maladaptive aspects of his life and making some useful connections with his past and his family. After several months his work inhibition began to take center stage, but he made no serious attempt to change the pattern despite the obvious threat to his job. The complaining and inertia became a stable aspect of the therapy.

He agreed to the use of a monetary technique. He had three assignments due in the next two weeks; he would write three checks to a favorite charity and give them to me. For each job finished on time I would return a check to him. After finishing the first on time and receiving his check from me, he was late for the second and third. When he told me he had missed the third deadline, he remarked, "Don't bother to send in those checks, there's no money in that account." This provided a fine opportunity to explore his contemptuous, grandiose attitude both toward work and toward me and my "little game." His work habits improved over the next six months, and his therapy concluded with improvement in his major areas of difficulty. In the use of the monetary contract there would have been gain no matter what his response. Another patient might have managed to meet the deadlines; such a novel experience would have had other useful results, perhaps new associations or new attempts to sabotage success.

Discussion

The way in which active technique works is a large question, touching on issues of free will versus determinism, the role of the therapist, and the mode of action of therapy in general, issues which are beyond the scope of this article. But some useful observations can be made.

Ferenczi's understanding of active technique involved the contemporary hydraulic theory of energy, which proposed that symptoms resulted from the blockage and redirection of libido from normal, genital pathways of discharge. Active technique was meant to manipulate this channelization by blocking or unblocking the channels in question. He stated his conception most clearly using a hemodynamic metaphor. "Just as in experiments on animals the blood pressure in distant parts can be raised by ligature of large arterial vessels, so in suitable cases we can and must shut off psychic excitement from unconscious paths of discharge, in order by this "rise in pressure' of energy to overcome the resistance of the censorship and of the "resting excitation by higher psychic mechanisms'" (1920, p. 197).

Recent writers have abandoned this concretely physical model. Wheelis (1956) has attempted an explanation of the effect of insight-oriented therapies relevant to active technique, using the usually neglected concept of *will*. He believes the normal therapeutic process has these steps: conflict-insight-will-action-character change. Insight leads to resolution of conflict through the belief that a new mode of behavior will offer partial gratification to both sides of the conflict. Beyond belief, an act of will is required to initiate the new way of behaving. Wheelis invokes a modified energic view, suggesting that in the act of will the ego adds the neutralized drive energy at its disposal to reinforce the compromise motivation. Whether or not we wish to use this energic concept, we must agree that some forceful motivating factor often tips the balance in situations of agonizing decision or in hard-fought conflict resolution. Even in the most expectant therapy, the therapist may provide this little extra push beyond insight, either by suggestion, by general attitude, or as a result of the patient's projections and identifications.

When active technique is employed, Wheelis' steps can be modified to read: conflict (stagnation in therapy)-will-action-insight-character change. The therapist can assist the patient's will to break through the inertia and initiate a new behavior, which stimulates the uncovering process. Action breaks through the last layer of repression or disavowal. Several mechanisms might explain such a phenomenon.

1. The new behavior provides concrete material to work on in therapy which makes the issues more immediate and relevant to the patient. For example, in the second case, the patient was instructed to carry out a typical symptomatic behavior pattern with its attendant attitudes. A patient who witnesses his or her behavior in such a way finds it hard to deny what is happening.

Action tends to unify the self-concept. When one acts, the whole self—mind, body, and any imagined internal agents—is called upon, as when a country is unified in the process of going to war. The notion of personal responsibility for acts or for inaction is then harder to avoid.

The action triggers reminiscences. As one thought leads by association to other thoughts and sometimes to insight, an action may lead to associated thoughts and feelings. A new action, or conscious desistance from action, is a new starting point for associations. Any change in a behavior pattern sets off ripples in new directions, as does a stone thrown in a different part of the pond. Moreover, a chain of associations is bidirectional; it may lead to an action, but the mind can recover the chain by going backwards from the action, even picking up tributary chains along the way.

Another important aspect is the effect on the therapist. Often when a therapy bogs down in a repetitive situation, a conspiracy develops to maintain the status quo. The therapist's unresolved masochistic or dependency needs may render the situation fairly comfortable. In other cases, the therapist, demoralized by the controlling power of an obsessive patient, may fall into a state of impotence, usually rationalized as patience or tolerance. Active technique can help to break this impasse, posing a challenge to the therapist, who in order to make use of the technique must overcome his own inertia.

In summary, active technique imposes an actual experience on the patient, which convinces by its actuality and intensity. It forces the patient and therapist into a more open interaction, which with accurate behavioral and psychodynamic analysis can be precise and well-aimed. The active intervention is an interpretation in action; it elicits the patient's symptomatic pattern as well as the dramatized interpretation of that pattern.

This approach involves some difficult questions. When should an active technique be imposed? How long should the therapist wait before deciding the therapy is stagnating? Countertransference may well influence whether he or she waits too long or not long enough. But such are the problems of any technique; the only help is adequate training and personal analysis for the therapist.

Another problem, of uncertain weight, is that, in the development of a hybrid technique, the advantages of each method may be lost instead of mutually enhanced. Some critics of the combined techniques have pointed out that the power of the therapist's neutrality is lost in the activity, and the power of the behavioral treatment is diluted by the patient's tendency to seek refuge in talk and pseudo-insight. The technique I am suggesting avoids this difficulty by preserving each method almost intact. Although there is some overlap, the therapy is analytically oriented until the active intervention and may return to that state afterwards.

Note

1 Previously published in Psychiatry (1981), 44: 133–140.

References

Bibring, E. (1954) Psychoanalysis and the Dynamic Psychotherapies. *Journal of the American Psychoanalytic Association*, 2: 745–770.

Birk, L. & Brinkley-Birk, A. W. (1974) Psychoanalysis and Behavior Therapy. *American Journal of Psychiatry*, 131: 499–510.

Eissler, K. R. (1954) The Effect of the Structure of the Ego on Psychoanalytic Technique. *Journal of the American Psychoanalytic Association*, 1: 104–143.

Feather, B. W. & Rhoads, J. M. (1972) Psychodynamic Behavior Therapy. *Archives of General Psychiatry*, 26: 496–511.

Ferenczi, S. (1920) *The Further Development of an Active Therapy in Psychoanalysis.* in S. Ferenczi, *Further Contributions to the Theory and Technique of Psychoanalysis.* Hogarth, 1950.

Ferenczi, S.On Forced Fantasies (1924), in S. Ferenczi, *Further Contributions to the Theory and Technique of Psychoanalysis.* Hogarth, 1950.

Frankl, V. (1960) Paradoxical Intention. *American Journal of Psychotherapy*, 14: 520–535.

Freud, S.(1914) Remembering, Repeating and Working-Through, Vol. 12. *Standard Edition of the Complete Psychological Works.* Hogarth, 1953–74.

Freud, s. (1918) *From the History of an Infantile Neurosis*, Vol. 17.

Freud, s. (1919) *Lines of Advance in Psycho-Analytic Therapy.* Vol. 17.

Gill, M. M. (1954) Psychoanalysis and Exploratory Psychotherapy. *Journal of the American Psychoanalytic Association*, 2: 771–797.

Glover, E. (1955) *The Technique of Psychoanalysis.* International Universities Press.

Haley, J. (1963) *Strategies of Psychotherapy.* Grune & Stratton.

Kernberg, O. (1980) *Internal World and External Reality.* Jason Aronson.

Segraves, R. T. & Smith, R. C. (1976) Concurrent Psychotherapy and Behavior Therapy. *Archives of General Psychiatry*, 33: 756–763.

Wheelis, A. (1956) Will and Psychoanalysis. *Journal of the American Psychoanalytic Association*, 4: 285–307.

Wolpe , J. & Lazarus, A. A. (1968) *Behavior Therapy Techniques*. Pergamon.

Chapter 2

The Behavioral Schema

An Integration of Modes of Learning

Introduction

In this paper I shall develop an integrated learning model as a way of understanding mental and psychotherapeutic processes. I take as a starting point the fact that there are many different types of psychotherapy, a phenomenon that in itself calls for an attempt at integration. What follows is an indirect approach, like various other "black box" approaches to mind. In this case, I look at the various ways in which we learn, and the ways in which we attempt to cure mental ills, and from the results I try to describe what kind of an entity the mind is[1].

Several writers have categorized the panoply of therapies; they number in the hundreds, and most of them, when practiced by good-hearted people, seem to work much of the time (Karasu, 1977). There are many ways to assign therapies to categories, but the one I shall use arises from the notion that therapy is basically a learning experience and therefor therapies divide up according to certain very different modes of learning, and that if we consider these modes we can develop an integrated approach to mental process, seeing connections between learning modes, types of pathology, and types of therapy.

Let us look at several kinds of statements that therapists make about patients. In my view, they represent different learning models:

1   We make statements of causality of a cognitive type. We say a certain behavior is caused by conflict of drive and proscription, by the patient's theories and fears of related consequences. An example is the dynamic explanation of a patient's reluctance to be successful, as the result of a compromise between his desire to surpass his father and his fear of retaliation if he were to do so. This is basic psychodynamic theory. Subtypes of the genre are those which see the compromise as between force vectors representing drives, which are linguistically represented, and those which see the conflict as between meanings, without the concrete notion of forces. Therapy is devoted to uncovering such conflicts so that

DOI: 10.4324/9781003399551-3

they become part of conscious knowledge, but what is uncovered is certain of the patient's theories about life, its pleasures and dangers.

2 We deal with the form of thought. Most specifically this is done in the recent developed cognitive therapy (Beck, 1976). With this kind of approach, the therapist focuses on stylistic elements in a person's thinking, such as pessimism, self-denigration and the like, as they perpetuate maladaptive behaviors and moods.

3 We make statements about internalization. For instance, we say a person is acting a certain way because her mother did so, or she is harshly critical of herself in the way her father was of her. We also speak of the splitting of the self and objects, along the lines of object relations theory. Here part-objects are seen as internal agents representing certain qualities —such as manic activity, criticism, seduction, rage —and these exist in a relationship with the self-representation or parts of it. These notions are of course expressed in linear cognitive language, but they describe a model in which there is an inner drama between players on a mental stage. Melanie Klein, Otto Kernberg (1966, 1982), and most recently Joyce McDougal (1985) describe this way of thinking.

4 We deal with the issue of conditioning. We see symptoms as results of the attempt to avoid anxiety or depression, learned patterns of behavior that have become quite stable through repeated reinforcement or, at least, non-extinction. For instance, a hand-washing compulsion can be seen as a behavior repeatedly rewarded by the experience of lowered anxiety immediately following each wash.

5 We see behaviors and traits as the result of biological factors, such as learning deficits, affect disorders, and thought disorders. Here the brain hardware is assumed to be malfunctioning in a way not necessarily modifiable through psychotherapy.

These are several disparate approaches that are not translatable into each other. Now I propose to make the following assumption: if therapies in all these modes are not interchangeable, yet they all have some success, they must be approaching slightly different forms of mental function. How can one conceptualize these different forms in a useful way? I would like to try seeing them as different modes of learning; this provides a single rubric to work under, in which the differences have some heuristic potential.

It will become apparent that I am using the term "learning" very broadly. For the purposes of this discussion, I consider learning to be any change in mental process resulting from experience. This is contrasted to change caused by maturational process. It is true, as Piaget and his colleagues have pointed out (Piaget, 1952), that both learning and maturation process interact in an indissoluble way. In an interesting description of the parallelism between maturation and development, Meyersburg and Post (1979) show how the myelination of various functional parts of the central nervous system match up with childhood stages of development as described by Freud, Piaget, Mahler and others. Once certain parts of the brain become myelinated, certain modes of learning become possible. However, in an enriched early environment the process of biological maturation is enhanced, and in a deprived environment it is retarded.

Now if we take these modes of learning as a group, we can postulate certain relationships between them, and we may be able to define pathological entities in terms of structures built of these relationships. In this paper I will present a schematic method for describing clinical phenomena which may be useful in integrating the various points of view. It involves a two-step mental process. First, I suggest that we reduce the amount of information we have to consider at a given time by focusing on a delimited field, represented by what I will call a "behavioral schema." Second, I propose that we bring to bear on this narrowed field some of the rich fruits of recent research, and that we do so by integrating four points of view, including the biology of the brain and three types of learning, the behavioral, the internalizing, and the cognitive.

I will begin by briefly describing a case that is admittedly more complicated than is common, but that I have selected because it illustrates some of the issues I have just mentioned.

Case Example

At the beginning of seven years of psychoanalytically oriented therapy, the patient was a second-year law student. He complained of moodiness, anxiety about school, paranoid, angry relations with teachers, and an avoidance of women because of. performance anxiety associated with sex. On interview he was appropriately dressed and well spoken, but mildly anxious and apparently uncomfortable. His mood was not depressed, and there was no history of vegetative signs. However, he reported occasional periods of low mood and anger if he was criticized by an instructor or slighted by anyone else.

We embarked on a course of twice-weekly therapy, which included interpretive interventions to contain his anger and to integrate genetic material; also useful were frequent interventions of a supportive, encouraging nature, making use of the positive aspect of the transference to validate his experience, and at times to help correct his distortions.

The therapy at first passed through a very difficult phase of rage and paranoid feelings about me. The instability of his personal relationships, his violent swings of emotion, and his tendencies to idealization, denigration, gross paranoid projections and lapses in reality testing would warrant a diagnosis of borderline personality disorder. After three years of this analytically oriented approach, the tumultuous nature of our relationship became much less violent; at the same time, his tendency to split and project grew milder. He was functioning at an associate level in a law firm; his professional life was running on course except for occasional bouts of suspiciousness, which he was able to keep to himself.

However, his sexual fear, indeed his inability to make contact with any woman, remained quite untouched by interpretation or, later, by direct encouragement. Finally, he and I agreed that he might find behavior therapy useful against this roadblock of anxiety, and I referred him to a behaviorist. This treatment, carried out quite skillfully, continued once a week for over six months concurrently with his psychotherapy; it led to some reduction in his anxiety and to some interesting feedback into our understanding of the transference, but it produced no progress in his problems about establishing any contact with women. At one point, we considered a consultation with a sex therapist, but he rejected the idea.

Although in retrospect I realized that an affective disorder was involved in his pathology, his usual state did not readily suggest depression; his anger and suspiciousness were much more in evidence. At times he would go through withdrawn periods, which began to look more like depression. Eventually, nudged by Stone's (1980) discussion of the affective spectrum associated with the borderline condition, and the fact that he had dropped into a more than usually depressed state, I began treatment with an antidepressant. After the first two drugs proved intolerable because of side effects, a third (imipramine) was tolerated long enough to show results. The results went beyond my expectations. His mood gradually improved over several weeks, he developed a sense of optimism about the behavior therapy, and he began to do the homework exercises more regularly than before. Now he became interested in sex therapy and went for a brief course. He began to make contact with women at work and dated several; in a few months, he began seeing one woman regularly.

The beginning of his sex life was associated with surprisingly few problems. Later he married, and in subsequent years his life has continued in a reasonably happy way. We have made two attempts to taper the antidepressant, both of which have resulted in a depressed mood, loss of concentrating power, irritability and traces of paranoid suspiciousness. During these times there were no vegetative signs and no potency problems.

This case poses a number of important clinical dilemmas and questions that the theories under which we operate do not answer in an integrated way. Issues such as these assail us every day:

1 How important are psychodynamics, compared with biological factors, as causes of his phobia regarding women, his depressed moods and his paranoid reactions?

2 Do we judge his noncompliance with assignments and his refusal to see a sex therapist as "resistance" in the traditional sense, or as the result of a biological affect disorder, or both? How much harm do we do to a

patient's self-esteem and to the therapeutic alliance when we interpret affect disorder as resistance, or when we make the opposite mistake?

3   Why was behavior therapy not helpful at first but more successful with the antidepressant?

4   If we had begun antidepressant treatment earlier in the therapy, could we have done without the behavior therapy, and/or the interpretive therapy; or were these approaches also necessary for his treatment once the severity of his phobic anxiety had been reduced by the drug?

5   In his early, sexually inhibited state he experienced a negative inter-nalized parent figure, a "hostile introject" who criticized him and dis-couraged him, and which seemed to be projected onto me and certain other authority figures. His negative image diminished in therapy prior to the drug trial; was this because of interpretation, or corrective emo-tional learning, or both?

6   Symptoms occurred predictably in anticipation of separations. This phe-nomenon diminished during the pre-drug period, but it improved even more after he began taking the antidepressant.

7   This case presents an interesting diagnostic dilemma that is often encountered in the more severe personality disorders, namely, is it pos-sible to tease apart the personality disorder from an associated, coin-cident or underlying affect disorder?

It will be tempting for the reader to criticize many aspects of the technique in this case, in terms of a possible impression that the treatment was interrupted by arbitrary and confusing changes. However, the therapy took place over 8 years, and the four additions to the ongoing psychotherapy took place during the last 4 years, each one after considerable deliberation. It may be that a more purist therapist could have produced the same results with a single technique, although that seems to me unlikely. But that is not the point. I have described this treatment because of what it suggests about learning and therapy *via different channels.* Current evidence suggests that it is possible to achieve the same or related results by alternate routes. For example, Reiser (1985) describes a case of a phobia treated by psychoanalytic means, and suggests that similar results might have been achieved with med-ication. Cooper (1985) describes a patient many of whose problems were successfully treated in psychotherapy, but whose residual panic disorder required a pharmacological treatment, a course similar to that of the case I have described here.

In any event, the case I have described combines in an unusual but illus-trative way the numerous issues we face when we contemplate a person's behavior and pathology in the light of the variety of models of the mind now available, and of the variety of possible treatment modalities. What follows is an attempt to make the problem more manageable.

The Behavioral Schema

When we listen to a patient's presentation of complaints, we can usually organize our thought around one or several problematic themes. In a short-term therapy, as described by Malan (1976), Davanloo (1978), and others, such a theme becomes the "focus" of therapy, and all other issues are avoided. However, in longer and more diffuse therapies it is useful, in one's own mind, to separate problem areas from the welter of material presented. Each focal area can be selected from what the patient presents as an ongoing train of behavior; each has a characteristic structure; each must be explained from more than one point of view. I shall call such a focal area a *behavioral schema,* a simply described phenomenon, which includes in its description a situation and a characteristic reaction to that situation. Sometimes we can reduce several schemata to one underlying schema, but this is not always possible or useful. Schemata often become part of the transference, especially in psychoanalysis, where the analyst becomes incorporated into the structure as an important element.

In the patient described, there are several schemata. One is his tendency when in states of anxiety to view authority figures as hostile and condemning, and then to react to them in a maladaptive, angry way, threatening his own success. Another is his fear and avoidance of women, so severe as to amount to a phobia. A third is his depressive, paranoid reaction to any experience of separation.

Once we have focused our attention on an individual schema, we have a manageable phenomenon, unlike the situation in which we try to understand all the patient's contents and discontents at once. Ultimately, we may assemble the various schemata into an integrated clinical picture, but that becomes much easier after we have analyzed the schemata one by one.

The four explanatory components in the system are these: 1) Biological: the contributions made by the brain as hardware—the inborn biochemical and neurological mechanisms; 2) Behavioral: the way in which the brain is programmed by the consequences of behavior in a reward and punishment system; 3) Internalizing: internal modifications derived from identifying with or from introjecting whole or part objects; 4) Cognitive: the mind's higher computational, symbolic functions, which allow for language, thought, planning, technical learning and culture.

I will now discuss these four elements in some detail, showing how they interact in explaining a given schema.

Biological

The brain itself does the work of learning, and we must consider it from several functional points of view. Certain built-in features are important to the clinician—learning capacities, inborn behavior patterns, and affects. The inborn behavior patterns have been described by the ethologists and developmental psychologists. Included here are the apparently innate attachment behaviors noted by Bowlby (1969), inborn levels of activity, passivity and sensitivity, sleep patterns, and growth and hormonal patterns. These inborn psychobiological factors cannot be reviewed here but are the subject of intense research summarized by Siever et al. (1985).

Learning capacities are to some extent innate but are modified by early experience, stimulation and deprivation. Piaget has shown that the ability to perceive, understand and operate upon the external world is a process that increases in complexity during one's early life. This has an impact on learning: earliest experience cannot be learned with the full complexity of adulthood; indeed, it may not even be registered linguistically but may be incorporated instead as somatic reactions and primitive behavior patterns.

For our purposes here we have to consider the brain as the substrate for all modes of learning and experience. In clinical work we are used to considering brain malfunctions as contributors to psychological disorders, i.e., metabolic, toxic, degenerative, developmental, and neurological factors. We treat these problems with biological, behavioral and training methods. To some extent psychotherapies have an effect on biological disorders: they may help developmental lags by training and modeling, and they may remove the damaging effects of depression and anxiety that usually aggravate the biological disorders.

It is also becoming apparent that biological structures contribute to the constitution of the defense systems and to the make-up of the unconscious. Joseph (1982) and Levin and Vuckovich (1985) have reviewed research suggesting that certain parts of the brain mature at different rates; in particular, the corpus callosum matures after considerable experience has been acquired by the two cerebral hemispheres, so that much right brain information is unconscious by virtue of the absence of any channel to the brain's linguistic centers. Findings of this kind will profoundly deepen our understanding of the connections between modes of learning and the biological understructure.

A basic system of particular interest to us is the affect system, which Magda Arnold (1970) describes as a biological system for evaluation of experience. Affects used to be conceptualized as resulting from the discharge of drives. Now, with more information-oriented theories, we find it easier to see affects as evaluators of information that become powerful motivators for action or inaction. Presumably, limbic system centers are the biological substrates that connect perceptions and behaviors with pain and pleasure as well as more complex feelings. Clearly, the limbic centers themselves are basic equipment, prewired. However, Kandel's work (1983) shows that even they may be modified by early learning so that certain affects may predominate. It suggests the possibility that an anxious childhood may lead to generalized anxiety in adulthood, and that depression and the welfare emotions may function similarly. Other research based on observation of infants, such as that by Stern (1983), indicates that although the capacities for certain affects are innate, they must be exercised and "attuned" in repeated countless interactions with caretakers.

The main idea here is that affects are also state phenomena, that they persist over time and influence the experience that coincides with them. What I mean is that the ambient affect will influence learning as it takes place, by for instance rendering the glass half full rather than half empty. Thus, the depressed child will have a different learning experience than a nondepressed child in approximately the same circumstances.

The clinical pathology identified to date as being related to the biological realm includes the learning disabilities, psychomotor disorders, affect disorders, panic disorders, and schizophrenia. Treatments include medication, remedial learning techniques, and supportive and expressive psychotherapies to varying degrees.

Behavioral

Behaviorist theoreticians have studied two forms of learning-operant and respondent conditioning. Operant modification, a basic form of causality in the living world, has been put to use by organisms as a mode of learning. It is a form of causality, unknown in the inorganic world, in which future occurrences of an event are influenced by the consequences of the event. We see this in its most fundamental form in the evolutionary process in which the future of a mutated gene is determined by the effects of that mutation. The mutation may be caused by a random event, but the survival and reproduction of the new gene complex depends on its influence on the organism's adaptation to the environment.

The behaviorist school has made a great deal of this process in understanding behavior, pointing out that random behaviors are reinforced or extinguished by rewarding or aversive consequences. The ethologists have modified this view to include the fact that much early behavior is not really random but is the result of internal programming; however, the operant principle still holds in the maintenance or discouragement of this behavior (Bowlby, 1969).

A related behavioral principle, that of respondent or classical conditioning, usually associated with Pavlov, holds that if two stimuli are simultaneous, the organism may come to respond to one as if it were the other. Kandel (1983) invokes this form of learning in his work with aplesia. He demonstrates a possible mechanism for laying down basic affect structures in early life experience. In experiments that "sensitize" the organism—a previously innocuous stimulus is given simultaneously with an aversive stimulus—he showed that physiological changes occur at the synaptic junction. In sensitized animals the presynaptic terminal is changed so that it can release increased amounts of a neurotransmitter. This suggests a physiological change underlying learning to avoid painful stimuli, as well as more general patterns of avoidance and anxiety.

The common feature of both types of learning is contiguity. In operant conditioning two events are serially contiguous, one immediately following the other; in respondent conditioning the two events are simultaneous. Even the simplest organisms can learn through this process, and it may be the earliest form of learning. The internalizing and the cognitive processes have been added as evolution has led to more elaborate cortical structures, but behavioral learning has not been jettisoned by any means. Greenspan (1975) has outlined some of the connections between the behavioral and cognitive levels, showing the complexity and far-reaching importance of these interactions.

In this schema, behavioral learning plays an important part, but a part which varies greatly. And, being essentially a nonverbal mode, it is the hardest to get at in the verbal therapies. It is likely that the earlier the origin of a problem, the more important is the role of conditioning. For example, if an infant finds that every time it suckles there is a kind of uncomfortable tension and not much milk, the suckling behavior begins to be only partially pleasurable, even eventually unpleasurable. Yet the baby is hungry and needs and wants to feed; the conflicts between appetite satisfaction and the painful frustration tend to establish a complicated reward/frustration situation that may well lead to problems later on.

Operant learning and reinforcement occur at two levels. One involves the outside world, the *external* reinforcer. This is what is usually meant by the term "secondary gain" from pathology; the depression, the phobia, the inhibition, is reinforced by a nurturing or attention-giving response from the patient's relatives and friends. The reinforcement is usually unintentional and may result from the pattern of response as much as the nature of the response. In another example, certain responses to a child's whining seem to encourage more whining. If a parent responds by cuddling the child in an inconsistent way, the whining may be enhanced on a schedule of "variable ratio reinforcement." This schedule is particularly difficult to extinguish because it fosters the expectation that multiple responses eventually lead to reward and it provides no one discriminative nonreward stimulus that clearly signals that further whining is futile. The *internal* reinforcer is closer to what Freud meant by the "primary gain" of an illness; every time a compulsive person performs a ritual, he or she is internally rewarded by an immediate drop in dysphoric tension.

I am here limiting behavioral learning to unconscious, nonverbal learning, which can be done by primitive organisms, and in human beings is mostly subcortical. It can be differentiated from a similar form of conscious learning—"empirical" learning. An example might be, "I will not take my car to the center of town because the last three times I did it I got stuck in traffic jams." Such learning, although it arises from experience, is different from behavioral learning and belongs to the cognitive realm.

Some forms of pathology may be more "behavioral" than others in that they have an essential continuous pattern of dysphoria followed by reinforcing relief caused by expression of the symptom. Among these are the psychosomatic disorders, which can sometimes be modified by biofeedback. Addictions, in addition to their genetic and sociocultural aspects, have a behavioral component: a recurrent vicious cycle of discomfort followed by the reward of relief through the drug. Other symptom disorders such as compulsions, fetishes, and the phobia of the patient described here may be maintained in the same way.

Internalizing

Internalization learning is the acquisition of forms or objects. As a mental event this mode of learning is different from both behavioral learning and cognitive apprehension of facts, theories and procedures. It seems to involve another kind of cerebral function, a direct apprehension of a gestalt, more spatially than temporally construed, more holistic than linear or discursive. In current descriptions of hemispheric lateralization, internalization learning may be predominantly a function of the right side of the brain. This learning involves the formation of mental representations, at first permitting recognition of objects and later allowing evocation of an image in the object's absence. By objects I mean ordinary physical things as well as psychological objects-the important people in one's early life.

Mahler, Kernberg and other object-relations theorists, have described the differentiation of the self from the object, and the internalization of the object, as a psychological entity. There are several levels of maturity in this process. The self and object may remain poorly differentiated, or there may later be a regressive dedifferentiation. The self may identify with objects, changing so as to resemble the object, or the self may introject the object, in such a way that the object retains some autonomy within the psychic apparatus.

The semi-autonomous introject is often an issue in therapy. Object relations theorists discuss the introjection of unintegrated, polarized good and bad parts of objects. Kernberg (1966), Modell (1968), and Meissner (1981) have written about the internalization of the transitional object relationship. The relationship in which the object is engaged in the self-regulatory processes and self-esteem development of the infant is internalized as the infant gives up the transitional object. With the introject there remains a sense of separateness from the ego. "The pathology of many patients can be aptly described in terms of the tendency for the introject to take over and dominate their experience of self so that it becomes mistaken for the self as agent" (Meissner, p. 26).

The self-representation arises from a complex of experiences, including the differentiation process, imitation and internalization. It also is influenced by how the person is treated as an object by others. Most dramatic in this regard is the development of gender identity from the experience of being treated as a boy or girl; social gender labeling sometimes takes priority over biological endowment (Person, 1980). Similarly, being treated as a "bad child" can induce a sense of identity as bad or worthless.

An important issue in practice is that the internalization process sometimes results in a self-system that is split, so that there may be several centers of motivation and ownership (Ogden, 1983). For this reason, this form of learning is central in the major personality disorders, particularly the borderline and narcissistic disorders. In psychotherapy, labeling and differentiating these parts of the self may help the patient integrate and unify various centers of the sense of agency.

How is internalization learning relevant to the case I described? It pertains to the "hostile introject," an apparently internalized parent figure who criticized him, discouraged him, and told him he was really a loser, and which was projected onto authority figures (including me, for a while), turning them into persecutors.

Cognitive

The cognitive is the brain's highest order of computational activity. Included here are language, factual and technical knowledge, expectation and judgment, thinking, planning and culture. Here is the text that the semiologically inclined analysts prefer to analyze. Here is one's life story, and here are the defenses that modify it. This sector includes the topographic entities of conscious and unconscious, both of which have cognitive content, possibly processed by different rules. In Lacan's (1968) terms, the unconscious language has a logic based primarily on metaphor and metonymy, a different logic from that of conscious thought but still a cognitive entity. Defenses are included here because they are part of the apparatus for organizing thought and expectation, often removing certain things from consciousness in order to avoid pain or imagined danger.

From this point of view the mind is a symbol processor. It proceeds from one symbol to another by certain rules of transformation and meaning. From other points of view the connections between symbols may result from influences other than primary or secondary-process connection. For instance, from the biological point of view, the connections are between neurons, and secondarily between meanings. But from the cognitive point of view, $2+2=4$ because of the properties inherent in the meanings of these symbols, not because of juxtapositions in the brain. From the biological point of view an individual says "$2+2=4$" because of neural connections made in the learning process, which in fact represents reality fairly accurately. If one had learned that the world is flat, one would say that because of similar learned connections.

In the cognitive world the meaning of symbols is present in the symbols, not in the biological substrate. In psychoanalysis, we unpack the symbols to find implications long hidden by defensive processes. This is the hermeneutic task of the analyst. In this procedure, latent meanings of one's symbol system emerge and one's life story changes and becomes consciously much richer. The endeavor is grounded in the analysand's output as a text, not in a biological reality. In analysis, learning in the other modes is translated into language and consciousness; some of this learning was "unconscious" by virtue of being in the nonverbal behavioral or internalization realm. Other content is unconscious because of defensive processes within the cognitive realm, the familiar techniques of repression and disavowal.

There is a conceptual division within the cognitive mode that is quite important clinically—namely, the division between content and form. Content refers to such outputs as facts, stories and conflicts. The conflict between one's desire to surpass one's mother and one's fear of retaliation is a part of content. So is the notion that one caused a parent's death by having angry thoughts. The form of thought refers to certain repetitive patterns in the way one thinks. This has been the focus of the present generation of cognitive therapists (Beck, 1976). At issue here are certain styles of thinking, such as extremism, negativity, predictions based on mood, and the like. Under this category one might include a tendency to see people as all good or all bad, a tendency to expect the worst of any situation, or a habit of reading negative thoughts in other people's minds. As the cognitivists have demonstrated, the forms of thought are quite dependent on affect; they are pushed in a negative, maladaptive direction by depression.

Let us now look again at the illustrative case. As to the form of his thought, it had a depressive, paranoid cast: selective attention to bad news; prediction and selective attention to maltreatment, especially by authorities; lack of confidence, with prediction of failure. The cognitive content included his life story of upbringing by a distant but apparently seductive mother and a subtly denigrated father, leading to theories of possible oedipal triumph and the threat of retaliation in case of any heterosexual success. He had intense memories of occasionally sharing his mother's bed as an adolescent and of a scene where his father took a swing at him and hit him in the groin; these memories contributed to and supported his theories.

Discussion

If we turn now to the case example and focus on one of the schemata—namely, the avoidance of sex—we may be able to see more clearly the elements that are important in maintaining the pathology and that offer a guide to its treatment. In the therapy, most of the first few years were spent in discussing the cognitive aspects, primarily the anxiety in interactions with women. His mother's seductiveness, alliance against the father, and subtle denigration led to fear of oedipal victory. His diffuse fear of competing with other men in any realm because of castration anxiety was also relevant. These seemed to be oedipal issues and were interpreted as such. The issue of separation was also extremely important, so that loss of a pre-oedipal object seemed to be threatened when separations occurred in the therapy.

As an influence of the internalization mode, the patient experienced difficult periods during the therapy, in which he felt I was an incompetent though frightening persecutor; at other times he saw me as a great source of help. I understood these alternations as related to shifts of focus within the internal object world, his self-representation shifting from that of a weakling persecuted by a bad maternal introject to that of a haughty, sadistic father figure who tortured me, and to that of a gratified child in the presence of a benign parent. To varying degrees all these internalized relationships supported his fear and inhibition with women.

On the operant level, he had achieved a certain equilibrium based on avoidance of sex, a phobia that was reinforced by anxiety every time he thought of trying to meet a woman. In treating this problem, the behaviorist tried a technique of aversion relief in which a mildly unpleasant electrical stimulus was interrupted when the patient entertained heterosexual fantasies; this treatment provided the opposite to the reward system the patient had previously developed.

Of great interest in this case is the fact that all three modes of learning were undermined by a chronic affect disorder that only partially responded to psychological therapies. The antidepressant appears to have altered the biological substrate so that learning could proceed in a different way. Most dramatic was the change in his ability to profit from behavior therapy; perhaps changes in neurotransmitter metabolism led to affective improvement, which in turn reduced the immediate aversive quality of heterosexual fantasies and increased the reinforcement value of the available rewards. This was mirrored on the cognitive level, where now the threats of punishment seemed less terrifying and the pleasures of sexuality could be seen as more inviting. At the same time the negative introjects were experienced as less malignant and powerful, and his self-representation as more estimable. However, it is important to note that the medication did not cure his symptom but changed the contingencies of information processing so that new learning became possible. The response to medication does not definitively answer the question of whether this is inherited brain condition or a syndrome induced by early experience. Either is possible, but apparently some very early learning leaves a stable biological condition that may require medication to change it.

Another still unresolved question is whether the medication benefits the patient by simply improving mood, so that everything goes better, or by directly affecting the symptom or defense mechanism. There is evidence both ways. Sometimes when a medication helps to resolve a depression, there is also improvement in other problems such as the phobia, the compulsion, or the bulimia. On the other hand, the mood may not improve even though another symptom gets better; this is sometimes seen, for instance, in the treatment of obsessive-compulsive patients with clomipramine.

In Figure 2.1 we see the schema, conceptualized as three modes of learning distributed equidistantly around the biological core.

This paper has two agenda that are necessarily interconnected. One is the narrowing of the field to focus on the behavioral schema; the other is the broadening of the realm of explanation that can contribute to an understanding of that field. This approach provides a different perspective from which to view the patient, a clearer base from which to assemble one's understanding and interpretations. It is not presented as the only approach one should use but as an adjunctive viewpoint; using it is a little bit like shifting from a longitudinal view of an object to a cross-sectional view.

The schema, then, provides a conceptual nexus for translation between biology and meaning. Brain mechanisms and the modes of learning are an

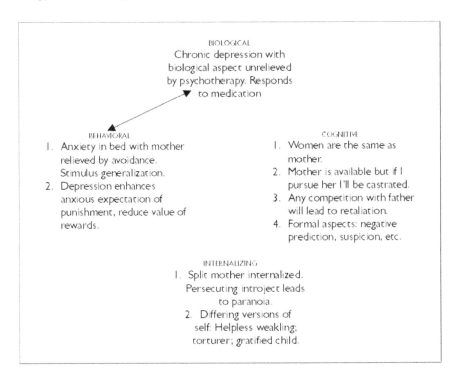

Figure 2.1 Possible relationships between modes of learning, anatomical areas, and kinds of treatment.

escalating series in the translation of biological events into meaningful events. Elements from each contribute to the present-day structure; by unpacking these elements, we may better understand the schema. A good way to take advantage of the schema is to examine it from the four points of view, one after another, in order to gain a grasp of the multi-determination; this helps to conceptualize the problem and often suggests imaginative solutions one would not otherwise have considered.

It is also interesting to note that there is some specificity in the relationships between the various modes and certain types of psychotherapy. Most specific is the use of behavioral therapies in treating behavioral learning pathology. At the internalization level several therapeutic modalities with different theoretical viewpoints deal with similar issues. Freudian theory makes use of the elements of ego and superego: Kleinian, the internal object representations; Jungian, the archetypes; and for Gestalt theory, the concepts of "top dog and underdog." The cognitive level is most relevant to psychoanalytic therapies and cognitive therapy. There is, of course, a great deal of overlap between modes and therapies. However, in some cases a therapy specific to one mode will fail if another mode is important in the patient's pathology; for instance, a patient with a phobia may get no help for that problem in psychoanalytic therapy but may do very well in a behaviorally oriented therapy. On the other hand, some behavioral problems are more reachable in psychoanalysis than in behavior therapy. For example, adult problems related to uncomfortable breast feeding in infancy may yield only to reconstruction out of the depths of a transference neurosis.

One other set of connections may turn out to be quite important —namely, the possibility of some specificity to the modes of learning. The nuclei of importance to affect are in the hypothalamus, the limbic system, and the locus coeruleus-norepinephrine system. Pure behavioral learning is primarily subcortical. Internalization seems to require gestaltic, nontemporal learning, mostly associated with the right cerebral hemisphere. Cognitive learning, especially logical linguistic thought, requires the left hemisphere. Although there is a great deal of overlap, especially in hemisphere specialization, these anatomical divisions lend some rationale to the learning categories I am describing. Figure 2 speculatively shows how these categories might fit into the schema.

The approach I have outlined can be compared to other multifocal systems. Freud (1915) and later Rapaport and Gill (1959) developed a set of meta-psychological points of view. Rapaport's version included five of these: genetic, dynamic, structural, economic, and adaptive. These meta-psychological points of view are different ways of understanding the same phenomenon—namely, psychic functioning in general. The modes of learning described in this paper, however, are descriptions of actually different activities of the brain, not the same function viewed in different ways.

BIOLOGICAL
Central Nervous System, Limbic System
Pharmacological

COGNITIVE | INTERNALIZING
Left Brain | *Right Brain*
Psychoanalytic therapy | Object relations therapies
Short-term therapy | Gestalt therapy
Cognitive therapy | Experiential therapies

BEHAVIORAL
Subcortical
Behavior therapy
Desensitization Biofeedback Assertiveness training

Figure 2.2 Possible relationships between modes of learning, anatomical areas, and kinds of treatment.

Also different is Waelder's (1936) "principle of multiple function." Waelder described the set of psychic structures all at the same level of conceptualization, leading to compromises among the different interests of ego, id, superego and the outside world. His theory is really about functions as purposes rather than as different brain modes.

Another model that takes a multimodal approach is that of Gedo and Goldberg (1973). This is a hierarchical, epigenetic model, which describes the infant developing psychologically over five stages, each with its characteristic mode of functioning. It is a historical ontogenetic model that follows the development from an infantile stimulus-response (behavioral) style to higher levels of psychological functioning. The learning model I have described is similar to theirs in spirit but focuses more on different modes of learning, which probably occur in different parts of the brain, each having its own timetable.

Finally, I should like to review some of the advantages that accrue from using the descriptive model I am describing.

1   In psychotherapy we sometimes get into a rut of unidimensional thinking about a patient. It is especially difficult to shift attention from a learning mode to a consideration of biological factors. This may be because of the traditional view that "reductionism" is undesirable, that it

undercuts the person's conceptual system and erodes the self. But when a patient's conceptual system is constantly biased by an affect disorder, or by cerebral learning dysfunctions, we will fail the patient if we ignore the brain. An appropriate medication may do what years of frustrating, demoralizing psychotherapy cannot do. It is my conviction that the use of this conceptual scheme helps us to shift between psychology and biology without falling into a dehumanizing mechanization. As Michels (1983) has pointed out, a full consideration of the patient must include adaptation" from both the semiotic and biological points of view. Even though psychoanalysis may be conducted as a debiologized search for meaning, the prescription of analysis and the evaluation of its success require a broader point of view.

2   It is encouraging to recognize the mutual interactions—the two-way street—between biological givens and psychological modes of learning. The common fear that everything will be reduced to biology, that in a dehumanized society all psychological ills will be "treated with a pill," can be allayed by awareness that the psychological therapies do have an effect on affect. Psychoanalysis may be the only effective treatment for some personality disorders and for the dysthymic and anxiety disorders that accompany and support the personality problems. As Brenner (1982) in fact points out, no analysis is complete without thorough attention to the patient's underlying anxiety and depression.

3   It is useful to think in terms of the various modes of learning and the techniques appropriate to each. When psychoanalysis is the method of choice, the various parameters of learning will be worked through on the verbal, cognitive level. If possible, this will be done using an abstinent approach, working through a transference neurosis in which the early versions of the person's behavioral schemata will be reexperienced and reintegrated. With patients in less intensive therapy, it is somewhat useful to attack biological or learning modes directly (Olds, 1981). We may treat the biological with medication, the behavioral with operant conditioning or biofeedback, the internalized with gestalt-style dialogues between imaginary characters representing internal objects, the cognitive with cognitive therapy techniques in addition to clarification and interpretations.

4   The use of a schema provides a systematic way to organize one's thinking about a patient and therefore can also be of great use in supervision. For a therapist at the start of their career, the multitude of explanations for pathology and for the effects of therapy can be overwhelming and confusing. The schema here described allows therapists to take each piece of pathology and dissect it in an organizing and integrated way. We can examine therapeutic interactions to see how they may be deconditioning, or permitting new identification, or producing new

understanding and insight. We can see how all of these interact with modifications in affect, sometimes in mutually beneficial feedback.

5   Finally, this method allows us to organize our data according to categories that could turn out to represent the stages of the evolution of human knowledge. The affective and behavioral modes may reside in MacLean's (1972) "reptilian brain," internalization seems to require a cortex but is prelinguistic, while cognition at the linguistic level is unique to humans. A system that integrates this hierarchy has potential for being both aesthetically and scientifically satisfying.

Note

1 Originally published in *Psychiatry* (1987), Vol. 50: 112–125.

References

Arnold,M. (1970) Brain function in emotion: A phenomenological analysis. In P. Black, ed., *Physiological Correlates of Emotion*. Academic Press.

Beck,A. (1976) *Cognitive Therapy and the Emotional Disorders*. International Universities Press.

Bowlby,J. (1969) *Attachment*. Basic Books.

Brenner,C. (1982) *The Mind in Conflict*. International Universities Press.

Cooper,A. (1985) Will neurobiology influence psychoanalysis? *American Journal of Psychiatry*, 142: 1395–1402.

Davanloo,H. (ed.) (1978) *Basic Principles and Techniques in Short-Term Dynamic Psychotherapy*. Spectrum.

Freud,S. (1915) *The unconscious. Standard Edition of the Complete Psychological Works*, Vol. 14. Hogarth, 1957.

Gedo,J. & Goldberg,A. (1973) *Models of the Mind: A Psychoanalytic Theory*. University of Chicago Press.

Greenspan,S. (1975) A Consideration of Some Learning Variables in the Context of Psychoanalytic Theory. *Psychological Issues*, Monograph 33. International Universities Press.

Joseph,R. (1982) The neuropsychology of development: Hemispheric laterality, limbic language, and the origin of thought. *Journal of Clinical Psychology*, 38: special monograph supplement.

Karasu,T. (1977) Psychotherapies: An overview. *American Journal of Psychiatry*, 134: 851–863.

Kandel,E. (1983) From metapsychology to molecular biology: Explorations into the nature of anxiety. *American Journal of Psychiatry*, 140: 127793.

Kernberg,O. (1966) Structural derivatives of object relationships. *International Journal of Psychoanalysis*, 47: 236–253.

Kernberg,O. (1982) Self, ego, affects, and drives. *Journal of American Psychoanalytic Association*, 30: 893–917.

Lacan,ISBN: J. (1968) *The Language of the Self*. Johns Hopkins University Press.

Levin,F. M. & Vuckovich,D. M. (1985) Brain plasticity, learning, and psychoanalysis: Some mechanisms of integration and coordination within the central nervous system. Presented at American Psychoanalytic Association, December 1985.

McDougal,J. (1985) *Theaters of the Mind.* Basic Books.

MacLean,P. D. (1972) Cerebral evolution and emotional process: New finding on the striatal complex. *Annals of the NY Academy of Science,* 193: 137–149.

Meissner,W. W. (1981) *Internalization in Psychoanalysis.* International Universities Press.

Meyersburg,H. A. & Post,R. M. (1979) An holistic developmental view of neural and psychological process: A neurobiologic-psychoanalytic Integration. *British Journal of Psychiatry,* 135: 139–155.

Modell,A. (1968) *Object Love and Reality.* International Universities Press.

Malan,D. H. (1976). *The Frontier of Brief Psychotherapy.* Plenum.

Michels,R. (1983). Adaptation: A reassessment. Presented at Association for Psychoanalytic Medicine, October 1983.

Ogden,T. H. (1983) The concept of internal object relations. *International Journal of Psycho-Analysis,* 64: 227–241.

Olds,D. (1981) Stagnation in psychotherapy and the development of active technique. *Psychiatry,* 44: 133–140.

Person,E. S. (1980) Sexuality as the mainstay of identity: Psychoanalytic perspectives. *SIGNS: Journal of Women in Culture and Society,* 5: 605–630.

Piaget,J. (1952) *Origins of Intelligence in Children.* International Universities Press.

Rapaport,D. & Gill,M. (1959) The points of view and assumption of metapsychology. *International Journal of Psycho-Analysis,* 40: 153–162.

REISER,M. (1985) *Mind, Brain and Body.* Basic Books.

Siever,L. J., Klar,H., & Coccaro,E. (1985) Psychobiologic substrates of personality. In H. Klar & L. J. Siever, eds, *Biologic Response Styles: Clinical Implications.* American Psychiatric Press.

Stern,D. (1983) Affect attunement. Presented at World Association for Infant Psychiatry, April 1983.

Stone,M. (1980) *The Borderline Syndrome.* McGraw-Hill.

Waelder,R. (1936) The principle of multiple function. *Psychoanalytic Quarterly,* 5: 45–62.

Chapter 3

Brain Centered Psychology

A Semiotic Approach[1]

Introduction

Now that the neurosciences are contributing so much to our understanding of brain function, it may be time to begin developing a brain-centered psychology. I mean a psychology on the same level of abstraction as ego psychology, or structural theory. In a sense this approach is an addendum to ego psychology, an attempt to make use of the neuroscience data to cover some of its weaker areas.

Psychoanalytic theory handles the notions of intrapsychic conflict, autonomous ego functions, and the general integration of the personality fairly well. But it has not adequately integrated the concept of affect, of the organic aspects of brain function, or some of the principles of learning and information processing. Consequently, some of the symptom disorders, learning disabilities, and psychotic disorders have engendered theoretical problems when it was found that they could in part be directly treated by biochemical manipulations. This fact can be included within current theory only by means of some awkward stretching. Our theory has also had to stretch in order to deal with the effects of other therapies that are not purely verbal, such as behavior therapy, biofeedback, and some of the gestalt techniques.

What we would like to do with a brain-centered psychology is to incorporate explanations for these formerly peripheral phenomena, while not losing the obvious advantages of our present modes of explanation. In discussing such a possible theory I shall in capsular form try to include: 1) an overview of the currently known interactions between brain and mind; 2) information processing as a basic concept; 3) semiotic theory as an approach to the problem of reductionism; 4) differential learning models and modes of psychotherapy; and 5) discussion of the above as a prolegomena to a brain-centered psychology.

I shall argue, in a rather speculative vein, that if we take information theory as a description of the nature of information, and that if we take sign systems as methods of conveying information within living systems, we may build a hierarchy from DNA to mind, which is less reductionistic than the

DOI: 10.4324/9781003399551-4

traditional hierarchy from atom to brain. In other words, we may build an evolutionary ladder which evolves through informational stages. Mental phenomena will be seen as a natural outgrowth of this progression, rather than a dualistically separate realm.

Mind and Brain

It has long been accepted that there is some connection between mind and brain, but it is the apparent discontinuity between the two which has been central to the Cartesian model, which we have inherited. Recently, however, we have been finding that phenomena once considered purely mental, such as will, emotion, cognition, even consciousness, result from neuronal processes.

Kandel's (1983) work is an example of the exciting research in this area. His by now well-known studies of the simple marine snail, *Aplysia californica*, have opened up the tantalizing possibility of a molecular alphabet of learning. He has demonstrated that in a simple animal, certain kinds of learning from experience are based on changes in the strength of connection at the synapse; there is a change in the number and activity of the vesicles containing neurotransmitters, and ultimately in the number of release sites at the presynaptic terminal, which alters the firing rate for the neuronal system. He suggested that an increase of activity in a withdrawal response (sensitization) could be related to certain affect dispositions in higher animals, dispositions to anxiety or depression.

Whether or not such a generalization beyond the single cell turns out to be warranted, Kandel's work shows something about the biology of learning, of the fact that when associative connections are made there is a physical change. As I shall argue later such a physical change can be part of a sign system.

Another important discussion of this subject is Morton Reiser's *Mind, Brain, and Body* (1985), which explores some of the possible connections between psychoanalysis and neurobiology. His conclusions have mainly to do with psychosomatic medicine, which is the most obvious point of mind-body connection. In the development of a stress-induced disorder he postulates a four-stage process: 1) the recognition and evaluation of danger; 2) transduction into a physiological process; 3) the activation of a central stress mechanism; 4) pathology in target organs and tissues. Here we have a connection between cognition and pathophysiological syndromes; the perceptual/cognitive apprehension of danger generates "signal anxiety," which works through the *locus coeruleus* to activate physiological systems leading to disease in genetically predisposed individuals. This is a "downward" connection from the cognitive world of meaning to the physical body, which is one of several crucial mind-body coalescences. We have been aware of this connection for years, however, and it is not incompatible with a dualistic approach. The "upward" connections have been harder to establish, always against the resistance of those who fear reductionism (i.e., that the mind is "merely" the result of neurobiological process). In other words, strangely, we have had no trouble with the fact that a close call on the highway can engender palpitations, cold sweat, and tremulousness; it is apparently easy to accept that an emergency should call forth a physiological emergency response. But that our most abstract thinking should be the product of neural mechanisms seems more difficult, threatened as it is by the philosophical notion of "category difference" as well as by our resistance to being considered "mechanical."

But the game is nearly up for this kind of resistance. More and more "purely mental" phenomena are being described as the result of neurological phenomena. Thompson (1986) presents an exhaustive collection of neurological research approaching the description of memory trace circuits and neural plasticity in the brain. I will not try to summarize it here, especially since at the present state of knowledge it is impossible to get an integrated picture of the brain's handling of memory. But there are complete neural diagrams possible of certain conditioned responses, including the brain nuclei and the types of neurons involved. We are tantalizingly short of integrating the whole system.

Information Processing

The potential usefulness of information theory to metapsychology has become apparent in recent years. Peterfreund (1971) developed an informational, biological model which made use of informational concepts and feedback control systems, replacing the by then outmoded notion of psychic energy as an explanatory term. Rosenblatt and Thickstun (1977) developed the model further, elaborating a motivational system theory, based on informational concepts. As part of their argument, they reviewed the history of psychoanalysis showing that even in Freud's several models there is an evolution from energy concepts to more informational ideas such as "signal anxiety." These two books produced viable and well thought out alternatives to libido theory in psychoanalysis. Possibly because they were ahead of their time, they did not have immediate impact on psychoanalytic theory, especially upon clinical theory, one reason being that for them, as for Freud in the *Project* (1950 [1895]), neurobiology had not progressed to the point where information theory could be used to maximal advantage. Now twenty years later, neurobiology has advanced in a spectacular fashion, and we begin to see both the need and the possibility for linking theories using informational concepts.

First to define *information*. At the most basic theoretical level, as described by Claude Shannon (1949), information is *structure*; in terms of the Second Law of Thermodynamics, it can be viewed as "negative entropy." Information is the production of order out of disorder, certainty out of improbability.

Thus, like physical structures, informational structures deviate from randomness. The house is less random, more improbable than the pile of lumber; similarly, the gene is more structured than a soup of nucleic acids, a sentence is more structured than a bunch of letters. Strictly speaking, information is not the structure itself; information is a measure of the reduction of improbability in any given message. An example is that more information results from the throw of a twelve-sided die than from the throw of a six-sided die; in the former toss, eleven possibilities were ruled out, while in the latter only five were eliminated. Another way of saying it is that in the larger die there were more possibilities so that the probability of occurrence of each one was smaller; the throw of the die then reduced a greater amount of uncertainty. Information is a property of a *system*, not of a given message; information is not to be equated with *meaning*. Information theory deals with two major issues. The first is the amount of information which can be carried by a given system, such as a die, an alphabet, a language, or a genetic code. The second is the maintenance of a message structure against the pull of entropy. During World War II Shannon was concerned with the transmission of information, for instance radio messages, and with the fact that message structures tend to degrade, because of static electricity, obstructions, and distance, in the same way that any other structure will degrade if it is not maintained. Genes are maintained by the strict rules of replication and cellular methods for gene repair, as well as by the destruction of mutants. Linguistic messages are maintained by many forms of redundancy, so that, for instance, in human speech, we can usually understand the message even in situations where we hear only half of the words spoken. Even so, in the game of "Telephone," in which a message is whispered from one to another in a circle of people, it is remarkable how fast the message can alter so as to be unrecognizable.

The point for our purposes is that information can be carried by physical structures. Such structures are used within a system to carry messages from one part of the system to another. This fact allows us to understand the connections between systems, particularly the relationship between biologic phenomena in the ascending path from gene to human culture.

Transfer by Code

In the evolutionary hierarchy there are several levels of development which are connected by a *coding* relationship, which transfers information between levels. The most basic level of coding is the genetic code. Here, a structure, the patterned sequence of nucleotides, carries a message for the building of a patterned sequence of amino acids, the protein molecule. The properties of the protein are completely different from those of the DNA molecule. The important connection between them is the information transfer. At the molecular level information is carried by physical shape and electrical polarity. The gene codon links with a certain amino acid because of its physical structure. Similarly, the antibody recognizes the antigen by physical attributes, in a key-lock fitting. The same is true of recognition proteins in one-celled animals, of neurotransmitters at their receptor sites, and of enzymes with the molecules they cause to interact. It is by means of information from the genes that the most complex organisms are built, and with the higher animals, the same principle of information transfer leads to quantum jumps in complexity.

Most of the intracellular and intraorganismic communication systems, referred to above, use molecules to carry information coded into physical structures. Primitive communication systems between organisms also use chemicals, as in chemotaxis, pheromones, and the sense of smell. At higher levels, communication can be mediated through sight and sound, in facial gestures, voice calls, and language. Now the point of all this is that there are several of these jumps up from the gene to language, and they are all by way of the coding. At these junctures there is a change from causality as we usually conceive of it, a discontinuity called by Pagels "causal decoupling" (1985). In other words, the relationship between levels is informational, whereas the relationships within a level are more classically causal. The relationship between nucleotides lined up on a DNA molecule is chemical; the relationship between transfer RNA and the protein is chemical but *in addition* it communicates a pattern which *informs* the protein.

This is the crux of the argument that mind and brain are the same thing, but the same thing looked at from two points of view. A description of brain events as physicochemical is a description of brain; a description of the same brain events as informational is a description of mind.

Semiotics

The use of structures as codes brings us to consider the *sign*. Semiotics, or the study of signs, has generated concepts which may be useful in defining a brain-centered psychology.

Semiotics has a surprisingly long pedigree, with certain concepts of current value originating in the Middle Ages. In fact, semiotic notions have formed a kind of parallel philosophy, often considered heretical, in opposition to the establishment thought of Aquinas, Descartes, and Kant. John Deely (1986) has provided an account of the development of semiotic thinking in the early Middle Ages. The definition of "sign," which persists, comes from St. Augustine in *De Doctrina Christiana*. "A sign is something which, on being perceived, brings something other than itself into awareness" (Deely, 1986, p. 12). The most complete development of the idea came in the seventeenth century with the Portuguese scholar John Poinsot (1632). The essence of this way of thinking is that signs may be objects—rocks, flags, words, or even ideas—but they are signs only insofar as they signify something else. Thus, an important distinction from mainstream philosophy was this: according to more familiar figures, such as Locke and Descartes, the mind directly apprehends ideas; this for Descartes is in the suprapineal gland mind. Poinsot and others, however, believed that the mind does not apprehend ideas, but entities which *signify* ideas. The mental phenomenon which makes me think of a tree, I might now call a representation or image of a tree; but my awareness is of a tree not of a representation. In my philosophical reveries I might think about representations, as I am doing right now; but in my imagination I am not conscious of going from representation to representation; instead, I am aware of the objects of representation. In current jargon, the brain event, say the firing of certain cells, brings to mind a tree or a concept; I have no direct awareness of the brain event. Even when a neurosurgeon electrically stimulates a certain memory cell, I am aware not of that stimulation, but of a vivid image from memory. This neurosurgical experiment, however, demonstrates that the brain has electrical events which *bring to mind* images or ideas but which are not images or ideas themselves. In theory the patient could even demonstrate it to himself by inserting the electrode, pushing the button, and seeing what "comes to mind."

This semiotic concept has led to an extremely valuable approach, via Peirce (1897) and contemporary semioticists, Sebeok (1986), Deely (1986), and others.

Now, we soon see that semiotics deals with the same material as does information theory. The two are parallel theories, one dealing with quantitative aspects, the other with qualitative. It is similarly important to note that signs too can exist only within systems. For instance, a pile of black clouds gathering on the horizon is just a pile of clouds. That pile becomes a sign only when there is an observer, for whom it could be a "sign of rain." Similarly, a serotonin molecule is just a bunch of atoms unless there is a receptor site. As Peirce defined it, a sign is "something which stands to somebody for some thing in some respect or capacity" ([1897]; cited in Innis [1985], p. 5).

With this in mind let us go back to our evolutionary hierarchy, and we can see that at every leap by way of code we find the same phenomenon: a physical structure with its own array of properties is *at the same time* an information carrier, or, more accurately, *it exists within a system whereby its structure conveys information*. The message is transferred "up the line" to a new structure with very different properties from the entity "down the line." It is meaningless to say that the RNA molecule and the coded message it carries are not the same thing. It is similarly meaningless to say that the brain event and the thought it generates are not the same thing. From a semiotic point of view there is a pathway from signifier or sign to signified or referent. The signifier is secondary to, dependent upon, and "up the line" from the signified. Thus, the RNA is the signifier for the DNA. The protein is in one sense the signifier of the RNA; it is also a structural entity with its own chemical properties; it acts as a carrier of a coded message when, by its physical shape, it enters into chemical reactions between other compounds; in a sense it acts as a signifier carrying the message originally generated in the gene. Analogously, thoughts, spoken words, and written words act as signifiers for brain events.

In normal brain functioning there is a chain of signs: a pattern on the retina stands for a pattern of light waves reflected from an object; a pattern of optic nerve transmissions stands for the retinal pattern, various relay points transmit the pattern to the striate cortex; a more or less permanent neuronal alteration acts as a sign of the transmitted pattern; when later activated, various output phenomena, visual images, conscious recognitions, or verbal descriptions act as signs of the brain alteration.

This directional pathway concept shows us another interesting thing about the brain, which in fact coincides with certain recent empirical findings. It is well known that when one steps on a tack, one withdraws quickly by reflex, some time before becoming conscious of the event. Even more striking is the recent finding (Libet, Wright, Feinstein, & Pearl, 1979) that when we make a deliberate decision, we become conscious of it milliseconds *after* we make it. Thus, all thinking is unconscious; consciousness samples what our mind has recently accomplished, so that we are aware of some of what is going on. If we go back to the question which is the signifier, the brain event or the conscious thought, it now becomes clear that the brain event is primary and the conscious thought is a signifier of it, most likely a secondary brain event in the amygdaloid- hippocampal complex, and other brain areas specialized for attention and self-awareness. Kissen (1986) provides an interesting account of such brain areas, describing an ascending spectrum from lower to higher centers, integrating levels of consciousness from simple arousal to alertness, focused attention, and self-consciousness. Conscious thoughts then are a kind of read-out, somewhat like the words on the screen of a computer monitor, which represent what has happened microseconds ago in the computer.

Integration

Information theory deals with the structured nature of information and the issues involved in preserving structure. It is a quantitative concept, and includes notions of *amount* of information a channel can carry. *Semiotics* deals with systems by which a structure may act as a sign, standing for something else. It deals with *what* the message is, the semantics of it; it is qualitative. Putting informational and semiotic concepts together, we can explain the hierarchy of coding systems which provide the basis for a general psychology. The crucial point is that physical phenomena provide coding operations which allow for information processing and retention otherwise known as learning. As we go from the gene up to communication as we know it, the information becomes increasingly medium independent. In other words, the message from RNA to protein is only useful in combining amino acids into proteins, which then have very specific functions. But at higher levels the message becomes abstractable. The message "War" could be relayed from tribal drums, via a semaphore system to a telegraph operator, all the while remaining the same message.

A more complete view of an information system includes the fact that in most systems there is an intermediary which is usually used to bridge a physical distance. In other words, we take a medium which can pass from sender to receiver, impress the coded structure onto it, then transmit it to the receiver, who then decodes the message from the medium. For instance, the sky-writer begins with some undifferentiated smoke, imposes a structure on it, the results of which we see from a distance, and then decode. An apparent anomaly here is the DNA-RNA system where there is no medium; the information goes directly to the RNA. Even here, however, we may have an apparent exception which proves the rule; the RNA functions as the medium carrying the gene's information to its ultimate consumer, the protein. In actuality the usual information system is really two subsystems, one involving the sender, the information, and the medium, and another involving the medium, the information, and the receiver. The intermediary, in semiotic parlance, is the *sign*; or, in the classic McCluhanism, "the medium is the message."

Learning Modes

Now, if the brain is an information processor ultimately designed to perceive and adapt to the world around it, we must consider two facts. One is that the world itself is noninformational; only when rocks, clouds, and raindrops are included in a living system do they become sources of information. So the brains of all organisms develop in order *to turn those things into information.* They do this first by converting certain elements of things in the world to information by transduction through organs of perception, that is, certain electromagnetic frequencies into colors and shapes in a visual system. They do not perceive everything—ultraviolet light, high-frequency sound—but they get enough to have a fairly accurate picture of the world. One form of information processing is the transduction of sensory stimuli to internal brain languages at specific storage centers, such as the occipital lobe's visual area or the parietal lobe's sensory areas.

When we look at higher animals, we find that not only do they process light, sound, chemicals, and tactile stimuli, and turn these into brain languages and storage; they also *integrate* these stimuli in importantly different ways. This is a central process of great significance. In a previous paper (Olds, 1981), I described a schematic approach to learning which recognizes these several "modes of learning" occurring in different parts of the brain. By learning I mean the integration of information beyond the sensory storage level and the storage of this integration. By storage I mean a more or less permanent change in the neural apparatus, this change becoming, in the language of this paper, a *sign* of a bit of learning.

The different kinds of learning, distinguished here as different modes of integration of sensory input, are quite important, and they represent major developmental advances up the evolutionary ladder.

Affect

Possibly the most pervasive mode of integration in all organisms is that of affect. In the earliest organisms, affect is represented by mechanisms for approach and avoidance, simple chemo- and phototropisms for instance. In higher organisms the affect system involves several limbic centers which participate in the *evaluation* of experience, thus providing the basis for motivation as well as appraisal of results (Arnold, 1970). Affect itself is a form of information; the affect capacities seem to be inborn, although their association with certain stimuli is an aspect of behavioral learning. As Kandel (1983) suggests, it is conceivable that the affect systems themselves may be modified somewhat by experience; in other words, anxiety or depression systems could be increased in sensitivity because of childhood experience.

Behavioral

The simplest form of learning, which must have evolved in concert with affect systems, is the behavioral, which is available to the most primitive organisms. Behavioral information underlies our notion of *causality*, which as Kant pointed out is one of the *forms* of thought, and which is indispensable for the survival of any creature. The *Aplysia* experiments have demonstrated several forms of behavioral learning including sensitization, and classical and operant conditioning. The learning process involves synaptic changes which essentially *record* the close temporal connections between stimuli, responses, and consequences. With classical conditioning, for instance, the cell increases its capacities for neurotransmitter release in response to closely paired stimuli; reinforcement occurs most strongly when the conditioned stimulus precedes the unconditioned stimulus by 0.5 seconds (Kandel, 1984). Now, in this system the conditioned stimulus (CS) becomes the *sign* of the unconditioned stimulus (US), and may therefore induce behavior appropriate to the US in the absence of the US. These connections are then stored as "predictive" connections. This process allows the organism to bridge a period of time to predict that "A" will likely be followed by "B," and therefore to be able to modify its behavior accordingly. In the process one event is associationally linked with another, and *also* linked with an *affect*, which influences which way the behavior will be modified. In the human the primary locus of behavioral learning is subcortical.

Internalizing

A third form of processing is the *internalizing* mode. Here, the information consists of gestaltic representations of objects, which are stored and manipulated. This seems to be the mode of learning most clearly the concern of object-relations theory, which deals with the internalization of whole and part objects; these become players in an internal drama, and may to some extent manifest themselves as ego and superego, as good mother and bad mother, and the like. Their development and maturation, described in particular by Kernberg (1966), play a major role in the emergence of the self-concept. They are not simply spatially organized percepts, they are complex percepts derived from all of the senses, which become internal centers of motivation and identification. In later life they become the structural sources for transference phenomena (for further support of this notion, see Watt [1986]). This kind of learning may be associated with the right cerebral hemisphere, in its gestaltic, affect-laden mode.

Cognitive

A fourth mode is the *cognitive*—the learning of facts and theories mediated by language. It is a uniquely human mode, since language is required. It involves our general learning and culture, including the theories of life entertained by neurotic patients. Since many of these theories, such as that underlying separation anxiety or unconscious guilt, are unconscious, some of the defense mechanisms reside here. Consciousness seems to require this mode, which is primarily located in the left hemisphere, with access to the language and speech centers.

The heuristic importance of these different learning modes lies in their usefulness in explaining some of the different ways the brain operates. The clinical importance of these different modes is that psychopathology in each mode may require a different kind of therapy, such as behavioral, experiential, psychoanalytic, cognitive, or pharmacological.

Each mode represents a particular kind of information integrated in a unique way. Each mode of therapy has aspects that are relevant to certain types of integration. With the behavioral mode, behavioral therapies directly affect the behavioral programs, usually reducing the expectation of punishment, as in phobias, or in the expectation of reward, as in compulsions and addictions. In other words, the previous relationship of the stimulus and the response is changed through desensitization and other modifying techniques. This is done not only in behavior therapy, but in psychotherapy as well. Schwartz (1987) shows some of the ways in which psychoanalysis alters behavioral expectations. Internalization systems are modified in psychoanalytic treatments, which make use of transference, as well as some techniques, such as Gestalt, which deal directly with dialogues enacted by voices representing internal objects. Elements in the cognitive mode, particularly repressed theories of the origins of one's suffering, are elucidated in psychoanalytic-therapies; certain automatic types of thinking, particularly depressive types, can be directly approached by the techniques of cognitive therapy. The affect system is often modified in any successful form of therapy; in addition, it sometimes can be approached chemically by psychotropic drugs, they themselves being structured information carriers which enter into the sign chains of the limbic system. It is clear that psychoanalytic methods have the potential for the broadest and most inclusive influence; but in certain cases a specific approach to a particular mode may be effective by itself, or in addition to a psychoanalytic technique.

Brain Storage and Representation

We could speculate how the system might work based on analogies to computers. Some neural event occurs, possibly something along the lines of Kandel's account of sensitization, in which a stimulus to a cell alters in a distinct quantum jump its capacity for neurotransmitter output. We may then say it has been "turned on" like a switch in a binary coding system. It then carries one bit of information which could be used as part of a larger informational pattern. In creating a *representation*, it could combine with other bits in a way similar to that in which the pixels on a video screen combine to make an image.

There are nondigital modes of communication, usually referred to as *analog*. The gestures and facial expressions, which convey affect states, are common to all mammals. Many species can communicate by making noises, although these noises may be adapted for the species by evolution, and tend to be fixed (i.e., bird songs and cricket chirps). Jones (1981) has referred to the affect system as a nonsymbolic, analog information-processing system. He refers to inner felt states such as hunger, thirst, and sexual interest as *needs*, and to the feelings arising from experience of the world and other people, such as joy, anger, and sadness, as *emotions*. All of these are continuous functions, like the resistance of a spring balance, or the height of the column of mercury in a thermometer. In his words they "measure" rather than symbolize. For our purposes here, we can say that affects do represent a different mode of information, an analog mode which cross-weaves with the other forms, including the digital form of language, to produce modulated, flexible kinds of meaning. In other words, the glass is half full or half empty, or one is bragging or complaining, depending on the ambient affect. This may be a little bit like the Chinese language in which the meaning is carried by an interaction between an analog system (pitch of voice) and the digital phoneme (for the complexity of levels and shifts between analog and digital communication, see Wilden [1972]).

Infant Observations

Now to look from phylogeny to ontogeny. In recent decades the scientific observers of infant behavior and learning have amassed fascinating and plentiful data on early experience. Piaget (1952) and Mahler, Pine, and Bergman (1975), among others, have erected major developmental systems based on such observations. Mahler's is the first psychoanalytically oriented system; it is derived from the hypothesized initial fusion of infant with mother, a fusion which evolves through phases of separation and individuation to mature individuality. The more recent work of Stern and his associates (Stern, 1985) has garnered more information, and now points to an alternative hypothesis, that the infant begins in a state of isolation but with systems for attachment, in Bowlby's sense, already intact, and with rapidly developing systems for establishing a core sense of self, and of a self in relationship to others. This self develops during the first three months, via a complex set of "amodal" felt experiences, not differentiated in terms of cognitions, actions, or perceptions. It then progresses to develop a "core self" and an interpersonal relatedness, eventually arriving at a state of verbal relatedness during the second year of life. The process of "affect attunement" in the infant's interactions with mother, and various other kinds of empathic response, assist the baby in its development.

We need not join the debate between these two hypotheses now, although Stern's arguments for the initial separateness of an immature mind, and the subsequent development of relatedness to others, seems to fit better with the informational tack I am taking here. How so? Stern, like Piaget (1952), shows this early brain functioning at first with ethologically inborn capacities, and then, as new capacities become available, learning new things in new modes. There may even be a recapitulation of phylogeny analogous to the above series of learning modes. For instance, weeks' old babies can learn to *behaviorally* (operantly) control sources of visual stimulation (Watson, 1979). Stern describes how later in the process of developing a core self and intersubjective relatedness, the child can internalize "working models" of the caretaker, which he calls RIGs or "Representations of Interactions which have been Generalized." The RIGs are representations which become the basis for *internalization*. Most likely certain RIGs become separated according to strong affect tones; this may be the basis of a similar system described by the object-relations theorists as splitting of self and object. Then, with the development of the verbal self we have the entry of the *cognitive mode* to the repertoire of learning.

Information and Evolution

As we follow the chain of life back to its primitive beginnings, we see two principles which seem necessary for life and which are repeated at different levels of complexity at various strata up to the most complex organisms. The first principle is that of *information/semiosis* which I have been discussing. The second is *evolution*.

The principle of evolution we may call the *operant* principle after its manifestation at the behavioral level. It has also been called the Law of Effect (Dennett, 1978; Broadbent, 1961). In the inanimate world there is nothing whose repetition depends upon its consequences. But at the first instance of life, the evolutionary principle of survival begins. The earliest proto-organism, thrown together by chance, with a system for reproducing itself, will reproduce if it is adapted to its environment; if it is not, it will neither survive nor replicate itself. From then on, all chance modifications of the genome will be rewarded by existence and reproduction if they success-fully fit the environment. The next stratum at which we see this principle is the behavioral; with operant conditioning, rewarded behaviors are reinforced and tend to become habitual, unrewarded behaviors are not. We see the same principle in the development of social organizations, skiing techniques, sci-entific theories, and the like, determining which ones will thrive and which will not. It is possible that some such principle is related to memory; that certain ones of the day residue are selected for long-term retention, while the majority are soon discarded. What constitutes "success" or "adaptation" for a memory is not well understood, but it probably will be at the heart of a successful theory of memory. We see that, in an important sense, evolution is itself a form of learning, appropriate to the biosphere, possibly the original model for all other learning systems.

If these principles are universal, they should be seen together at the earliest stages of life. That apparently may be the case. Tomkins (1975) has described what he calls a *metabolic code*. The most primitive version is the signal of the absence of a nutrient; if a nutrient is absent, the metabolic chain is inter-rupted, and there is a bottleneck and a consequent build-up of the immediate precursor. This build-up is a "sign" of the lack, which becomes the initiator of some form of response. An example is a variety of slime mold *(Dictyos-telium discoidium)*, in which, when nutrient levels fall to the starvation level, there is a block in the metabolic chain, which leads to a build-up of cyclic-AMP, which then diffuses into the surrounding medium. "This substance serves as a chemical attractant that causes the aggregation of a large number of myxamoebas to form a multicellular 'slug'" (p. 762). Thus, at this primi-tive level, a mechanical event, and the resultant build-up of cyclic-AMP, evolves into a kind of *sign* of the lack of nutrient. The organism responds to this sign by an action, one which has apparently been proven operantly suc-cessful for its adaptation and survival. At this level the process is quite mechanical; the presence of the cyclic-AMP catalyzes the reaction which leads to the cellular aggregation. But this is true of most signs at the sub-linguistic level. For instance, a hormone or a transfer-RNA molecule carries a physical key-lock message, which works by simple physical interaction.

Cybernetic systems make use of the two life-principles I have just descri-bed. In a biological negative feedback system, there is 1) the maintenance of an adaptive state; for instance, overproduction of insulin → depressed blood sugar → reduction in insulin output; and 2) the excess or deficit acts as a *sign* of the departure from homeostasis. Tomkins speculates that in multicellular organisms, certain cells became specialized to communicate, to other cells, messages about the nutrient level in the external environment. They even-tually evolved to be able to utilize neurotransmitters for intercellular com-munication, now making use of the fact that intracellular cyclic-AMP increase leads to neurotransmitter release for communication with other cells.

Consciousness

As I have described above, consciousness may be a read-out phenomenon, grafted onto the work of the brain, which selects some of the results of brain activity. There are a number of reasons why much of what happens in the brain does not become conscious. The standard defenses, described by Anna Freud (1946), which keep information out of consciousness, such as repres-sion, displacement, denial, and projection may work as she suggested, with a kind of censorship occurring in the brain which has learned that certain thoughts, images, or memories are too aversive or too threatening for con-sciousness to bear.

There are other reasons why some memories do not reach conscious awareness. One reason is described by Joseph (1982); it is that there is a developmental sequence in the brain, which renders some early experience unavailable to the left brain, and hence language and consciousness. Some experience occurs before the child has learned language, and therefore any relevant memory traces exist as vague sensations, motor responses, and pos-sibly psychosomatic phenomena. Another important factor in unconscious-ness is the fact that several years' worth of experience occurs before the maturation of the corpus collosum, so that even after the beginning of lan-guage there are developmental barriers between the two hemispheres. Joseph points out that the left hemisphere develops its connections with the motor system before the right hemisphere, and that the right hemisphere connects sooner and more extensively with the limbic system. Thus, certain early experiences may be stored in the right hemisphere, with its connections to the limbic system, and result in vague, affect-laden experience without words.

There is a great deal else which is necessarily unconscious, as a review by Kihlstrom (1987) suggests. He summarizes the research into activities that are not necessarily conscious, such as: 1) automatic processes, such as driving to work; 2) the subliminal perceptions which may remain unconscious but influential in mental activity; and 3) the effects of hypnosis. The picture which emerges shows a brain with millions of things going on at once, only a fraction of which can become conscious. More and more, consciousness seems to be a derivative, almost nonessential activity of the brain.

What then is the purpose of consciousness? Some of the split-brain research has led to some clarification of this issue. Gazzaniga (1978), Sperry (1979), LeDoux (1985), and others have performed numerous experiments elucidating the different functions of the isolated cerebral hemispheres and have derived some illuminating theories about consciousness. In some experiments a post commissurotomy patient cannot name objects presented to the right hemisphere, but can later point to them and select them from a group of objects. With one patient, if items were presented to his right hemisphere, he would not be able to name them using his left-sided language function. But he could rate these objects as to how much he *liked* them.

Consciousness seems to be a kind of central processor, which allows for integration of the various modes of experience, and a form of feedback system so that the individual can continuously evaluate his or her interactions with the world. If psychotherapy leads to an expansion of that feedback system, that may be an important aspect of the benefit derived.

Dualism versus Monism

The information/semiotic model makes a useful contribution to the argument opposing dualism and monism. The argument deals with the question: is the mind simply a product of the brain or is there something ineffable added to the brain's activities? The classic Cartesian dualist notion is that the mind is separate from the brain, and although it may be dependent upon the brain, their activities cannot be equivalent.

The debate over these two positions is a major philosophical issue, much too large to do justice to here. In thinking about the matter, we are confronted with the everyday feeling that mind is one thing and brain is another; we can see and experiment with body and brain, but mind we experience in a different way. Philosophically there are good arguments on both sides, but in the end the dualist is left in Descartes' position of postulating two different kinds of reality, and thereby being in a scientifically indefensible position. The monist, although supported by the respectable notion that there is only one reality, is faced with the apparent duality inherent in experience.

Dualist Arguments

An example of a dualist position is Edelson's (1986) argument that, although we proceed from one idea to another, that cannot be the *same as* proceeding from one brain state to another. Edelson contends that psychoanalysis and neuroscience are *autonomous* sciences, despite the fact that any given mind state requires a certain brain state. The point, for him, is that the rules of passage from one brain state to another are independent of the rules of passage from one psychological state to another. This is similar to Popper's (1972) argument that we must consider three "Worlds." World 1 is the physical and biological realm, World 2 is the scope of psychological or mental processes, and World 3 is the realm of abstract ideas, mathematical laws, and scientific theories. World 3 is a kind of independent reality, existing in a realm of abstraction; the truths involved were true long before the brain ever existed, and therefore are necessarily separate from brain.

Another version of the dualist argument is that there is something *emergent* from brain activity which accounts for mind's activity, namely that subjective consciousness, especially self-reflection, is a property which can theoretically be said not to be reducible to brain states, but to emerge from highly complex brain activity. Emergence is a useful concept, taking an important role in recent discussions of the theory of *chaotic systems* (Gleick, 1987). Chaos theory attempts to explain the unpredictability inherent in complex systems on the basis of the massive number of initial variables, and the extreme sensibility of a system to infinitesimal changes in these initial conditions. In such a system it becomes impossible to know exactly where you are starting, and therefore doubly impossible to know where you are going. The classical example of a chaotic system is the weather, where prediction for more than a few days is impossible. Another classical system is the brain where attempts to model it on the chaotic-system paradigm may be relevant to current connectionist models of brain activity (Skarda and Freeman, 1987). Emergence theory is extremely useful in explaining the novel, unpredictable capacities and properties of complex systems. In dealing with the notion of freedom of action it is useful, and it may be one explanation of our subjective feeling of a distinction between mind and brain. It leads to a quantitative distinction and a *functional dualism* (Churchland, 1986).

It interposes between brain and mind von Neumann's notion of the "complexity barrier"; in other words, it preserves the mind—body split. Information theory, on the other hand, while not incompatible with the emergence theory, leads to a *qualitative* distinction within a monistic system.

Monist Arguments

Most monists believe that there is only one reality, and that what we call mental events can be "reduced" to brain events. Churchland (1986) makes the analogy to the reduction of optical theory to electromagnetics. At one time light and electromagnetics were thought to be different phenomena governed by different laws. Once it became clear that they followed exactly the same rules, the distinction disappeared. The monist feels that ultimately mental events will be similarly reduced to be seen as *the same thing as* brain events.

The information/semiotic model presented here makes one contribution to this argument. It is a monist position in that it does not require more than one kind of reality. It says that brain events and mind events are the same thing, that mind events *are* brain events insofar as they are informational. Even the apparent difference of light and electromagnetics is explained. Light may be the same as electromagnetics, but it is not "light" until it becomes a part of an information system, transduced by a sensory system which then uses it to interact with the world. This model may also provide a rejoinder to Popper's system. The abstract objects of World 3 are sign systems. The "law of gravity" or the value of "pi" are *signifiers* of brain events which have computationally integrated incoming stimuli from the world.

Summary

Let us review the argument in its rudiments. At the beginning of the process of evolution, information came into existence simultaneously with a *system* for information processing, a system with a sender and a receiver. With the first such system, which could perpetuate itself, the operant or evolutionary principle came into existence, and living systems proceeded to evolve.

Once this process had begun, information-using intermediaries became possible, and hence the principle of semiotics, in which one thing, in an informational system, can stand for another thing.

The modes of learning are different ways of integrating incoming and stored percepts into *affective* (evaluation of experience), *behavioral* (temporal connections between events), *internalizing* (internal object gestalten), and *cognitive* (symbols and language) - semiotic systems.

The apparent gaps in the evolutionary hierarchy, which lead to dualist explanations, are really *informational* jumps, not the violations of causality which the classical dualist argument would suggest.

The result is a monistic system where *brain* and *mind* are two terms for the same thing. The entities we attribute to mind, such as words, thoughts, and motives, are *signs* of central brain events, which themselves are signs of stored information.

Any physical event or object (a neurotransmitter, a trio of nucleic acids, a sound pattern) is simply a meaningless event or object unless it is part of a system designed to use it as a sign. It is the *system* (brain system, gene system, language system) which determines that a physical event is also a semiotic event. Dualist theories arise because of a lack of appreciation of this distinction.

Conclusion

What is the point of adding yet another name for the psychology of the human organism? How will "brain" be a better focal point than "ego" or "consciousness," or "self"? There are several reasons which I find convincing.

When we take an abstraction, such as "ego" or "self" as our starting point we prejudice our clinical studies, and clinical practice, in the direction of disorders at the level of that abstraction. When our only access to the brain was through words, then a verbal abstraction might have been the best place to start; at the state of the science of his time, Freud was forced to use the verbal route when contemporary technology made the ideas of his *Project* not practicable. As technology has advanced, many more disorders of the brain have become treatable much more successfully by other than verbal means. At the same time, certain disorders have become more clearly psychoanalytic issues, as we have been able to separate them from the more biological disorders. The point is that, when we deal with the abstract entities, we are dealing with output phenomena; to concentrate on disorders of ego function or the self may be like focusing on the fever in pneumonia rather than on the underlying organic infectious process.

Ego psychology confronts us with the age-old homunculus problem, which has always troubled philosophers. The major philosophical difficulty is that of the infinite regress; is there an ego inside the ego? The conceptualization of a central agency tends to imply certain spatial concepts, such as an ego inside the mind, over against a superego and id; these spatial notions are particularly offensive to many, since mind is a functional not a spatial concept.

For Freud, the organization of defenses implied an organizer, the ego. Curiously, his earlier model, the topographic one, did not require an ego, but was a brain which maintained a barrier against unacceptable mental content. When he confronted the problem that there are unconscious defenses, he had to postulate an ego which was both conscious and unconscious, and which maintained defensive boundaries against the id. Anscombe (1986), in an article on ego and will, confronts the issue of the *sapient* ego, the ego which guards consciousness. Such an ego, in order, for instance, to set up defenses against unacceptable input, must be a little brain unto itself which can appraise the input fully. This is the result of a "bottom up" approach in which the percept is fully understood and then rejected; that is, "seen" before it is "not seen." Anscombe suggests a "top down" approach, derived from the finding that tachistoscopically presented stimuli of emotional valence— *cancer, breast, swastika*—reach consciousness later than neutral stimuli. The conclusion drawn is that the subject recognizes these stimuli as belonging to anxiety provoking *classes* of words, before they are fully recognized in their individual meanings. In other words, there may be a censoring process, similar to that in Freud's topographic model, in which received percepts are classified by emotional valence before final decoding from generic to specific meaning. The functions of the ego, as our neurophysiologic knowledge grows, are becoming more diffusely spread over the brain, and do not appear to be the work of a central agency. The Libet et al. (1979) finding about the delay between unconscious brain work and conscious awareness has altered our commonsense view of the ego as the central agency which is aware of choices and initiates behavior, and has rendered the integration of behavior more unconscious and more diffusely organized. This position is further strengthened by studies of so-called Parallel Distributed Processing (Churchland, 1986; Rumelhart & McClelland, 1986), which show that the same percept is represented in many different brain loci and that the entire brain is constantly carrying out countless processes simultaneously.

These findings have led to a major change in our conceptualization of the human mind. In a sense the brain becomes the ego; philosophical problems of dualism, of the homunculus, and of reductionism do not disappear but can be looked at from a different, and possibly heuristically enlightening perspective. It is also interesting that Freud himself was closer to the present picture when in 1897 he noted that defenses may be "multi-locular" (Freud, 1897).

The brain events under discussion are the central events in the, psychology of mind. *They are in one sense simply a nexus in the* chain, from external event to sense datum to perception, which then proceeds to output signifiers such as words, gestures, and thoughts. But their peculiar position puts them in the role of information processor. The brain events themselves may be modified, by *learning* from new percepts, or by rearrangement of old percepts, or by *modification* from within the brain, through affect changes or other metabolic changes via disease, hormone shifts, and pharmacological agents. When they are so modified, the signifiers they generate will also change. The brain event has only one parallel in history, although it will have another parallel in the future. I am speaking of its condition as a plastic signifier. It is capable of becoming a signifier, and then modifying itself and the information it carries. The parallel in the past is the gene; the parallel in the future is the computer. The modification of information in brain circuits is a speeded-up version of evolutionary change, through DNA modification; the computer may eventually do it even faster.

The model that I have described does not pretend to be all-inclusive. As a metapsychological construct, it might be considered another "point of view." In his theoretical work, Freud (1915) described three metapsychological points of view, the "dynamic, topographical and economic aspects" (p. 181). Subsequent writers (Hartmann, Kris, & Loewenstein, 1946; Rapaport & Gill, 1959) have added two others, the *genetic* and the *adaptational* points of view. These viewpoints allow explanation from deep, underlying principles, these principles not susceptible to translation into each other. For instance, the topographical point of view describes the mind insofar as it is internally divisioned, whereas the economic point of view describes the effects of the flow and counterflow of energy; these are not incompatible but they are different. We may now be able to add a sixth point of view, the *neurobiological*, namely that which *describes mental activity from the point of view of its reliance on neural function and physiologically describable malfunction.*

It is important that our metapsychology relate to the scientific Zeitgeist in a nonanachronistic way. If it is our theory that we are helping the patient to exorcise demons, or rechanneled libido, or reorganize the ego, or reintegrate the brain, it makes a difference, and in the present era the last of these is more credible. It may be that the low points of the acceptability of psychoanalysis have been those times where it has drifted away from accepted scientific models of mind.

Finally, we must ask about the *clinical* importance of this shift. In many respects clinical theory is like the civil service, which does not change much with changing administrations, or in this case changing metapsychology. The practice of psychoanalysis and its derivative psychotherapies have changed in only minor ways despite the changes in theory from topographic theory, to structural theory, to object-relations theory. Then again, there *have* been some important changes. For instance, there have been changes, for certain diagnostic groups, in the degree of abstinence or activity on the part of the therapist. There have been major modifications derived from our understanding of "primitive defense mechanisms" of the object-relations theorists (Kernberg, 1966). There have been important changes, too, in our choice and prescription of type of therapy based on our recently more refined diagnostic criteria. We do not prescribe psychoanalysis for the same patients we used to. And our diagnostic definitions themselves have received increasing support from our new knowledge of brain structure and function. How will a brain-centered psychology affect our clinical theory? I believe it will in several important ways.

First, The notion of the brain as an information processor, rather than an energy regulator, has led us to think more in terms of learning models and of therapy as a learning process (Marmor, 1974; Karasu, 1986). This does not mean that therapy is didactic in the sense of teaching history or golf. It means that in therapy we aim to modify the programs by which the patient learns and organizes experience. We also may modify the very hardware that uses the programs. Our conceptualization presents a rather smooth hierarchy from brain to words, involving several coding steps, and at least two types of processing, analog and digital. In a sense the whole system is biologized, since there is no coding or signifying independent of biology, and there is a clear continuum from the learning to constrict the bronchioles in the face of stress, and the learning to repress thoughts of aggression or sexuality, and the learning of the facts of world history. We become more comfortable with the notion that psychotherapy can help with psychosomatic illness, that it can modify brain biology as well as modifying a patient's self-concept and even his or her life story. Psychotherapy is now more frequently seen as a *biological* treatment, for theoretical, not just pragmatic reasons (Mohl, 1987).

Second, I think that we are beginning, as we adopt a brain-centered model, to appreciate the interaction between information processing and state factors. Until recently we have considered psychodynamics and affect state to be relatively independent of each other; or, more accurately, we have not focused on the necessary integration of the two. But it becomes clear, as we follow patients for any length of time, that our psychodynamic formulations can be colored by the current affect level of the patient. For instance, a patient whom we consider to be possessed of a success phobia, because he cannot be sufficiently assertive in pursuing his career, may change radically when his depression clears, and he becomes naturally more assertive. He may still have neurotic conflicts, but the previously diagnosed castration anxiety may now appear to be less important. A similar finding is that the symptom disorders, such as phobias and compulsions, often get worse when the patient becomes depressed.

Third, different kinds of therapy, including the somatic therapies, can be seen to be on more of a continuum than is now the case. The learning paradigm mentioned above gives us a rationale for integrating somatic and verbal therapies. As the psychotherapists and the psychopharmacologists have grown further apart, and as the teaching of psychotherapy has waned in perceived importance, we see constantly the repetition of errors caused by mutual ignorance. Some patients receive lengthy, ineffective psychotherapy, which would be much enhanced by medication; and others receive only medication, when chronic personality factors clearly require intensive psychotherapy.

Fourth, psychoanalysis can be seen as the tip of the semiotic iceberg. Free associations are the prime example of semiotic interaction, of one thing standing for another, in this case by way of causal logic, metonymy, and metaphor. The psychoanalytic dialogue represents a constant interplay of the verbal, digital signs, and the affective, nonverbal analog signs. The transference provides for a channeling of the associative flow into the archetypal symbology unique to each patient. The system I have described allows us to consider this psychoanalytic dialogue as a biological event, now taking account of the fact that sign systems are biological systems, and vice versa.

Notes

1 Originally published in *Psychoanalysis and Contemporary Thought*, 1990, Vol 13, No. 3.: 331–363.
2 Dr. Olds is Assistant Clinical Professor of Psychiatry, Columbia College of Physicians and Surgeons, New York; Faculty Member, Columbia Psychoanalytic Center for Training and Research.

References

Anscombe, R. (1986) The ego and the will. *Psychoanalysis and Contemporary Thought*, 9: 437–463.
Arnold, M. (1970) Brain function in emotion: A phenomenological analysis. In *Physiological Correlates of Emotion*, ed. P. Black. New York: Academic Press.
Broadbent, D. E. (1961) *Behavior*. Totowa, NJ: University Paperbacks.
Churchland, P. S. (1986) *Neurophilosophy*. Cambridge, MA: MIT Press.
Deely, J. (1986) *The coalescence of semiotic consciousness*. In: Frontiers in Semiotics, ed. J. Deely, B. Williams, & F. E. Kruse. Bloomington, IN: Indiana University Press.

Dennett, D. C. (1978) *Brainstorms.* Cambridge, MA: MIT Press.

Edelson, M. (1986) The convergence of psychoanalysis and neuroscience. *Contemporary Psychoanalysis*, 22: 479–519.

Freud, A. (1946) *The Ego and the Mechanisms of Defense.* New York: International Universities Press, 1966.

Freud, S. (1897) *Letter to Fliess, May 31, 1897.*Standard Edition, 1. London: Hogarth Press, 1966.

Freud, S. (1915) *The unconscious.* Standard Edition, 14. London: Hogarth Press, 1957, pp. 159–215.

Freud, S. (1950 [1895]) *Project for a scientific psychology.* Standard Edition, 1, pp. 283–397.

Gazzaniga, M. S. (1978) *The Integrated Mind.* New York: Plenum.

Gleick, J. (1987) *Chaos.* New York: Viking Press.

Hartmann, H., Kris, E., & Loewenstein, R. M. (1946) Comments on the formation of psychic structure. *Psychoanalytic Study of the Child*, 2: 11–38. New York: International Universities Press.

Innis, R. E. (1985) *Semiotics: An Introductory Anthology.* Bloomington, IN: Indiana University Press.

Jones, J. M. (1981) *Affects: A nonsymbolic information processing system.* Paper presented at the Annual Meeting, American Psychoanalytic Association.

Joseph, R. (1982) The neuropsychology of development: Hemispheric laterality, limbic language, and the origin of thought. *Journal of Clinical Psychology* (special monograph supplement), 38: 4–33.

Kandel, E. (1983) From metapsychology to molecular biology: Explorations into the nature of anxiety. *American Journal of Psychiatry*, 140: 1277–1293.

Kandel, E. (1984) Is there a cell-biological alphabet for simple forms of learning? *Psychological Review*, 91: 375–391.

Karasu, B. T. (1986) The specificity versus the nonspecificity dilemma: Toward identifying therapeutic change agents. *American Journal of Psychiatry*, 143: 687–695.

Kernberg, O. (1966) Structural derivatives of object relationships. *International Journal of Psychoanalysis*, 47: 236–253.

Kihlstrom, J. F. (1987) The cognitive unconscious. *Science*, 237: 1445–1452.

Kissen, B. (1986) *Conscious and Unconscious Programs in the Brain.* New York: Plenum.

LeDoux, J. E. (1985) Brain, mind and language. In *Brain and Mind*, ed. D. A. Oakley. New York: Methuen.

Levin, F. M. & Vuckovich, D. M. (1985) Brain plasticity, learning, and psychoanalysis: Some mechanisms of integration and coordination within the central nervous system. Paper presented at American Psychoanalytic Association meeting, December.

Libet, B., Wright, E. W., Feinstein, B., & Pearl, D. K. (1979) Subjective referral of the timing for a conscious sensory experience: A functional role for the somatosensory specific projection system in man. *Brain*, 102: 193–224.

Mahler, M. S., Pine, F., & Bergman, A. (1975) *The Psychological Birth of the Human Infant.* New York: Basic Books.

Marmor, J. P. (1974) The nature of the psychotherapeutic process. In *Psychiatry in Transition*, ed. J. Marmor. New York: Brunner/Mazel.

Mohl, P. C. (1987) Should psychotherapy be considered a biological treatment? *Psychosomatics*, 28: 320–326.

Olds, D. D. (1981) The behavioral schema: An integration of modes of learning. *Psychiatry*, 50: 112–125.

Pagels, H. (1985) *Perfect Symmetry: The Search for the Beginning of Time*. New York: Simon & Schuster.

Peirce, C. S. (1897) Logic as semiotic: The theory of signs. In *Semiotics: An Introductory Anthology*, ed. R. E. Innis. Bloomington, IN: Indiana University Press, 1985.

Peterfreund, E. (1971) Information, Systems, and Psychoanalysis: An Evolutionary Biological Approach to Psychoanalytic Theory. *Psychological Issues*, 7 (1/2).

Piaget, J. (1952) *The Origins of Intelligence in Children*. New York: International Universities Press.

Poinsot, J. (1632) *Tractatus de Signis: The Semiotic of John Poinsot*, trans. J. Deely. Berkeley, CA: University of California Press, 1985.

Popper, K. (1972) *Objective Knowledge*. Oxford: Clarendon Press.

Rapaport, D. & Gill, M. (1959) The points of view and assumptions of metapsychology. *International Journal of Psychoanalysis*, 40: 153–162.

Reiser, M. (1985) *Mind, Brain and Body*. New York: Basic Books.

Rosenblatt, A. & Thickstun, J. T. (1977) Modern Psychoanalytic Concepts in a General Psychology. *Psychological Issues*, 11 (2/3).

Rumelhart, D. E. & McClelland, J. L. (1986) *Parallel Distributed Processing: Explorations in the Microstructure of Cognition*. Cambridge, MA: MIT Press.

Schwartz, A. (1987) Drives, affects, and behavior—and learning: Approaches to a psychobiology of emotion and to an integration of psychoanalytic and neurobiologic thought. *Journal of the American Psychoanalytic Association*, 35: 467–506.

Sebeok, T. A. (1986) The doctrine of signs. In *Frontiers in Semiotics*, ed. J. Deely, B. Williams, & F. E. Kruse. Bloomington, IN: Indiana University Press.

Shannon, C. (1949) *The Mathematical Theory of Communication*. Champaign, IL: University of Illinois Press.

Skarda, C. A. & Freeman W. J. (1987) How brains make chaos in order to make sense of the world. *Behavioral & Brain Science*, 10: 161–195.

Sperry, R. W. (1979) *Consciousness, free will and personal identity*. In *Brain, Behavior and Evolution*, ed. D. A. Oakley & H. C. Plotkin. New York: Methuen.

Stern, D. (1985) *The Interpersonal World of the Infant*. New York: Basic Books.

Thompson, R. F. (1986) The neurobiology of learning and memory. *Science*, 233: 941–947.

Tomkins, G. F. (1975) The metabolic code. *Science*, 189: 760–763.

Watson, J. S. (1979) Perception of contingency as a determinant of social responsiveness. In *The Origins of Social Responsiveness*, ed. E. Thomas. Hillsdale, NJ: Lawrence Erlbaum.

Watt, D. F. (1986) Transference: A right hemisphere event? An inquiry into the boundary between psychoanalytic metapsychology and neuropsychology. *Psychoanalysis and Contemporary Thought*, 9: 43–77.

Wilden, A. (1972) *System and Structure: Essays in Communication and Exchange*. London: Tavistock.

Chapter 4

Consciousness

A Brain-Centered, Informational Approach

Introduction

This paper is the second in a series exploring the nature of a brain-centered psychology. In the first paper (Olds, 1990) I developed the idea of a psychology that would consider the brain as its central organizing concept, in lieu of previous abstractions such as ego, id, or internal objects. The rationale for this change is to organize all of our thinking about mental agencies, mental process, and psychological function in general with reference to brain processes. The goal of such a psychology, not fully realizable as yet, is to ground all mental processes in biology in a manner resembling that of Freud's early hopes. The model is an information-processing one, in which information and semiotic functions serve to bridge the gap between brain and mind[1].

I here pursue this idea further in discussing the phenomenon of consciousness. Once this model is developed, I will try to show that such a model places the psychoanalytic concepts of the unconscious and of psychoanalytic therapy in a different light, bringing them into line with current research in brain function and biology. The ultimate aim of such an endeavor is to ground psychoanalytic theory in a currently relevant scientific context.

Writing about consciousness is a kind of quicksand. The topic is vast, the history of thought about it is nearly infinite, and the relevant research findings are accumulating faster than one can write. This paper provides a view of selected issues relevant to a brain-centered psychology, and at the same time relevant to psychoanalysis. I will pursue the following sequence: 1) A condensed account of the history and definition of the term consciousness; 2) A discussion of consciousness in terms of information theory and the notion of re-representation; 3) A discussion of the evolution of consciousness and its part in the larger context of human evolution; 4) A brief description of the currently known neurobiology underlying consciousness; 5) An exploration of the relevance of the preceding issues to the psychoanalytic explanations of defense and the effects of psychoanalytic therapy.

DOI: 10.4324/9781003399551-5

History

The idea of consciousness has not always been with us. Among the ancients, there was little idea of consciousness as we think of it. The idea of the divided self in the sense of an internal homunculus or soul controlling a body had not yet developed. The Greeks had many different theories of mind, so it is difficult to generalize, but a popular conception involved a monistic system of psyche. Events that we might call unconscious, mythic cultures usually attributed to divine intervention, to a god inducing a dream figure to appear to a human, or to a god inducing irrational behavior. With Plato appears a more modern idea: the appetitive, lustful faculty and the spiritual faculty are subordinated to the rational faculty; except in sleep, when the lower faculties escape from rational control and may bring dreams of monstrous behavior. Here we find a sense that forbidden wishes may originate from within; yet even Plato gives us no concept of consciousness and unconsciousness or any notion of self-awareness and introspection of the modern sort. The Middle Ages return to a more mythic approach—intrusions by God, influence by the Devil, and the like.

The word consciousness, according to Whyte (1960), begins to appear in the seventeenth century in Europe. Descartes took the long-established split between divine soul and mortal body and secularized it to render a duality between mind and body, which we have inherited. This dualism has become part of our "common sense," with the resulting contradiction that within our apparently unified universe are two kinds of substance. The intuitive sense that there is a "self" or "mind" over against a body is impossible to remove from our daily thinking, where this contradiction does not seem to matter. In scientific thinking we can ignore the split until we come to psychology. Here the problem will not go away.

This dichotomy has also pervaded the thinking of psychoanalytic theorists. From the topographic model, where the mind was simply split into an executive consciousness and a drive-influenced unconsciousness, to the structural model, where the executive ego had its own unconscious element, this dualism returned in different guise. One of the aspects of the Freudian revolution troubling to traditional philosophy was that one had to confront the fact that the unconscious, with its feet in the clay of *res extensa*, could influence the commonly conceived nonmaterial conscious self. Freud saw consciousness as an organ different in type from the rest of the mind, although not necessarily of an immaterial type. He connected consciousness and perception as organs that could receive sensible qualities but did not store memory traces. In the Project (1895), he called this the omega system; in later writing he (1900, p. 615) named it the perception-consciousness system, which received sensory information from the outside world but which also had an inner view as the "sense organ for the perception of psychical qualities." He related its internal aspect importantly with "word-presentations" as opposed to unconscious "thing-presentations" (see Natsoulas, 1989), a prescient understanding in view of the current emphasis on the importance of language to consciousness.

The fact is that in the early part of this century consciousness was given scant attention. For the psychoanalytic movement the development of the theory of the unconscious was of more pressing interest. On the other hand, in the world of academic psychology, important work on consciousness was begun in the nineteenth century by major figures, such as Wilhelm Wundt and William James; but it came to a halt with the hegemony of behaviorism. Well into the 1940s, "consciousness" was an unscientific form unworthy of research attention. In the 1950s, however, such diverse workers as Broadbent (1958), Lashley (1951), and Chomsky (1957) broke the behaviorist grip, and the study of consciousness is currently of major importance.

Recent advances in neurobiology and information theory have generated new models of mind in the psychoanalytic realm, that have eschewed the Freudian drive theories underlying the earlier dualistic system. All the versions of the Freudian model included id-generated psychic energy, orchestrated by "higher" agencies that control and civilize behavior, rather like the Platonic model. In later versions, as Rosenblatt and Thickstun (1977) have pointed out, an informational nuance crept in under the name "signal anxiety," really a bit of information that warned of danger and the need for inner defensive measures. Peterfreund's informational model (1971) and Basch's paper on communication science (1976) have been major influences in the recasting of psychoanalytic theory.

Dualistic models still exist. It is my view that such models severely strain credulity, requiring as they do two kinds of substance, and render any psychological system incomplete. The behaviorists, wrong-headed as they now seem, did perform the service of unifying the split by legislating consciousness out of consideration. My endeavor has been to instead use the concepts of information and semiotics to explain why the split is only an apparent one. I have discussed this at length in the previous article: I will briefly review the arguments later in this paper, as I try to include consciousness in an information-processing model.

Definitions of Consciousness

Definitions of consciousness are strongly influenced by one's theory of consciousness and vice versa. Consciousness is one of those complex concepts which draws one into a vicious cycle of definition and redefinition.

Consciousness is often defined by what it is not, by various kinds of unconsciousness, the most basic of which is the opposition to stupor, coma, or sleep. At another level we oppose it to vague states of inattention such as trance, fugue, or even distraction. A third is based on awareness. One may be aware enough to be engaged in a familiar activity, such as driving, or cooking, but simultaneously thinking about something else. At a higher level one may be focused fully on a task that is new or difficult without being "self-conscious." Then, usually at the top of the consciousness hierarchy, we place self-consciousness, wherein I am aware of what I am doing and notice the fact that I am doing it. I will deal here with the last three of these definitions, all involving awareness and self-awareness; they have a reflective or recursive aspect, which makes them unique, and which I call re-representation.

We can define consciousness in terms of content or in terms of process (Rosenblatt, 1990). The content definition deals with what is or can be included. The Freudian model included the currently conscious, the potentially conscious or preconscious, and the unconscious. The unconscious also must be divided between the dynamic unconscious, the contents which cannot be brought to awareness for defensive psychological reasons, and those which involve brain and body functions, such as motor and autonomic regulation. The content definition is a functional one, which addresses the "what" and the "why" of consciousness. The process definition relates to the "how." This would ideally include a neurobiological explanation; but we are not yet ready to do this. My hope here is to use an informational model to lay some of the groundwork for future speculations about this process.

The Role of Consciousness in Information Processing

Essential to our discussion is the idea that the brain is an information processor. Claude Shannon (1949) formulated an information theory that has become standard as the basic theory of communication systems. The theory uses the laws of thermodynamics as a model for informational structures and permits a kind of quantification of information by use of the concept of entropy; like any structure, information bears an inverse relation to entropy.

A corollary to this theory, which was important to Shannon, is the fact that messages are structures that tend to degrade, as in the game of Telephone. All effective information systems have methods for preventing this degradation. For instance, in human language there is a great deal of redundancy so that one can often understand a sentence even when one hears only half the words. Electronic messages have several tricks for reducing error, such as retransmission or providing digit counts. Or, in other communication systems, sending the same message by different media can be effective, such as using both blinking-light Morse code and semaphore between ships at sea. One purpose, then, of sending a message more than once—re-representation—is for validation.

An example of a system without a re-representation device, which is consequently a poor system, is a dial telephone. If I dial a number and no one answers, I have no way of knowing if I dialed the wrong number, or if indeed no one is at home. I may do a primitive verification trick and dial again; but a much better system is a phone with a digital read-out that shows just what numbers I dialed.

Validation in Biological Systems

Let us consider biological information systems to see if they contain examples of re-representation. One example might be the way enzymes organize the pairing of nucleic acids in making copies of DNA molecules. At one end of the enzyme the pairings are made, at the other end the sequence is checked for errors and these errors corrected. This also is a re-representation system, a kind of proof reading of the gene.

With cybernetic biological systems, the re-representation is a feedback sign to the governing entity. For instance, blood-sugar exists in the blood; it also becomes a sign of its own level by being counted, compared to standard, and thus stimulating an error correction. Or, a flying bee keeps re-representing its distance from the hive and flying toward it to correct for the error (distance).

Representation as Sign

Let us clarify the idea of "representation." In my previous paper, I proposed that the theoretical discipline of semiotics has something to offer in explaining mind-brain interaction. The theories of Poinsot (1632), Peirce (1897), and Sebeok (1986) converge on the idea that the sign is ubiquitous in all living systems. Basically, these theories suggest that all life depends on the ability of one thing to stand for another. An amino acid stands for a codon in an RNA molecule, an RNA molecule stands for a DNA molecule, glucose concentration stands for a certain metabolic state, etc. With respect to our current interest, brain events (more or less permanent cellular modifications) stand for percepts and by so doing can "store" them in memory. Other sign systems can stand for these brain-storage events. Human language is one such system. I mean that words, expressed in appropriate syntax, stand for memory traces stored in the brain. We may say they carry the information for the purpose of communicating it to others. Similarly, gestural language, sign language, writing, music, and others are systems for translating brain events into signs that may be transmitted. My thesis is that consciousness is one such sign system; it is a sign system in which cellular events in the consciousness system re-represent cellular events that have recorded information in the nonconscious brain.

Consciousness as After-the-Fact

Let us pursue the idea that consciousness is part of such a re-representation system. Traditionally, consciousness has been placed in the position of initiator of behavior, the decision maker, the center of will. The work of Libet et al. (1983) brought this idea into question by revealing that conscious awareness is after the fact. It is well known that a reflex withdrawal after stepping on a tack will be followed by consciousness of that act. But Libet and his colleagues demonstrated that even with an active spontaneous decision a readiness potential in the brain can be detected almost a half second before conscious awareness of the decision. So, all computations and cogitations would seem to be initiated by the nonconscious brain; some of these are fed into the narrow stream of consciousness.

The conclusions derived from this finding are at first glance distressing. It suggests that we do not make conscious decisions; therefore, the whole system of personal responsibility seems to be in jeopardy. But in fact, the conclusion is almost self-evident even without the experiment of Libet et al. If we think of the alternative to this conclusion, namely, that consciousness can be a cause of brain activity, then we have to accept that consciousness is uncaused or comes from outside the brain; this assumption forces us into a dualist position.

Also, we have to remember that the Libet et al. experiment represents a microscopic view—the events taking place in 500 milliseconds. When we make any decision that really counts, that has any moral implications or touches on issues of responsibility, the time frame is much longer. A prolonged dialogue takes place between brain and its self-monitoring consciousness; it should be possible to hold the entire person responsible for the result.

This leads us to think about some other curious aspects of consciousness. One is that when we speak, we can be conscious of the words we speak, we can even explain how we constructed the sentence (in retrospect), but we cannot be conscious of our use of syntax as we are speaking the sentence. Another related fact is that most thinking and reasoning is done outside of consciousness. Research psychologists of the Wurtzberg School understood this as far back as 1900. In Karl Marbe's experiment, reported in 1901 (discussed in Jaynes, 1976), subjects were asked to lift two weights, one in each hand, and place the heavier one in a designated spot. It was clear that the instructions were consciously received, the result was consciously perceived, but the act of judgment could not be retrieved by any amount of introspection.

Similarly, the most creative complex decisions are not made consciously. Kekulé's solution to the benzene-ring problem involving his snake dream, and Poincaré's dazzling insight into Fuchsian functions while stepping onto a bus, are examples of this phenomenon.

Evidence suggests then that consciousness is a re-representation device. The brain replays some of the results of its activity—later and in a different medium. Subsequently, in replaying a scene from memory, one becomes aware of what one has learned and can then make corrections. This capacity is similar to the computer monitor, which, like the telephone read-out, tells me what I have just typed. If I did not have the monitor, I would not be sure of exactly what I had written. I could perhaps print it out, but if that printout had to be my final draft, I would be typing with much anxiety and loss of efficiency and speed.

Let us look at this phenomenon a little more closely. What needs feeding back? If we follow the computer metaphor further, in its function as a word processor we can find primitive analogies to some thinking processes. In terms of feedback, the monitor shows me what I have just typed. I can make corrections in spelling, punctuation, as well as in the meanings of sentences, paragraphs, even the concept of the whole manuscript. In other words, I may make changes in the signs themselves (correct spelling errors) or in the meanings I wish to generate (changing the words). The monitor, however, is only a part of the feedback loop; the human operator is the most essential part. The computer cannot write a word by itself.

To go one step further with this analogy, the computer screen displays only the results of the machine's computations. We do not see the computations themselves. If a computer were designed so that each computation, presumably done in machine-language symbols, were represented on the screen, and that the process was slowed down sufficiently so one could see it, there would be considerable time and space between each final character on the screen. Consciousness seems to be a series of tips of icebergs, discontinuous frames showing the results of computations. It may be that the mind turns them into a continuous experience, as it does with the frames of a movie film.

Feedback and Re-Representation

One of the essential principles of living systems is that all processes are governed by feedback loops, which themselves include sign systems. Genetic processes are governed by the "feedback" principle of survival. Within organisms, metabolic processes such as glucose metabolism, hormone regulation, and muscle control all remain in balance because of negative feedback. In fact, for a process to work, the feedback is as important as the process itself. Without proprioceptive mechanisms, muscular action becomes chaotic. Disruption of hormonal feedback systems can lead to death. Manipulation of the feedback system can also be useful in certain circumstances—for instance, in altering the output of endocrine systems, in using hormones to slow the progress of cancers, or in manipulating neurotransmitter levels with psychotropic drugs.

If feedback systems are ubiquitous, then we can enquire whether they have something to do with consciousness. With perception, a multichannel input from the senses is organized and routed to consciousness so that we are aware of our immediate experience. In the loop of input-output the conscious representation is itself a feedback phenomenon, which the brain takes into account in forming the next action or response. Analogously, when we recall an image from memory, again representing it via multiple channels, often with attendant affect, the conscious representation acts as the next input to the brain. It is the sign to the brain representing what the brain has just accomplished.

The interesting thing is that this re-representation is a highly selective linear stream out of the massive parallel-processing brain. Mandler (1988), in discussing consciousness, stresses that the conscious stream is not only narrow and selective but that it is a constant process of construction, of putting together the multiple input trains into an ever-changing complex. The point for our purposes is that the selection is for items of interest for feedback. It is a sampling of brain activity, not of the whole of reality. It resembles a diagnostic device like that of taking one's pulse to see if one is doing an adequate workout. Similarly, an airline pilot, instead of looking out the window, may observe his instruments for read-outs concerning the position or altitude of his aircraft.

Consciousness does not "look out" through the eyes (and other senses); it represents what the brain has assembled from using all the senses. The choice of what to represent consciously is a puzzle that tends to generate a circular argument. It is conscious because it is deemed important; it is important because it is conscious. Ultimately, we need a mechanism to explain how importance is evaluated and how importance leads to consciousness. The currently exciting neural-net models of the mind (Campbell, 1989) suggest possible mechanisms involving alterations in connection strengths of certain complexes to put them over a hypothetical threshold to consciousness. In this kind of model, that event itself—the becoming conscious—alters relationships in proximal or "associated" complexes, which may then be boosted over the threshold.

As to the reasons for the supraliminal importance of conscious contents, we have to assume that certain hierarchies exist. In the realm of content there may be ordering in terms of survival value, instinctual importance, interest, fantasy, etc. With respect to structural qualities of perception there are other "attention-getting" criteria, such as intensity of stimulus, novelty, or dissonance. We can only surmise the reasons for choosing a particular conscious item, and we often do just that in psychoanalytic therapy. Lichtenberg (1989) has described motivational systems underlying content hierarchies.

Neurobiology of Consciousness

As I mentioned in attempting an initial definition of consciousness, we think of the term on a hierarchical series of planes. And these planes all have neurological correlates. Kissen (1986) describes the known circuits that are considered responsible for the functioning at the different levels.

The most basic definition of consciousness opposes it to such states of unconsciousness as sleep or coma. From the neurophysiological point of view this basic distinction is quite complex. There are thought to be two primary activating systems in the brain stem, one mediated by norepinephrine, the other by acetylcholine. The nor-adrenergic system involves two anatomical structures—the reticular activating system, which drives basic states of arousal, and a subdivision of that system, the locus coeruleus, which organizes states of attention. The other activating complex, the cholinergic system, stimulates the brain but does not generate alertness; this is the mechanism that is active in REM sleep. At a higher level, there is a general awareness system that mediates an awareness of experience and surroundings, as opposed to focused attention. This involves a system which includes—and apparently links—parts of the hypothalamus, the thalamus, and the basal ganglia (globus pallidus and putamen). Damage to parts of this system can produce such syndromes as akinetic mutism in which there is wakefulness but minimal reaction to any stimulus, or the thalamic syndrome of Dejerine-Roussy, in which emotional reactions to stimuli are grossly exaggerated or diminished. Thus, the brain centers at this level are necessary for an integrated but unfocused sense of being in the world, along with a general affective sense of one's condition.

Self-Awareness System

When we come to the most "advanced" capability of consciousness, which we may call a self-awareness system, we have to deal both with a high level of consciousness and the idea of self. Self is a concept that has filled many volumes; here I will limit my discussion to the minimum and deal with it in relation to our information-processing model.

Several neurological deficit syndromes have led us to clarify and refine what we mean by conscious self-awareness. The best known such deficit is that arising from splitting the brain by cutting the corpus callosum. Such lesions have led to the discovery of specialization of functions in the two hemispheres, the results of which are by now generally known (Gazzaniga, 1978). Of most interest in the present context is the fact that visual information fed to the isolated right hemisphere alone will not enter any kind of self-awareness; the person will deny seeing anything. At the same time experiments have shown that the object is perceived and registered at a certain level. Although the person cannot name the objects, she can point to them or rate them according to feelings about them, such as whether she likes them or not. In one experiment, the picture of a nude man was presented to the isolated right hemisphere of a woman. She said she saw nothing, but at the same time she blushed and giggled. In such situations we have to assume that the person receives the images up to the level of the right parietal cortex, and that there is some sense of self in relation to the objects. But the last step into the linguistic brain is missing. Self-awareness seems to require that step.

The work of Mountcastle et al. (1975) and Mesalum and Geschwind (1978) has elaborated on other complex connections underlying the focused awareness of the self-awareness system. Experimental lesions of the posterior-inferior area of the parietal lobe in monkeys lead to an inability to focus attention on the contralateral side. In humans cerebrovascular damage to the same area leads to the unilateral neglect syndrome in which the patients cannot even conceive of anything of interest on that side of the body, or in the world, that would be perceived in that visual field.

The "self-system" seems to involve integration of many inputs at the posterior inferior parietal lobe—by routes from the other association cortical areas, from the limbic system and brain stem. This is a major integration point of somatosensory and affective input; the sense of one's body appears to be central to the sense of self. The important conclusion from the research into the neglect syndromes is that the self-system is as essential to focused awareness as are the intact perceptual systems and lower awareness systems. To focus on objects, they must be seen as significant to a self. Mesalum and Geschwind (1978) have concluded that the self-system is somewhat more localized in the right brain than in the left. According to this definition of self, selfhood exists in all mammals; if it is obliterated a neglect syndrome will follow. So, the sense of self developed early in evolution, long before consciousness in human terms. This self exists on conscious and unconscious levels, integrating proprioception, sensation, and affect into a central entity, which becomes a center of significance and mediates the importance of all experiences.

As we review the neurobiology, it becomes possible to imagine that the mechanism of consciousness involves certain brain centers. It may be that there are multiple centers, perhaps even a diffuse distribution. But in the discussion to come let us accept that conscious events are brain events, involving discrete areas of the brain, without worrying about exactly where they are. To conceive of consciousness as a sign system allows us to proceed without exact anatomical knowledge.

The idea of a sign system also helps with the distinction between consciousness and self-consciousness. Consciousness has to do with re-representing percepts and memories selected from the brain's vast storehouse. Self-consciousness has to do with re-representing those signs which refer to the individual as an object and as a center of significance.

The idea of a "consciousness center" that re-represents brain events in a feedback loop by way of selective integration, is, I believe, useful heuristically, although it does not land us in conceptual utopia. Vexing complexities arise immediately. One is the when of consciousness. If consciousness is a reflective loop or feedback system, does consciousness of a percept or a memory occur at the instant it reaches the hypothesized consciousness center or when it l;;kreturns to wherever in the brain it originated? Another question is what chooses the contents of consciousness, the whole brain, or the consciousness center? If we say the whole brain, we seem to be begging the question, since the brain, in order to know what to flash into consciousness, must be aware of it already. Contrariwise, the consciousness center is in the same position. These are problems that have long plagued the notion of the "sapient ego."

The answers, emerging from neural-network theory and related philosophical writings, suggest that the brain functions in a modular fashion, with "multiple partial homunculi" (see Dennett, 1978). The general idea is that if we have specialized homunculi who are not simply miniature versions of the self but are specialized members of a team that "knows" more than its individual members, we do not have the problems of infinite regress, and, in this case, who chooses what becomes conscious. The parallel-processing brain sends certain items to the consciousness system, which is itself a brain area specialized for re-representation (see Anscombe, 1986; Gazzaniga, 1985).

Consciousness in Evolution

If we look back through the history of evolution, we may be struck by a phenomenon that has interesting similarities to consciousness, namely, the REM state in mammals. In his book Brain and Psyche, Winson (1985) describes an evolutionary leap in brain ability. The most primitive order of mammals, the monotremes, are mammals in that they have a four-chambered heart, are warm blooded, and suckle their young; but they still have a reptilian vestige: they hatch their young from eggs. Another striking thing about them is that their brains are larger and more convoluted for their body size than those of much more intelligent animals further up the evolutionary tree. Noting that the monotremes, unlike later-evolving marsupials and mammals, do not have REM sleep.

Winson postulates that REM sleep is an efficient organizer of brain activity, a mode of "off-line processing" of information; this efficiency may allow for a relatively smaller brain. He theorizes that in sleep, mammals re-represent complex behaviors, possibly as a form of rehearsal or of maintaining skills, perhaps the forerunner of the "fantasy rehearsal" currently popular among athletes. Normally the motor system is paralyzed during REM states; if this paralysis can be surgically prevented, the animal will move its body as if it were running and leaping.

The point for our purpose is that the REM dream may be the first evolutionary instance of cerebral re-representation. This is not the same as recognition memory such as exists in a reptile, enabling it to recognize stimuli, learn tasks, and follow elaborate operant procedures. In such an animal an engram in the brain is activated by the recognized stimulus; but we presume that the reptile cannot call up a fantasy of that stimulus and run through an action sequence in fantasy. With the behavioral learning of such creatures, the memory consists of a recognition of a stimulus followed by the responsive behavior. With the mammal's REM state, on the other hand, the episode can be expressed in representative form, without the behavior.

Let us speculate that the ability to re-represent in image or trial-action form is an achievement of lower mammals and that it may be analogous to what we call consciousness. The next evolutionary stage would be the ability to do such imaging and trial actions in a waking state. Apparently other primates can perform complicated tasks and can plan complex strategies. For the chimpanzee who fetches a box to climb upon in order to reach the banana, it is likely that some kind of cerebral trial action took place in forming the action strategy.

Thus, there is a phylogenetic line of self-consciousness-like phenomena. The most primitive organisms have biochemical feedback systems, such as those which represent glucose levels, hormone levels, and response to antigens. With more overtly informational processes feedback is still required. In an animal communicating through facial or bodily gesture, in the fashion Darwin described, there must be internal feedback systems to let the animal "know" it is generating the right gesture, as well as the external feedback from those who receive the signals. Such feedback systems are unconscious, for the most part. With language we must hear ourselves speak to know what we said; this too may be more or less conscious. Self-consciousness is like all the other forms of feedback in that it is a re-representation with certain additions including an owning, a self-reference, or self-responsibility.

Language and Consciousness

How necessary is language to consciousness? Given the split-brain experiments that show patients having perceptions by way of the right hemisphere, but showing no evidence of consciousness of them, language seems to be necessary (Gazzaniga, 1978; LeDoux, 1985). However, a commonsense objection arises. One can imagine visual scenes without the need for language; in fact a scene image may be so elaborate as not to be fully describable in words.

Gazzaniga (1985) describes experiments that show that in even those split-brain patients who have some right-brain language ability, it is the left brain that is better able to call up scenes in imagination. If this capacity is a left-hemisphere phenomenon it may be related to language, and the following hypothesis emerges: that the imaging capacity was an evolutionary precursor to language. In other words, the functions necessary to language, such as re-representation in a linear sequence, analogous to a spatially imagined sequence and involving a linearly ordained logic, required an advanced imaging capacity. This becomes even clearer when applied to written language, which makes full use of the power to imagine visual symbols in a sequenced, syntactic order. Thus, it seems that consciousness, in order to be fully rigged, requires both the imaging and the linguistic capacity.

We are now in a position to guess at an evolutionary series leading to consciousness as we know it. First were biochemical feedback systems, then, with motile organisms, proprioceptive feedback systems. With early mammals we have a primitive visualization system operating in sleep, the REM dream state. Next comes a capacity to visualize scenes and form strategies, from the behavioral map that allows a dog to find its buried bone to a complex strategy that helps a chimpanzee to reach a banana. The awake visualization becomes subspecialized into the language functions in the dominant hemisphere, this final set of systems making up the basis of our consciousness system.

Co-evolution With Other Functions

Having focused so far on the re-representation aspect of consciousness, we must now confront the fact that consciousness as re-representation exists within a group of functions that probably co-evolved, each one necessary for the functions of the others. We have related consciousness to the self, to language, and to society. It is probable that in order to have any one of these we must have them all. As they developed in tandem each must have synergized with the others, leading to a system inextricably bound with the development of the individual in society.

We may be able to discern at least four of these functions:

1   1. The imaging function has the longest genealogy. It evolved as an advanced form of re-representation, following a history that includes biochemical feedback, proprioception, the REM dream, and advanced imaging systems.
2   2. Another is the self function, also with primitive origins but becoming more complex as the organism has advanced and the imaging function allowed for a self image.
3   3. A third is the empathic function, most likely a late developer. Humphrey (1984) theorizes that consciousness of one's own feelings is helpful in judging or predicting the feelings of others. This ability might give one a selective advantage in the community.
4   Fourth, and presumably the latest to emerge, is the language function.

The possibilities for synergy among these evolving capacities are striking. The imaging function allows for an enhanced sense of self, for the sequencing aspects of language, and for the empathic placement of others in predictive simulations of behavior. The self function orients oneself in one's fantasies, allows for empathy, adds to the development of syntax, the subject-object basis of grammar. Empathy allows for images of others to resemble those of self, enriches the sense of self as it is differentiated from others, helps predict behavior, and may help uncover deceit especially that conveyed by language. Language, in addition to its dramatic advancement in communication providing the basis for advanced civilization, allows for the experience of consciousness (as evidenced by the split-brain experiments), stabilizes the self in a linguistic system, and allows for much more elaborate empathic communication.

Defenses: Interference with Re-Representation

As an evolved capacity, we have concluded that re-representation is apparently very useful. The question must arise, why do we so frequently interfere with it?

It is not immediately obvious why we should need to repress memories. It may be, however, that the brain, in order to work efficiently, must protect itself from excessive affect. If we can truly re-represent without motor action, as in fantasy rehearsal, it seems that we should be able to do it without overwhelming affect. However, the two types of separation represent very different processing problems.

In evolution, the perceptual system has a long history of division from the motor system. In reflex behavior we say there is no separation; action follows percept with no intermediate processing and no choice. As time has gone on, however, higher organisms have been able to perceive and then make use of intentional systems, having some choice in how they will make use of the perceptions.

It is as though we have been able to achieve trial action but are only partially successful at "trial affect." The brain is wired so that every percept comes with some affective loading. Unlike action, which is an output phenomenon and therefore can more easily be separated from input, affect is part of the input. The information-processing task is that much more difficult because the affect must be isolated after it has arrived packaged with the percept. The defenses are used in various ways to make this disconnection. Why? One reason may be that internal information processing is difficult when there is no separation. Certain affects are themselves aversive. The memory of a trauma brings with it a flood of painful affect which, in the absence of defenses, would be overwhelming, precluding any further thought or planning. The repertoire of defenses seems to be a graded set of methods for keeping consciousness as free as possible from overwhelming emotion and frenzied reaction.

The individual's motivation to defend against negative affect is operantly conditioned—avoidance results in less pain. This process of affect avoidance can be maladaptive, and can lead to symptoms. However, in terms of evolutionary adaptation and natural selection, the defenses may be useful in the overall scheme of information processing. Defenses are analogous to the muscle paralysis of REM sleep; they have evolved to allow for conscious function at least partially independent of affect.

The idea of consciousness as a feedback loop helps to clarify this conceptualization of defenses. For one thing, the fact that it is a loop means there is an efferent and an afferent limb. We could predict that there may be blockages possible with respect to each limb.

Repression and the other defenses devoted to keeping ideas and their attendant affect out of awareness may represent a functional interference with the transmissions to the consciousness center. When certain mental content has reached the consciousness center and is on its way back, it may reach a state of awareness but be disavowed or split. This leads to interesting questions. If we could time defenses in an experiment similar to that of Libet et al., would we find disavowal tending to occur some milliseconds later than repression?

The Function of Psychotherapy

Being able to separate and repress affect and allow for unencumbered thinking in a crisis has evolutionary advantage. In fact, it is no doubt beneficial to a social organism to repress and otherwise defend against various impulses that would be disruptive—Freud's (1930) model of civilization. In many people these defenses may be excessive; they can become chronic maladaptive aspects of personality, leading to problems in information processing throughout life. The results of childhood conflicts may be kept out of consciousness; they become set in place with no opportunity for revision. Once repressed ideas can enter the conscious stream, they can enter into a process by which conscious ideas are fed back into the preconscious mind and can be evaluated in relation to the person's adult understanding of the world.

In this light psychoanalytic therapy is an advance in social evolution that helps some individuals to succeed better than they otherwise would. A common rationale for therapy is that we use the defensive systems when they are needed in childhood, but that when their usefulness has passed, we may be crippled by them. Therapy is then required to help undo the obsolete defenses. The development of psychotherapy could be seen as a social development, similar to prolonged child care, the use of clothing, and certain urban amenities. It exists in the tradition of most of the world's religions, although most religious techniques tend to reenforce defenses rather than try to undo them. In societies in which life is much harsher and more dangerous than in the twentieth-century West, the defenses remain necessary more than they do for us; or it may be that different defenses are required. In societies with surplus capital, leisure, and time for reflection and creativity, the undoing of certain defenses may release consciousness and expand it, to adaptive advantage.

Psychotherapy is an analog of consciousness, a kind of re-re-representation, which involves a projection of dynamic unconscious structures onto the analyst, who reflects them back. Of course, other things happen in therapy by way of internalization, new behavioral learning, and cognitive restructuring (Olds, 1981). These things happen because the analyst takes the next step beyond consciousness.

The analyst or therapist, in taking a neutral, nonjudgmental role, is performing a function similar to the feedback function of consciousness itself, allowing for information to be brought into the discourse with the affective aspect temporarily reduced. In fact, this is never entirely possible. But in a successful therapy such a condition may be approached as the patient begins to trust the analyst's noncritical stance and realizes the therapist is benignly neutral.

Discussion

To summarize, in the process of evolution we have developed information systems devoted to processing and error correction, which have certain things in common. These systems allow for an escape from the constriction of behavioral learning and performance, in which behavior is learned always on the hoof, in the process of action. We may surmise that the dream is the earliest example of this "off-line" processing, where representations can be brought into some state of awareness, but with the capacity for enactment cut off.

Then we have consciousness, where a similar process can occur in the waking state. Here representations can be reviewed with the motor system disengaged at a higher level—the muscles are ready for action, but controlled by conscious (or unconscious) decision processes; in addition, the affect system can be more or less decoupled by use of the defense mechanisms. This allows for self-consciousness, conscious planning, fantasy rehearsal, daydreaming, and all the many products of imagination. The third great system in this series, which also makes use of behavioral decoupling, is psychotherapy, the method of repair. In motorcycle repair, it is useful in making a diagnosis, and in fine tuning, to run the engine in neutral, uncoupled from the wheels. In therapy we do something similar. Psychoanalysis is the most obvious in this regard. We ask the patient to lie on a couch, and put the muscles at ease, consistent with a waking state. Then the analysand is to disengage from normal practical goals and allow the mind to wander and follow its "free associations." In fact, even the normal "observing ego" is told to relax, as well as the observing superego. These functions are handed over to the analyst, with the purpose of allowing free association unfettered by even self-observation. This technique—while never fully realized in that there is never perfect trust or complete relaxation—allows for the revelation of the unconscious structures or inner constraints that guide thought and action. Analysis is a kind of meta-self-consciousness, with the analyst playing a temporary role of the meta-self.

Consequently, consciousness itself is a kind of model for psychotherapy, particularly the psychoanalytic varieties of therapy. If consciousness is the repair mechanism for the behavioral repertoire, therapy is the repair mechanism for consciousness.

If we accept this view, its implications have importance: We do not need the homuncular aspects of ego and self psychology. We do not need to postulate an ego or a censor or a superego, except as virtual entities representing certain clusters of functions. We do not need a sapient central organizer. It means that psychotherapy is a treatment for the brain. Consciousness reveals the effects of our work. By undoing defenses, we alter some of the information that the preconscious brain has to deal with; this may result in the brain's allowing more and different material into consciousness. This change allows a wider range of phenomena to enter the feedback stream and hence may lead to a greater freedom of action.

In a brain-centered model we see the organizing entity as entirely preconscious. The organizing entity is the brain itself. The brain seems to be a conglomerate of many semi-independent modular units, which organize themselves in a way as yet not understood. Consciousness is one of the brain's many output phenomena. Other such phenomena include motor actions, visceral responses, words, and dreams. The parallel-processing brain does thousands of tasks simultaneously. Each of its output processes is characterized by a reduction to a linear series. With motor activity there is a coordinate stream of action in a chained sequence. Proprioception gives us instant feedback regarding our progress along the chain. Conscious thought is the selective activation of a stream of current percepts, recalled images, or thoughts. This stream represents what has just happened in the brain, and acts like a video monitor. Each image or thought that becomes conscious acts as another input to the brain. Consciousness is a kind of proprioceptor of the thought process, a way of the brain's informing itself what it has just accomplished.

What are the implications for our theory of therapy? One result is an integration of our techniques. The verbal, behavioral, and pharmacologic therapies can be seen as altering different kinds of input to the preconscious process (Olds, 1981). I am not implying that there should be changes in psychoanalytic technique. In fact, this model gives considerable theoretical support to the analytic method, especially its empathic, reflective aspects. However, this theory does imply that psychoanalysis is one of several modes of modifying a person's pattern of information processing, and that a combination of psychoanalysis with other treatments may in some cases be desirable.

In semiotic parlance conscious thoughts, words, and actions are signs of brain activity; they represent a sign system by which the brain talks to itself.

They are also part of a sign system in the interpersonal world, in the culture in which one lives. In this conceptualization, neurotransmitters, pharmacologic agents, autonomic responses, words, and gestures are all aspects of sign systems; they can all act as inputs to the brain in its preconscious activity.

If we expand on the feedback-loop notion this point becomes more emphatically clear. If consciousness involves a brain center that integrates information from several brain systems—cognitive, behavioral, and affective—then a therapy that promotes a freer flow and widening scope of unconscious brain contents into consciousness will alter all these systems. Schwartz (1987) points out how the altered expectations of the analytic situation—the neutrality, abstinence, "containing" environment—alter a host of associational connections, connections between ideas, habits, behavioral expectations, and affects. Analysts tend to view what they do as mostly verbal, but the analytic experience is a global change in experience, with immediate effect on mood, reactivity, and opportunities for response. These lead to biochemical changes in the affect system, to habit changes in the behavioral system, and cognitive changes in the systems of internalization and verbal learning. Some of these changes open up the afferent limb to the center of consciousness, some the efferent limb. In neural-network theory any chemical alteration in the neurotransmitters involving affect or in those mediating other kinds of learning must modify the stream into and out of consciousness. Just lying on the couch will make a minuscule change in affect, which will modify the ensuing chain of associations. Similarly, any action of the analyst, including any interpretation, since it is carried out in an otherwise low-noise atmosphere, will also alter the stream. As this process leads to a deepening transference process, its course changes even more, and new defended-against and/or forgotten material catches the "mind's eye." The stream of consciousness becomes diverted like light waves around a planet, bending toward the transference.

Note

1 Originally published in *Psychoanalytic Inquiry*, (1992), Vol. 12: 419–444.

References

Anscombe, R. (1986) The ego and the will. *Psychoanalysis & Contemporary Thought*, 9: 437–463.

Basch, M. F. (1976) Psychoanalysis and communication science. *Annual of Psychoanalysis.*, 4: 385–421. New York: International Universities Press.

Broadbent, D. E. (1958) *Perception and Communication*. London: Pergamon.

Campbell, J. (1989) *The Improbable Machine*. New York: Simon & Schuster.

Chomsky, N. (1957) *Syntactic Structures*. The Hague: Mouton.

Dennett, D. (1978) *Brainstorms*. Cambridge: MIT Press.

Freud, S. (1895) *Project for a scientific psychology. S.E.*, 1.

Freud, S. (1900) *The interpretation of dreams. S.E.*, 5.

Freud, S. (1930) *Civilization and its discontents. S.E.*, 21.

Gazzaniga, M. S. (1978) *The Integrated Mind.* New York: Plenum.

Gazzaniga, M. S. (1985) *The Social Brain: Discovering the Networks of the Mind.* New York: Basic Books.

Humphrey, N. (1984) *Consciousness Regained.* New York: Oxford.

Jaynes, J. (1976) *The Origin of Consciousness in the Breakdown of the Bicameral Mind.* Boston: Houghton Mifflin.

Kissen, B. (1986) *Conscious and Unconscious Programs in the Brain.* New York: Plenum.

Lashley, K. S. (1951) The problem of serial order in behavior. In *Cerebral Mechanisms in Behavior*, ed. L. A. Jeffries. New York: Wiley.

LeDoux, J. E. (1985) Brain, Mind and Language. In *Brain and Mind*, ed. D. A. Oakley. London/New York: Methuen.

Libet, B., Gleason, C. A., Wright, E. W., & Pearl, D. K. (1983) Time of conscious intention to act in relation to onset of cerebral activity (readiness potential): The unconscious initiation of a freely voluntary act. *Brain*, 106: 623–642.

Lichtenberg, J. D. (1989) *Psychoanalysis and Motivation.* Hillsdale, NJ: The Analytic Press.

Mandler, G. (1988) Problems and directions in the study of consciousness. In *Psychodynamics and Cognition*, ed. M. Horowitz. Chicago, IL: University of Chicago Press.

Mesalum, M. M. & Geschwind, N. (1978) On the possible role of neocortex and its limbic connections in the process of attention in schizophrenia: Clinical cases of inattention in man and experimental anatomy in monkey. *Journal Psychiatric Research*, 14: 249–259.

Mountcastle, V. M., Lynch, J. C., & Georgopoulos, A. (1975) Posterior pariental association cortex of the monkey: Command function for operations within interpersonal space. *Journal of Neurophysiology*, 38: 871–908.

Natsoulas, T. (1989) Freud and Consciousness: IV. *Psychoanalysis & Contemporary Thought*, 12: 619–662.

Olds, D. (1981) The behavioral schema: An integration of modes of learning. *Psychiatry*, 50: 112–125.

Olds, D. (1990) Brain Centered Psychology: A semiotic approach. *Psychoanalysis & Contemporary Thought*, 13: 331–363.

Peirce, C. S. (1897) Logic as semiotic: The theory of signs. In *Semiotics: An Introductory Anthology*, ed. R. E. Innis (1985). Bloomington, IN: Indiana University Press, pp. 1–23.

Peterfreund, E. (1971) Information, Systems, and Psychoanalysis. *Psychological Issues*, Monograph 25/26. New York: International Universities Press.

Poinsot, J. (1632) *Tractatus de Signis: The Semiotic of John Poinsot*, tr. J. Deely. Berkeley, CA: University of California Press.

Rosenblatt, A. (1990) Discussion of this paper at the Annual Meeting of the American Psychoanalytic Association, May 1990.

Rosenblatt, A. & Thickstun, J. T. (1977) Modern Psychoanalytic Concepts in a General Psychology. *Psychological Issues*, Monograph 11. New York: International Universities Press.

Schwartz, A. (1987) Drives, affects, behavior—and learning: Approaches to a psychobiology of emotion and to an integration of psychoanalytic and neurobiologic thought. *Journal of the American Psychoanalytic Association*, 35: 467–506.

Sebeok, T. A. (1986) The doctrine of signs. In *Frontiers in Semiotics*, ed. J. Deely, B. Williams, & F. E. Kruse (1986) Bloomington, IN: Indiana University Press, pp. 35–42.

Shannon, C. (1949) *The Mathematical Theory of Communication*. Chicago, IL: University Illinois Press.

Whyte, L. L. (1960) *The Unconscious Before Freud*. New York: Basic Books.

Winson, J. (1985) *Brain and Psyche: The Biology of the Unconscious*. New York: Doubleday.

Chapter 5

The Physicality of the Sign[1]

This chapter is a semiotic expansion of a paper discussing consciousness from an information-theory point of view (Olds, 1992). I began to see this issue as important when I was trying to understand the contribution of neural network theory to psychology. The neural network endeavor—also known as connectionism—has demonstrated that all information processors are not equal, nor is all information. It was once assumed that a Turing machine, basically a linear computer like we have on our desk-tops, could handle any kind of information. But as computer science has become more sophisticated it is clear that there is a relationship between the nature of the information and the type of hardware that can best process it. The easiest example is the fact that linear computers are excellent for mathematical processes, but they cannot do any sort of pattern recognition nearly as well as a parallel computer.

Similarly, it may be that certain kinds of signs are better at carrying some types of information than others. A musical note for instance uses vibrations in the air, and we use transducer mechanisms in our ears to achieve the subjective experience of music. Let's contrast such a sign with a visual sign. A written word or a bronze letter can act as visual symbols, but they can also be used physically to point to something. The printed word on a page could be used to point but would not be good at attracting attention the way poking someone in the back with the bronze letter would.

Once we focus on this as a semiotic issue there are many interesting questions we can raise. The question relevant to the current topic is this: how does the physical nature of brain signs make the brain's function possible, and how does it make consciousness possible.

In speaking of the *brain sign* I am assuming that a physical event of some kind makes a more or less permanent alteration in some neurological structure, and that the resulting configuration acts as a *sign vehicle* coding for stimuli from the environment. It is not yet clear just what this alteration is, although one concept currently in vogue is the *neural network*, a structured set of connections among neurons. I will speculate that the physicality of such brain signs make them uniquely able to produce the recursive representational phenomenon which is consciousness.

DOI: 10.4324/9781003399551-6

In brief what I mean by consciousness is a state of awareness, awareness of what one is doing or thinking, and an extension of that to self-awareness. This of course is in one way a circular definition. It arises from the neurologist's practice of defining various levels of central nervous system activity, a hierarchy from "aroused" through "awake, alert, attentive, aware, and self-aware". What I am talking about here is the self-reflexive aspect of consciousness, which is so difficult to further define, because we still do not know what it is in neurological terms. Despite this gap in our knowledge of brain function, I want to speculate that brain signs, being made of neurons, and because of their physiological, biological properties, can lead to consciousness. So, let us talk about neurons, their connections, the growth of the cortex and consciousness.

Brain Signs

I'll deal with the brain sign under four headings: the neuron, the synapse, the cortex, and the peculiar properties of language.

1. *The neuron.* Every one-celled animal has the property of electric polarization across the semi-permeable membrane, which is its self-boundary separating it from the outside world. As cells aggregated to form multi-cellular organisms, some cells were specialized to be able to catastrophically depolarize. This allowed for an electronic avalanche to pass from one end of the cell to the other. In order to generate such an avalanche, the cell wall must have the ability to open itself to calcium ions, which flood in, triggering the wave-like depolarization. Once the cell can do that, all you have to do is be able to elongate the cell to make it like a telephone wire and provide it with many branching dendrites to connect with other cells. The development of these connections seems to be an important aspect of learning.

2. *The Synapse.* Another crucial aspect of nerve function is the synapse. At the synapse the depolarization of the upstream neuron causes the release of neurotransmitter, which passes over to the downstream neuron and causes it to depolarize. Thus, signals are relayed from one neuron to the next.

The way the nervous system develops is not fully clear. One thing is that synapses which are *used* get stronger and those unused fade away. Learning is this differential strengthening. When we learn there are anatomical changes in the brain.

The physical sign-vehicle that takes the message from one nerve to the next across the synapse is the neurotransmitter. This has a physical shape which allows it to fit its receptor site like a key in a lock. The neurotransmitter is an interesting kind of sign-vehicle. It can function in two main modes. It can operate between synapses, over very short distances. And its activity can be terminated by breaking it up using an enzyme, or it can be sucked back into the neuron which spewed it out in the first place. But, since it is a durable molecule, it has a second mode; you can squirt it into the bloodstream and it will be distributed through the body, over great distances causing dramatic bodily changes. For instance, when the adrenal gland pours out adrenaline, very similar to the nor-epinephrine at the synapse, the whole body goes into fight or flight mode. Furthermore, since these molecules have distinct shapes, the modern pharmaceutical industry has been able to make drugs which mimic or prolong the action of various transmitter molecules, with all sorts of effects on the nervous system.

It is worth noting that a very recent discovery has made this picture of the synapse even more complicated. It seems that two usually poisonous gases, nitric oxide and carbon monoxide, are also neurotransmitters. But gases are not like the commonly known neurotransmitters. They do not carry information by way of iconic shape, but simply by flow according to the laws of gases. They are undifferentiated as to shape and behave more like electrons in circuits. This property may turn out to enhance the position of the neural *network* (a circuit) as a sign-vehicle.

3. *The Cortex*. Now if we go from the cellular level to the whole brain level, we note that the evolutionary advance through primates to human has involved a dramatic increase in brain size—most of this increase being in the cerebral cortex. As the cortex has developed it has been able to accomplish many things including more elaborate forms of communication. We have taken gestural expression beyond its use by the apes. We have developed a system of expression mostly of affect, using facial movements, gestures and tones of voice. And we have developed language and speech (Donald, 1991). The nature of speech may give us another hint as to the origin of consciousness.

4. *Speech and Consciousness*. In all purposive body activities, there is a feedback loop which tells us what we just did, and measures it against the goal. With gestural language, for instance, we have proprioceptive mechanisms to tell us if we are making the right gesture or not. Now if the sign system is the aural system of speech there are at least two feed-back systems. One is the proprioceptive system which regulates the vocal chords and pharyngeal structures. The other is hearing oneself speak.

The uniqueness of speech lies in the fact that I hear myself talk in the same way another person hears me. So that in speech there is an implied otherness, unlike the other modes, where the feedback remains allied to the neural structures that generate them. Because of this the experience of language learning implies an *other*, and thereby implies a split within the self. When one hears oneself speak one is aware of speaking as the subject, and of hearing, as if one is the listener, the object for the other subject.

Dennett (1991) refers to this external loop as providing the basis for a conversation with oneself. He proposes an imaginary evolutionary scene where hominids had simple dialogues in which one asked for help from another, to solve a problem, or to find something. On one occasion the individual asked the question and there was no one there. He heard himself and then heard himself answering his own question. He then realized this talking to oneself could be useful, and the inner dialogue of self-consciousness was born.

Neurons and Computers

Now let's go back to the neuron and see how the structure of a neuron suits it as a sign. All that neurons do is conduct electrical impulses. But they don't do that like copper wire. They do it by a physiological, active, carrying process, expending energy. The neuron is a biological cell which develops and prunes its thousands of synapses with other cells. This complex of inter connections is mainly what differentiates neurons from any computer hardware yet devised. There is no computer that can have a set of units which sends out branching connectors to its neighbors near and far. In fact, the elements of a linear computer are not really physically connected. The electronic signs which store memory are binary signs on an electronic disk. They just sit there. The computer has a set of rules, a program which will give it step by step instruction how to go from one sign to another. With neurons in a brain, they reach out and connect on the basis of experience and associational learning. The neural network model of the connectionists does something like this: on the basis of experience a neural network will strengthen or weaken connections between elements.

Sense Organs and Semiosis

The nerve firing is itself not necessarily a semiotic event. *Patterns* of nerve discharges (most likely neural networks) can be semiotic events if they are included in a semiotic system and are interpreted in that system.

In the interaction with the world, there are many different kinds of neurons each specialized to turn an external phenomenon into a sign. The retina takes in visual images, distributes them to specialized neurons, adapted to individual gestalten, diagonals, etc. Or certain nerves in the skin and mucous membranes turn certain physical impacts into signs. These neurons have to be physically adapted to transmit a certain kind of sign, a sign of light touch, heat, pressure.

Thus, the human nervous system is a complex of specific kinds of information carriers or sign vehicles. But the point is that the firing of a specialized neuron can be a sign of the existence of its percipient. If the incoming information has a spatial or temporal shape, and if the sensory system is somatotopic, the brain can use the system to recognize spatial patterns. Thus, there is a similarity in the visual and touch systems. Stimuli which may be suited for special cells come in, but there are many such cells, and they can mirror the spatial pattern of the stimulus. With chemoreceptors, they cannot be arranged in spatial organizations. Smells don't come in discrete patterns like visual and tactile stimuli. They are more like sounds, which have special cells for each piece of the frequency range. But there is no attempt to arrange them spatially, only temporally.

Evolution and Problem-solving

Now how does such a system lead to consciousness? In a linear computer we could build in a re-representation system, which would represent what the computer is doing. We do that—the monitor. But the monitor is for the human operator. If we are building an automaton we will try to dispense with that operator. The machine will operate itself. If it moves its arm, it must know where its arm is, and where it is in relation to its goal. Let's say its job is to pick up all the cubical objects in the room, and to pile them together. Its program will have some instruction like "Object in visual field a cube—yes or no? If yes enact *pick-up* program, if no, go to next visual field". Here we have a kind of analog of consciousness, but it is built into the program. The central processing unit actually goes from instruction to instruction, and at certain branch points, makes a "decision." Neurons do not have such a system. If we follow the connectionist model, we do without the central processing unit and without the elaborate program.

Let's say we teach a monkey to put all the cubes in a pile. It will do so in order to get the reward we used in the training. The monkey has no notion of "creating a pile of cubes". It is simply following an instruction to get a reward. But the setting up of this associational pattern was done not by internalizing a program, but by the strengthening of synapses between neurons. This produced a new association between cubes and food in the behaviorist paradigm. Where is consciousness? There must be a constant self-monitoring especially if there are difficulties to overcome, such as avoiding shocks, jumping over barriers, etc. We must assume that when the behavior is easy and repetitive, the animal may do it almost automatically. But when challenges are met, there are branch points where decisions must be made.

Now let us go to a pongid, such as a chimpanzee. We don't teach it to pile up the cubes. But we put a banana too high for the animal to reach. A smart chimp will take the cubes and pile them up and climb up to get the banana. This is the basis of the claim that consciousness exists when there is a problem, a claim probably originated by William James. If this is true then it appears that consciousness is a temporal phenomenon in a linear stream, a little analogous to the linear computer's decision-branch points. It may occur at times where two streams converge requiring a decision. So that in other mammals, consciousness may be rather episodic, being an extra brain effort at sorting out the possibilities.

If we think of it this way consciousness becomes a linear rather than a spatial phenomenon. Consciousness is where cleverness lies. As the cortex increased in size mammals began to solve more difficult problems. It may be that the use of that higher cortex *is* consciousness. Not it and a projection to somewhere else. As the problem-solving cortex became larger, it developed a larger memory for events in the past, for past solutions to problems, etc. With the advance of culture and elaborate social structures, we may say that everything became a problem and the higher cortex was constantly in use. Consciousness is simply the use of the highest cortex. There is to some extent a "bringing it all together" in that cortex in order to solve problems. This means that it must attend to current states and compare them with other states, future goals, past failures, desirable and undesirable affects, etc.

Now, with the classic example of driving along and having a conversation, or daydreaming to oneself, what happens. The driving is handled by lower automatic processes, and the mind is devoted to things which present problems. In human discourse it is *all* problem; one must listen, and compose responses, etc. With fantasy, we have the posing of problems and solving them in the fantasy. The forming of a narrative is a problem. It requires this highest faculty. One is not necessarily self-conscious during a fantasy, but one can become so at any time. People have repetitive fantasies, which they suddenly "find" themselves in the middle of. It may be that even fantasy can be automatized. Fantasy may be a generalization of the insight capacity that apes have—the ability to visualize a future state of affairs.

When we go from lower mammals, to primates, to humans, as the cortex becomes larger, it can engage in creative process, solving problems small and large. At the level of dogs and rabbits the cortex can solve some problems, such as how to get out of a fenced back yard. At higher levels, in social life, there are many more novel situations, and the cortex is enlarged to handle them. At this point it can generate its own problems when there are none in the immediate outside world. Sitting bored on a stalled bus, one my make patterns in the upholstery, fantasize about fellow passengers, worry about money, anything.

This constant activity may be generated by cyclical wave processes in the brain, which keep one running from one association to the next along the synaptic connections which exist. In psychoanalysis, in free association, one's brain runs along these well-worn grooves, often at a low level of consciousness. The analyst's interventions often jolt the patient and demand a new look, a creative solution. This too leads to new synapse formation.

Summary

There are several aspects of human biological *brain signs* which have accumulated to produce consciousness as we know it.

1 The neuron is a kind of plastic sign-vehicle. It can connect with other neurons forming neural networks which store information.
2 These networks themselves are plastic and form other connections with each bit of new learning. These changes render the brain capable of recombination which leads to creative processes.

3 This problem-solving ability has come into constant use with the advent of the human's enlarged cerebral cortex. The occupation with problem solving, fantasy formation and language provide the brain with an endless and continuous supply of problems to solve.

4 Consciousness is not a simple all or nothing phenomenon. An individual has different levels of consciousness depending on wakefulness, attention or self- reflection. And, there have been changes as species have evolved. We assume reptiles have a representation of the world available to their sense organs which can be called consciousness. As organisms evolve, we theorize that with mammals, apes and humans, the complexity of consciousness becomes greater.

5 The physicality of signs is relevant at the following levels:

a Sense organs are physically adapted to receive certain kinds of information—sound frequencies, light frequencies and patterns, touch, etc.

b Brain signs, or neural networks, which store information are plastic and can lead to learning new things about the world.

c At higher levels internal representations and image formations allow for trial modification in fantasy, which is effective in problem solving.

d Juxtaposition of such fantasies with images of the self lead to a higher and more self-aware state in humans and possibly in some primates.

e The physical nature of gesture and sign is light mediated, and therefore line-of-sight and no good in the dark. Audible signs can go around corners and can be used while visual attention is devoted to other survival tasks. Audible signs can be digitalized into phonemes and can be heard by the self as if the speaker is the other. This can lead to language and to the levels of consciousness familiar to us.

Note

1 Previously published in *Semiotics* (1992) Vol. 9: 166–173.

References

Dennett, D. (1991) *Consciousness Explained*. Boston, MA: Little, Brown and Company.

Donald, M. (1991) *The Evolution of the Modern Mind*. Cambridge, MA: Harvard University Press.

Olds, D. D. (2004) Consciousness: A Brain-centered, Informational Approach. *Psychoanalytic Inquiry*, 12: 419–444.

Chapter 6

Connectionism and Psychoanalysis[1]

Connectionism is the collective name for a group of metaphoric and practical models of mind. These models, also named "neural network" systems, or "parallel distributed processing systems" (PDP) are currently generating great excitement and intellectual ferment in the worlds of cognitive psychology, philosophy, and cognitive neuroscience. The excitement is caused by several aspects of the models. One is that they appear to be able to simulate some activities of the brain and promise to give insight into the ways the brain processes information. Another is the suggestion of practical applications, such as expert systems for pattern recognition, language learning, baggage sorting, and other extremely complex processes.

The purpose of this paper is to discuss connectionist modeling of the mind, and to try to relate it to our usual psychoanalytic concepts. I believe that there will be some modifications in the way we think of these concepts, modifications that will bring metapsychology closer to current concepts of brain and mind. Although few psychoanalysts have ventured into the field of connectionist theory, Forrest (1992) has presented a synthesis for psychiatrists, and Palombo (1992) has integrated his dream research with the neural network model. Galatzer-Levy (1988) has used an analogy to simulated annealing and the connectionist "Boltzmann Algorithm" in understanding the psychoanalytic process of working through.

Among the issues in psychoanalytic theory that might benefit from a new model of brain function are: 1) the historically significant dualist theory of mind; this has influenced psychoanalytic thinking by yielding various other dualities—conscious/unconscious, ego/id, mind/body, thing presentation/ word presentation; 2) How does the brain process information, and what kinds of information? How can they be integrated, and how is psychoanalysis useful in this integration? And (3) What is the nature of psychoanalytic technique? What are the roles played by empathy, transference, free association, and dream work? What is the relative importance of here-and-now transference analysis compared to uncovering of childhood memories? How do we compare historical and narrative truths?

DOI: 10.4324/9781003399551-7

A new theory of mind, based on a new model of brain function, should at least give us some new insights, and new approaches to these questions. This paper aims to outline how connectionism may be useful to this end. My purpose is to show that entertaining this paradigm can provide us with the pleasure of looking at our old theories from a new vantage point. I shall explain the model at an elementary level and give a sampling of the questions we might address.

The Connectionist Model

First, we must define and discuss the notion of neural networks. Litowitz (1991) describes the connectionist model as part of the "third wave" of modern cognitive science models. Beginning in the 1950s, the early cognitive psychologists, influenced by Chomskian linguistic theories, studied information-processing systems using symbol manipulation, usually by serial computation. Such a system required a computer operating with a set of rules for manipulating symbols. An artificial intelligence machine of that generation could be programmed and crammed with data, which it could then retrieve. It could work as a data processor, a word processor, or an expert system such as a system for making a medical diagnosis based on an input set of symptoms.

In the second wave, overlapping with the first, attention was focused on processing of set pieces—schemas, scripts, and frames. Here a system could be programmed with a kind of narrative script, which was a somewhat more flexible program allowing it to answer a multitude of questions. An example is Shrank's *restaurant script*. This program represented various aspects of a restaurant, the notions of menus, waitresses, food, silverware, and the multiplicity of logical relations among them. You could then ask it questions, the answers to which might be implicit in the logical relations. If you asked where would the food be eaten, it would say on a table. Who would return cold soup to the kitchen? The waiter. This kind of system was again limited by the information plugged into it. If an unusual question came up, such as an argument over the bill because the food was burnt, the computer would not have the flexibility to generate an answer as to whether the person ate the food or not. It had the limitation of any expert system based on rules; one can inform it with a finite number of rules; reality always comes up with instances that do not quite fit. An amusing example of this kind of script in action is the tax law. It attempts to cover every contingency, but very soon after such a law is instituted, people find situations that are not explicitly covered. The judicial establishment spends its time fine-tuning the instrument to deal with an endless number of novel situations.

The third generation has developed machines that not only manipulate data, but can *learn*. Laboratory models presaging this general approach go back to the 1940s, although the term "connectionism" was first coined in

1982 by Jerome Feldman, a computer scientist at Berkeley. Decades before that, however, McCulloch and Pitts (1943) wrote a cornerstone article, "A Logical Calculus of the Ideas Immanent in Nervous Activity." They put forward the idea that electronic models of neural networks could compute and learn. Subsequently, Hebb (1949) suggested a possible mechanism for such learning, namely that the continuous activation of a connection between two neurons would strengthen that connection.

Another milestone in the development of the concept was Rosenblatt's (1962) invention of the "perceptron" a neuronlike learning device. In Campbell's (1989) description:

> In June 1960 the first perceptron was unveiled amid considerable publicity and fanfare. It had an eye made of photoelectric cells that scrutinized letters inscribed on cards, and passed messages about what it saw to an array of 512 units randomly hooked up together, which in turn sent the message on to a set of response units. The perceptron made a guess as to what letter was on the card. If the machine made a wrong guess, it was punished by having the weights responsible for the mistake weakened. After several punishments, and as a result of trial and error, the perceptron made the correct choices.
>
> (p. 169)

The perceptron, at first introduced with excessive enthusiasm, soon proved unable to live up to inflated expectations and fell into early obscurity. The computers we have grown used to—the von Neumann serial computers— entered their heyday in the 1970s. However, in the past decade, connectionist models, using the concept of neural networks, have emerged again and have become a major source of explanations and models for artificial intelligence research and psychology. Much of this work has been done by the PDP Research Group under the leadership of David Rumelhart, James McClelland, and Geoffrey Hinton. The basic text for current connectionist thinking, *Parallel Distributed Processing: Explorations in the Microstructure of Cognition*, was written by Rumelhart, McClelland, and other members of the group (1986).

The elemental neural net model is a structure of neurons, or hypothesized neuronlike nodes, which can take in information and—in an interactive mode—make guesses as to correct responses. When the system makes an error, it tries again with the same stimulus, having made an alteration in certain connection strengths, particularly in those connections most "responsible" for the error. Once it comes up with the "correct" answer, this set of connection strengths—possibly analogous to a web of synaptic connections in animal learning—is saved in the system and represents a kind of learning. This sounds like the perceptron, but the current models are much more complex, having "hidden layers" interposed between the input and output nodes. Another difference, which at first makes the whole field seem unfathomable, is that the networks are usually not built of electrodes and photoelectric cells. Instead, they are *simulated* on linear computers. They really are virtual entities, "what-if" objects, which, if they were built and functioned to specification, would "learn" as they do in their simulated enactments on computers. The reason for this is that the technical problems of making the massive number of connections, which would be required in a true connectionist machine using silicon and wires, have not yet been solved. In the meantime, computer scientists and cognitive scientists are making use of what they can learn from the simulations.

A major weakness of the earlier *schema* models was a kind of inflexibility and difficulty in attunement to a natural environment. The beauty of a connectionist system is that it learns and can adapt to its environment in a trial-and-error fashion. Errors are fed back through the system (which is why one popular model is called a "back propagation" system). An organization of millions of such nets, interrelated in some as yet mysterious way, could conceivably have brain-like properties. It would require no central processor. It would interact with the world, and learn in a mode similar to classical conditioning. For instance, it might be a model of the way we learn language— by trying words and syntactical structures, being corrected many times until we zero in on the pronunciation or grammatical use accepted in the immediate environment. It may also be a model for complex pattern recognition, for example the recognition of faces, of voices, or Bach.

Earlier I mentioned the tax law, which attempts to write an exhaustive set of rules, but constantly runs into exceptions. The immense establishment of accountants, lawyers, and courts is in fact a kind of connectionist system for feedback of error corrections into the law.

Mines and Rocks

Let us consider an example of a currently available device which demonstrates the properties of a connectionist system. This is a program designed to distinguish mines from rocks on the bottom of a harbor. The scenario involves a submarine with a sonar device attached to a network that can be trained to make the distinction. Figure 6.1 is a schematized and simplified representation of the system. The instrument sends out a sonar burst and, when the echo from an object returns, analyzes it into different sectors of the frequency spectrum, yielding a graph representing the energy at each frequency range. These values are fed into the neural network consisting in this case of 10 input units, four intermediate or hidden units, and two output units. Each input unit feeds a signal representing the power of its segment of the frequency range to all the hidden units. The hidden units, by virtue of their combined connection strengths, finally activate one of the two output units indicating that the object is a mine or a rock.

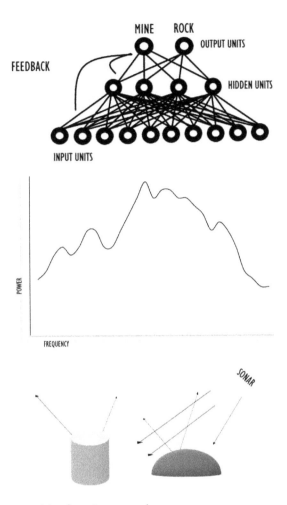

Figure 6.1 System training for mines vs rocks.

The system is "trained" by exposing it to a large number of mines and rocks and having it "guess" which it is. At first it will answer on the basis of randomly disposed connection strengths among the many units. When it guesses wrong, the computer on which it is running will automatically, in incremental fashion, adjust some of the connection strengths. In other words, each connection strength "responsible" for the error will be enhanced or diminished by a small incremental amount. The exposure is repeated on each test mine or rock until the system generates the correct response. The whole process may take thousands of trials, but can be done rapidly on a computer.

The learning consists wholly of the adjustment of connection strengths so that they end up generating correct results on the test items. Once trained, the device should be able to generalize its results and distinguish mines and rocks it has never encountered. The important thing that distinguishes it from serial computer expert systems is that in the neural network there are no explicit *rules* that lead it to designate a mine or a rock. What is in the system is a cluster of connection strengths, which, when it receives an echo, it "relaxes" or "settles" into one of the two possible solutions in a process of "multiple constraint satisfaction." It can become a system as accurate as the best-trained ears of a sonar operator. (For a fuller description of this system, see Churchland, 1988).

We can see a similarity here to the biological system of operant conditioning. In the biological method behavior is shaped by differential rewards and punishments to randomly generated responses to stimuli. In both systems behavior is learned as a result of *consequences* of previous behavior. For the rat that finds that pushing one lever results in food and pushing a second lever leads to an electric shock, the food lever will soon be the exclusive favorite. The consequences are mediated by the animal's pain and pleasure systems. In the connectionist model the *consequence* of error is a direct manipulation of connection strengths, without the mediation of an animal's complex value and reward system. But the process is ultimately quite similar.

Neural networks bear little physical resemblance to actual neurons. But it may be that connectionist networks actually do simulate the *functions* of certain biological neural structures. At the present time, though, they are simply artificial intelligence systems that mimic certain neurological functions and can accomplish simple perceptual and computational tasks. In so doing they provide models which psychoanalysts might use as metaphors for psychic function.

Models as Metaphors

Let us think for a moment about the history, within the psychoanalytic canon, of models of the psyche. In Freud's early model, involving the theory of libido, the physical model was a hydraulic machine or steam engine. This produced a mechanism for motivation, in which instinctual "pressure" followed laws similar to those involving fluid under compression. The notion of force passed directly into the notion of instinctual "drive," a notion that made intuitive sense to anyone who had ever experienced a wish, a compulsion, a phobia, or a sexual urge. The continuously rising sense of pressure, relieved by the expression of the symptom, made a fair model of the symptom disorders that were the subject of Freud's early interest. Hence the properties of energy flow in a steam engine were transferred to the concept of human motivation.

The next model, corresponding to the topographic psychic system, retained the notion of libido and force fields, but also developed the notion of an ego or inner demon which refereed between forces in conflict. This model combined libido and information; the ego sensed not only forces, but meanings. We now had a more intelligent steam engine which could use information "signals," such as "signal anxiety," to help in directing the energy. This model was possibly like some of the early computers which used water pressure and flow as analog devices to handle information.

With the emergence and explosive development of the electronic linear computer, a new paradigm was born in which energy became a given—undifferentiated electricity from the plug in the wall. The only thing of importance was information. Such a model of the mind dominated popular as well as professional thinking into the 1980s.

Enter now the connectionist model. Information is still key, but the mode of handling that information is as different from the linear computer as *it* was from the steam engine.

One potential problem with this model is that very few people, including most psychologists, have even a sketchy understanding of the prototype. Neural net theory is very abstract, and to really understand it involves considerable mathematical sophistication. Does that mean it cannot be a model? It never has before. Many libido theorists probably did not know a great deal about steam engines; they made conceptual use of the properties that interested them. This is even more true with the early computer model; very few analogizers know a mother board from a RAM, nor do they care. The way we *imagine* the machine handles information is what counts.

The point is that what gets transferred from one realm to the other is a set of *properties* we attribute to both entities. These properties, which may be shared by neural nets and by actual brains, can illuminate our conception of mental processes. In fact, there is a curious mutual metaphorizing going on:

> Our strategy has thus become one of offering a general and abstract model of the computational architecture of brains, to develop algorithms and procedures well suited to this architecture, to simulate these procedures and architecture on a computer, and to explore them as hypotheses about the nature of the human information processing system. We say that such models are *neurally inspired*, and we call computation on such a system brain style computation. Our goal in short is to replace the computer metaphor with the brain metaphor.(Rumelhart, 1990, p. 134)

Properties of the Neural Net System

What characteristics of the connectionist system will be of interest in reconceptualizing underlying psychoanalytic theories? In this paper I cannot attempt to be exhaustive in relating the model to analytic theory. My main object is to invite the reader to entertain the ideas and relate them to some of our age-old questions. Below is a short list, somewhat arbitrarily chosen, but representing some of the theoretical issues that interest us:

1   There is no central processor.
2   There is no need for a dualist conception of mind.
3   Homunculi are conceived differently than before.
4   The conscious/unconscious division is understood differently.
5   Free association takes on new importance.
6   Dream theory may have to be recast.
7   Perception takes on central significance.
8   It may provide us with a way to conceptually integrate the different modes of psychiatric treatment, including psychopharmacology.

No Central Processor

As we have grown to appreciate that the brain can do thousands of things at once, and as we have built "connection machines"—parallel computers that can do something similar—we have had to confront the notion of the central processor.

Throughout history the human mind has been able to reflect on itself as a unified subject, the object in the mirror, the object of introspection. One usually thinks of oneself as *one*, and language is based on the unitary subject, the *I*. The soul is one; the self is one; the ego is one. As an internal apperceived entity, from a psychological point of view, there is nothing wrong with this concept. In fact, it is a necessity for normal functioning, and various kinds of pathology arise when such unitary self-perception is absent or compromised. In forming a theory of mind, however, this way of thinking leads to the notion of ego or self as central organizer. This produces the paradoxes involved with the ego having an ego, of infinite regression. Then there are the problems of the "sapient ego," where, in maintaining defenses, one sees a repressed idea before "not seeing" it (Anscombe, 1986). During the hegemony of ego psychology, the central organizer was key to mental functioning; the ability of the mind to synthesize and develop hierarchical systems of values and behavior was the measure of mental health.

Underlying Freud's theories and the subsequent theories of ego psychology was a motivational system based on libido or psychic energy. As Rosenblatt and Thickstun (1977) pointed out, the energy model has gradually given over to an information-based model. "Signal anxiety" may have been the first term that was more informational than energetic, and since its introduction the hydraulic metaphor has waned in importance. With the development of a more information-based model, the basic structures of ego psychology remained in place, most notably the ego. The simultaneous development in the last three decades of the serial computer provided a ready-made metaphor that required little tinkering. A serial computer needs a central processing unit, and such a machine served as a model of our mind.

However, as computers developed into "supercomputers," the limits of serial processing became apparent. With certain processes, such as mathematical computations, or any logical computation where one step must come before another, serial computing is required. But with a busy machine like the brain, many things go on simultaneously. If, for instance, there are a thousand operations taking place, including all the activities devoted to proprioception, body posture, autonomic regulation, digestive processes, hormone regulation, perception through the senses, emotional reactions, and if all these processes had to go through one central processor, one can imagine the bottleneck. One might suggest here a central processor, which itself had a thousand channels, like the railroad switchyard control station that supervises traffic on many tracks. But then this controller itself must be a parallel processor, and its central processor would also have to be parallel, so we would not have made much theoretical headway.

The first and possibly most striking conclusion from the connectionist model is that in its computational processes the brain cannot have a central processor such as exists in a linear computer. There seem to be multiple activities going on in the brain, and the entities involved in these activities appear to organize without a central organizer. Gazzaniga (1985) describes a multiple modular system that operates up to a very high level. For example, some computational resources for language, and for spatial relations, are segregated into the left and right hemispheres, and their independent functioning can be appreciated by studying patients with lesions of the corpus callosum.

Dennett (1991) has proposed a generally convincing and well worked-out model of this sort, which he calls a "multiple drafts" system. In his model of mind there are homunculi upon homunculi which combine and integrate pieces of information to yield a complex but self-organizing model of consciousness. For the psychoanalyst this will relate to developmental theory: how are the various functions of the self integrated and organized? And, it may well have something to offer in thinking about the pathology involving internal conflicts between apparently semi-independent centers of motivation and value, from neurotic conflict to multiple personality.

There is No Need for Dualism

Having said all this about distributed processing, we still have to confront the fact that we *seem* to have a central processor, a subjective sense of self, which is intimately connected with *consciousness*. Indeed, the phenomenon of consciousness seems to make the existence of a central processor obvious and necessary. This is in fact the heart of the Cartesian dualist model of mind. That a dualist model is unnecessary, I have argued in a previous paper (Olds,

1992), in which I presented an information-processing-based system. In this model consciousness acts as a *re-representation* device by which the brain can represent to itself its own workings. Any information processor needs to verify its output, and the brain is no exception. Thus, consciousness may play a role similar to that of a computer's monitor. This allows for the verification of the process at many levels—at the level of the words and phonemes themselves, and at other more abstract levels of the ideas and their linguistic expression. Consciousness is an *output* of the brain, in the same sense as motor actions, thoughts, words and songs. The work of Libet and his colleagues (1983) suggests that consciousness occurs shortly *after* the brain event that it signifies. Thus, consciousness is not an executive organ, but a monitor of the brain, or, more accurately, a system by means of which the brain monitors itself. For example, I can use a mirror as a monitor to comb my hair, but it is I who combs the hair, not the mirror. Similarly, I use the computer monitor, or in a typewriter, the typed page, to keep apprised of what I have just written; the monitor itself does nothing but re-represent the information in the computer's active memory.

Now the important thing is that consciousness is necessarily *linear*. Just as with motor action, I can only do one, or maybe a few separate motor acts at the same time (walk and chew gum). With conscious thought, I can usually focus on one thing and maybe keep track of one or two other activities (talk and drive a car). But this stream is basically linear in comparison with the thousands of things the brain does simultaneously. Thus, out of the multiplicity of simultaneous brain events, a narrow stream is winnowed, and this is indeed a bottleneck. It is a *selective* monitoring, culled from the millions of items in the preconscious, which could become conscious, and the more millions which are in the dynamic unconscious, and in the brain's non-conscious, the autonomic and motor patterns.

The illusion of dualism derives from the experience of self-monitoring in which an "I" seems to be over against and distinguished from the rest of the brain processes. Mind is equated with consciousness, and is seen as of different stuff than brain. But this monitoring system is a brain process like any other, its only functional difference being that it is a linear process.

To go back to the impact of the connectionist model, we see that it proposes the brain as a self-organizer, putting into conscious awareness things that carry greater "weight," in order to subject them to the self-reflective aspect of its computational power.

Homunculi

We have already seen that the notion of the ego as a homunculus, a little bus driver within the mind, is plagued with the problem of infinite regress. Recent authors have, however, rescued the more generic notion of homunculus, recognizing that the concept is useful. Dennett (1978) points out that a homunculus can be a respectable entity as long as it is not omniscient. That is, if a homunculus handles a single brain function, but is so specialized that it knows little of the whole brain's activity, then it becomes a team player rather than an all-knowing executive. The brain becomes a group of specialized members.

This analogy brings to mind one of the evocative devices used to explain neural networks, namely the analogy to a small human group. Let us say that we have a group or committee which is to make a decision by having its members shout "yes" or "no." Complicating matters is the fact that some people can shout louder than others so that they may contribute more to the decision; in addition, some members may have higher rank or influence than others so that their opinions count more even when they are speaking at a normal level. Loudness is analogous to the connectionist term "activation," and rank or importance is analogous to the term "connection strength."

With this model, an answer to a question, or a decision, or a recognition, is arrived at almost by consensus politics. The model is more one of a settlement or a committee vote which is not necessarily unanimous. The analogy can take us farther if we liken the members to specialized homunculi; each is an expert in one thing, no one knows all about all things, and it is the group that comes to a decision.

This is all to emphasize that central authority is always "delegated" by the group. There is no built-in central organizer, on the model of the ego. In a sense, in the ego model, influence flows "outward" from the autocratic leader to the rest of the group. In the connectionist model, influence flows "inward" from the whole group to its specialized members. For better or worse, this model is more "democratic" than its predecessor.

The value of playing with such analogies is that it helps render connectionist theory less strange and abstract. The feeling of familiarity brings us a little closer to understanding.

Conscious/Unconscious

The division between the conscious and the unconscious now begins to hark back to Freud's early topographic model, where there was the conscious mind, and a sensor between it and the unconscious acting like Maxwell's hypothetical demon. That the demon should have its own intelligence and "know" what should be allowed through the gate was a weakness in the system which forced Freud to postulate an ego with both conscious and unconscious aspects.

The connectionist model, after removing the central homunculus, leaves us with a group process in which repression is the result of a consensus. The brain becomes the organizer, with consciousness a self-monitoring output phenomenon. The brain has certain rules about what items are forbidden to consciousness; for example, it might determine that memories with a certain level of negative affect will not be let through. We are, in effect, equating the ego with the brain, and making consciousness one of the brain's output vectors. That which is flashed in consciousness then becomes one of the many *inputs* the brain has to deal with, along with sensory input and input from memory and the visceral system.

Now, with the welter of other ideas in the preconscious, how are certain items chosen for rerepresentation? Here we have to postulate an associational flow in the brain which utilizes certain hierarchies, such as survival value, intensity, and novelty, as criteria that put certain contents at the head of the line. And why are certain items repressed and kept permanently out of consciousness? It may be that the brain works more efficiently when the affect load is kept within certain bounds by selective ignorance.

We frequently see the need for the higher-level modulating defenses. This is true in primitively organized patients who lack such defenses; with provocation they readily become overwhelmed and lose the capacity for adaptive judgment. The same is often true in cases of severe trauma where even the strongest defenses may collapse, leading to major psychic disruption.

Evolutionary biologists propose another reason for the development of certain defenses. Nesse and Lloyd (1989) suggest that repression is adaptive for individuals in that it allows *self*-deception, which then helps with deception of others; the deception of others may yield some adaptive gain for certain individuals. In other words, self-deception is part of a larger interpersonal system that balances honesty versus deception in the functioning of a social network.

As to the mechanism of repression, Jones (1993) presents a sophisticated discussion in terms of modern neurobiological models, including the connectionist model and Edelman's system of "neuronal group selection." As an example, this author points out that one neural net can inhibit another and could do so on the basis of connectivity with negative or overwhelming affects systems. Another example is the possibility that the absence of connection to facilitating neural nets may block a net from consciousness.

Free Association

The neural net theory could have been invented to explain free association. The notion of associational learning, and the clustering of associations in a person's discourse, seem at home in this conceptualization. The metaphors that the neural theorists use to model the phenomenon are difficult to understand, but seem quite apposite. The most popular metaphor is one based on a "rubber sheet" geometry, the so-called Boltzmann Machine (Pagels, 1988). The model is a bumpy rubber sheet with many hills and valleys, the valleys, in the metaphor, representing "energy minima." As with real hills and valleys, a ball would find a lowest point and sit there. The closest we come to a model is one described as a "momentumless ping-pong ball" which, when it lands on this bumpy surface, soon finds a lowest point and comes to rest. It is momentumless, so we do not have to worry about it bouncing or being thrown afar by its own momentum. In a neural network, electrical energy minima are achieved without any such thing as momentum.

This model works nicely with the notion of free association. When an energy minimum is achieved, it alters the electrical conditions in its vicinity so that some other entity is boosted over a threshold and falls to another minimum, generating a continuous cascade. In other words, *all* thought is free association. However, in order for thought to be organized and adaptive, this free-rolling process must be channeled in a hierarchical system. Thus, associations are usually under the control of such guidance systems as perception of the external world, immediate survival needs, perceived importance, logical or nonlogical connections, or emotional values. Other biases with negative or inhibiting effects may lead to repression and other defenses.

Lying on a couch and trying to follow a rule to say "whatever comes to mind," represents an attempt to allow thoughts to flow into consciousness with some reduction in the influence of hierarchical constraints, such as those imposed by engaging in a task, or dealing with the facial expressions of the analyst.

Certain states *channel* associations in predictable directions. The most obvious is that of mood, which will place a constant pull on all thoughts. Another may be the regressive effect of the analytic situation. Whatever that effect is, it seems over time to allow the patient to recover memories and even to reexperience some aspects of childhood. Whether this is truly regression in the several senses that Freud meant it, or is merely the patient's becoming comfortable and trusting, and with time able to explore more memories, is not always clear.

One thing that becomes apparent when we think in these terms is that every brain event exists in a swarm of other events, neighboring or otherwise connected nets, which provide the immense *context* surrounding each and every thought. Even perceptions go through a complex process of being screened for affective relevance and reassembled from sensory data before they reach consciousness. Free association is interesting for its own sake, but also for the context surrounding each item. Any association carries with it implications of mood, of recent history, of self- and object identity issues. One thing we do in analysis is unpack this package of context. If we see an association as a sign of multiple brain events, which are themselves signs of percepts and stored memories, we see the analytic field as incredibly rich with possibilities. (See Kris, 1982, for a discussion of the "constraints" on free association.)

Our technique is designed to allow these associations to eventually flow into patterns, influenced by the patient's early history. As these patterns become structurally similar to the narrative of the past, we are able to reconstruct some version of that past which is stored in memory. By naming and describing these patterns we may produce *insight* (Shapiro, 1979). Each pattern represents a well-worn track in the brain, namely a set of connections among nets, which generates a repetitive pattern of response and behavior. Making the pattern conscious does not always change things, especially when the patient retains an ability to disavow it and disconnect it from the sense of self. But it can make a difference, in that some of the unconscious criteria which supported the pattern become conscious and therefore must come in conflict with other conscious values and criteria. It could be said that certain very high-connection strengths, which produced a certain rigidity of category and behavior, are weakened, leading to more flexibility.

Consistent with the paradigm is the idea that the *analyst* has neural networks highly trained to recognize regularities in the analysand's associations. The process of listening, sensing patterns, reporting them to the patient, collaborating in coming to understand still larger patterns, may also be described by the model.

Dreams

The understanding of the biology of dreams has taken dramatic leaps in recent years. Crick and Mitchison (1983) see dreams as part of the disposal process of useless memories. Hobson (1988) describes dreams as random excitations of brain during REM sleep, excitations caused by periodic pontine-geniculate-occipital (PGO) waves which proceed randomly through the brain. Winson (1985) views dreams as a late evolutionary advance beginning with the marsupials. It coincided with a reduction in brain size in relation to total body weight, suggesting that dreams are useful in information processing, making the brain more efficient. In mammals it may be that dreams represent rehearsals of basic adaptive behaviors, such as sexual activity, search and predation for predators, and other exploratory behavior in nonpredators.

Reiser (1991), in a review of dream theory, has integrated some of these ideas into a coherent model. He suggests that during the day many experiences, both conscious and unconscious, produce thought patterns which are near threshold but do not quite make it to consciousness. In the REM state, the PGO waves radiate through the brain as Hobson suggested, and somewhat randomly push some of them over threshold. From the point of view of a psychoanalyst, this process is not purely random: the liminal items represent aspects of the day's experience, and their sequence in dreams represents the way they have been connected in memory. Dreams may not be the only road, but they are *a* road to the patient's meaning structures. (For a difficult but mathematically sophisticated connectionist discussion of dreams, see Antrobus, 1991.)

Reiser's model fits rather well with the neural net notion. Dreams become a kind of free association in a certain sleep state. In this state sensory input, motor output, and the potential proprioceptive input from motor output are all missing. The hierarchical rules are much less in effect, defenses may be reduced, and the passage from idea to idea may be less controlled, or may be controlled by different constraints—for instance by metaphor, metonymy, or phoneme similarity.

Palombo (1992) presents a connectionist model of the condensation in dreaming. He makes use of the ability of a connectionist system to take a partial image and superimpose it on a more complete image, or to bring forth into the dream a conflation of several images which may have common structural elements.

The model that is developing does not match up completely with Freud's notion of the dream as a censored, disguised, or symbolically represented wish, although such wishes may play an important part. The censorship and the need to preserve sleep postulated by Freud would seem to be unnecessary factors in this system. The newer model suggests that manifest content may be a direct expression of what is on the patient's mind. The dream elements, as the elements in any free association, may have symbolic connections and referents. But we now recognize more than before the importance of manifest content and day residue. For instance, Cartwright (1977) discovered that the dreams of women in the throes of divorce have a preponderance of material referring to the current life crisis. Marcus (unpublished) tabulated the dreams of medical students throughout their training and documented a consistent and predictable progression in the dream content.

Perception versus Conception

We may recall Kant's dictum, "Concepts without percepts are empty; percepts without concepts are blind." This remark points to the two major foci of the study of mind, *cognition* and *perception*. Science has alternated between emphasis on one and then the other. For Freud the inner cognitive processes driven by psychic energy—following ingrained patterns—were primary; the perceptual systems were secondary, easily fooled by the inner forces. Early artificial intelligence, although replacing energic notions with informational ones, still viewed the symbol-manipulating computer as paradigmatic. The problem of how to feed data to the computer was ignored, especially since the simulation of sense organs proved much more difficult than the simulation of logical systems.

With the connectionist shift, attention has moved to perception. Pattern, face, and voice recognition are perceptual tasks. They make up the connection between the self and the world, and they lead deep into the psyche. Perceptual processes now seem to be in center stage. We may say that *Homo Sapiens* has been transformed in the scientific mind to *Homo Percipiens*.

Psychoanalysis has moved in a similar direction. In the early analytic model, more importance was placed on inborn tendencies and on the enactment of early-instilled conflicts—the playing out of inner programs. In the past decade analysis has begun to place more importance on the interpersonal field, where perception is more important than program. Thus, we tend to emphasize issues involving empathy, transference, and expressive interaction.

Transference was once thought to be a perceptual distortion, rendering current objects identical to or similar to early internalized objects. Now we may see transference as a kind of perception; to say it is a distortion would be like saying vision is a distortion. As a form of perception, it is of course subject to error, as is vision. But the formation of early templates that provide a stable expectancy system and a stable ground of internal objects is a strength of interpersonal perception. Problems may arise in later life if processes of accommodation, in Piaget's sense, do not allow for flexibility and modification of expectations so that new objects can be seen clearly and their behavior predicted accurately. Slap and Saykin (1983), in their model of the *sequestered schema*, have described a system compatible with this concept. The unconscious, sequestered schema assimilates but does not accommodate; new percepts are assimilated into old repressed, unchangeable schemata and are treated as if they are represented by these unconscious prototypes. Transference involves this misperception and the interpersonal behaviors resulting from it.

Empathy can also be seen as a complex form of perception, readily understood in connectionist terms. Like face and voice recognition, it provides a perception of the other's feelings, and the sense of the other's subjectivity, in current philosophers' jargon, "what it is like" to be the other person (see Nagel, 1974). In so doing it relies on conscious mechanisms, projective mechanisms, and unconscious mechanisms working in parallel for rapid acquisition. The sense of the other's conscious state is a highly adaptive phenomenon and may play a part in forming the self. According to Humphrey (1984), the sense of self-consciousness was adaptive for early hominids because it allowed one individual to be aware of his own mental states, which gave him an indication of what the other might be feeling or thinking. Self-consciousness provided the advantage of prediction of others' behavior, which enhanced the political skill and therefore the individual's survival in an increasingly complex hominid culture. Thus, self-consciousness plays a part in empathy, a type of complex pattern recognition, which also involves verbal and nonverbal cues in simultaneous perfusion.

There is one more important thing about pattern recognition: it is the basis of transference as well as of self-consciousness and insight. Insight becomes the recognition of patterns about oneself. Such recognition requires a decentering, in the Piagetian sense. It is difficult to recognize a pattern when one is immersed in it. For instance, before Galileo, people assumed the earth to conform to the evidence of their senses, to be in the center of the universe. Anyone in a "decentered" position outside the solar system could have seen the pattern in an instant. Galileo figured it out by calculations concerning the movements of other planets, and was able to imagine the structure. It is similar for the individual in the orbit of his own personality. It is often easiest to see the complex pattern of self with the help of another. A therapist can describe the patterns, and this may contribute to a new view of self. In psychoanalysis a deeper process occurs in which the analyst and patient become immersed in the web of the transference. Seeing one's way out of that can be very difficult. The analyst must be constantly decentering in order to see the transference-countertransference pattern. As the patient learns this process, he or she identifies with the analyst's function, and can carry on the process of self-analysis.

Clinical Relevance

What difference will it make if we try to understand the brain in connectionist terms? From the point of view of cognitive psychologists, it may allow for more accurate and heuristically valuable models of mind. But of what use will it be to the psychoanalyst, who proceeds in a trained and intuitive fashion, usually uninterested in the details of brain function?

We do not yet know all the implications of this model. It will take time to work them out. But in general, an expert has a broader and potentially more creative grasp of a subject if it is understood in its basic scientific context. The orthopedist who understands bone metabolism and physical stress dynamics will have a broader range than the technician who has simply learned the technique of setting bones and casting them. Similarly, in psychology, as each model of mind more closely approaches an accurate model of brain function, the expert is provided with a more sophisticated view of the subject. This will not make up for a lack of clinical intuition and skill, but it should enhance whatever skill is present. And, of course, it should inform psychological research and lead it in more creative directions.

It is also important for psychoanalytic theory to maintain its comprehensibility in terms of the rest of the scientific culture. One reason that psychoanalysis lost some of its scientific respectability in recent decades is that it lost touch with the rest of science.

The Behavioral Schema

There may also be a more practical payoff, namely a better understanding of the different kinds of therapy available for the ills of the mind. In a previous article (Olds, 1987), I developed the notion of a "behavioral schema," a system for organizing four modes of learning: affective, behavioral, internalizing, and cognitive.

The *affective* refers to largely biological, inborn mechanisms of evaluating experience. It performs the adaptive function of deciding which experience is favorable and which unfavorable to life and well-being. Its locus of operation is primarily the limbic system, where we postulate that the orchestration of several nuclei imprint experiences with evaluation (Basch, 1983; Lichtenberg, 1989; and Hadley, 1989).

The *behavioral* is the simplest form of learning as we usually think of it, and is available to all motile organisms. In this form of learning there is a pairing of stimulus with response, in fact usually a pairing of stimulus with affect, where the connection made is usually one of temporal contiguity. It organizes the world so that the organism can have a set of stable expectations about the environment and a repertoire of behaviors with predictable consequences. There are several types of behavioral learning. One is *classical conditioning*, in which the organism is passively exposed to two stimuli, so that one stimulus begins to stand for the other. For instance, in Kandel's (1983) experiments with Aplesia, shrimp extract develops a learned equivalence to an electric shock and elicits the same response. A second form is *operant conditioning* in which the animal at first acts randomly, and then learns that certain responses will lead to the avoidance of pain or the gain of a reward (Skinner, 1953). A third behavioral form might be called *kinesthetic learning*, the learning required to perform skilled, not necessarily inherited, motor sequences, such as stalking prey or riding a bicycle. The behavioral types of learning seem to involve subcortical areas and the vestibulo-cerebellar system (Frick, 1982; Levin, 1991). As mentioned earlier, this mode maps nicely onto the backprop connectionist model.

The *internalizing* mode of learning involves the processing of gestalt representations of objects and self-representations. This higher form of learning is available to humans and possibly to higher mammals. It involves the internalization of whole or part objects which, in turn, play a part in the development of the self-representation. It is probably best described in the object-relations theory of psychoanalysis. Since the internal objects are heavily affect-laden and to some extent spatial and nonverbal, we think of the right brain as essential to their formation. In connectionist terms, these internalized objects may be the "prototypes" or generic objects that form the basis of our experience in the social world.

The *cognitive* mode is the uniquely human type of learning, usually involving language. In this mode we learn all our facts, theories, and rules of behavior. In its expression it probably is centered in the left hemisphere.

All behavior represents an amalgam of these modes of learning, but we can recognize a primacy of one system or another in various behaviors, traits, and disorders of learning. Thus, the *affect* system, almost by definition, has primary importance in the affect disorders; there can be a limbic system dysfunction independent of perceived reality, so that a depressed person will greet an event with sadness and apprehension, while a manic person will greet the same event as an opportunity for celebration. The *behavioral* system seems to be involved particularly in certain symptom disorders, such as inhibitions, phobias, compulsions, and addictions; certain behaviors or avoidances are reinforced by reduction in anxiety. The *internalization* system seems especially important in some of the personality disorders, particularly the narcissistic and borderline, where there is pathology in the way that important primary objects are taken in and incorporated into the self-concept. *Cognitive* errors seem important in high-level neurotic pathology and intrapsychic conflict, such as success phobia, certain theories about the wrongness of pleasure, and the like. This pathology can usually be expressed verbally in some maxim, such as "If I succeed in life, I shall be punished."

Each of these modes seems distinguishable from the others and may have a different anatomical locus. How they come together to determine behavior may best be explained by a connectionist model. Each one deals with a different *kind* of information, which must be translated into a common language in order to be integrated. Such integration may occur in a brain process analogous to a neural net. For instance, when we combine pharmacological treatment with psychoanalytic treatment, we have to imagine a common ground where the language of chemical molecules interacts with the language we speak. This may be the strongest rationale yet for the use of multimodal therapies.

Supervision

Another human activity that seems intuitively to fit the connectionist model is the achievement of expert knowledge. It is known that experts come to conclusions by rapid "intuitive" processes unlike the rule-based logical reasoning that one might expect. In the supervision of psychotherapy and psychoanalysis, we usually start out by establishing certain rules and basic programs for how to deal with a patient, certain definitions that help distinguish that treatment from social conversation, physical diagnosis, or skill training. By the time a therapist is an analytic candidate, the few basic rules are quickly learned intellectually. But the ongoing process of supervision is a recurrent feedback to the candidate of subtle nuances: "Instead of what you did, I might say it this way ..." or, rarely, "That was excellent, I can't think of a better move in that situation." Seldom is a rule invoked. It is a slow process of multiple corrections and rewards, similar to the "training" in a connectionist system. By the time the analytic education is far advanced, there is a more or less integrated model based on the candidate's own personality and gifts, the inputs of several supervisors, much reading, and many lectures. The end product, although recognizable as analytic technique, bears the marks of the "multiple constraints" produced by all these influences, rendering the technique unique.

Conclusion

The connectionist system is complex and abstract, and it is not the final chapter in the study of the mind. It provides us with a metaphor that links the explanatory power of the computer with the complexities of the brain. The connectionists' assumptions about the workings of the brain feed their construction of "naturally intelligent systems." These systems in turn become metaphors to help in theorizing about brain function. This may be one of the first occasions in science where there is such a mutual interaction of models. For psychoanalysts watching the progress of this interaction, there will be much to learn.

The metaphor suggested by the connectionist endeavor is not entirely new to psychoanalysts. Schafer (1970), long before connectionism became popular, developed the analogy, "mind as government." In his classic paper reviewing the work of Hartmann, he confronted the need for a model that would encompass what we know about mind, would improve on the force-and-energy model, and would fit the concept of mind that Hartmann developed. In describing the model, he refers to issues mentioned in the metaphor of the *social group* mentioned above.

> Those who govern are concerned with both the internal processes and organization of the government and its relation with neighboring governments... They have to reconcile conflicting interests so far as they can and draw lines as to what is permissible or safe. Those who govern must also generate their government's own strength from within, though they may also increase its strength through external alliances: they must generate the government's means, which include its finances and its traditions, national goals and pride.(Schafer, 1970, p. 443)

In applying this metaphor, Schafer was challenging the biologists to come up with a theory that would satisfy the needs of this kind of model, including the issues of central regulation, internal conflict, aggregate function, and multiple constraint satisfaction. The connectionist paradigm is a response to this challenge.

Note

1 Originally published in the *Journal of the American Psychoanalytic Association* (1994), Vol. 42: 581–611.

References

Anscombe, R. (1986) The ego and the will. *Psychoanalysis and Contemporary Thought*, 9: 437–463.

Antrobus, J. (1991) Dreaming: cognitive processes during cortical activation and high afferent thresholds. *Psychological Review*, 98: 96–121.

Basch, M. F. (1983) Empathic understanding: a review of the concept and some theoretical considerations. *Journal of the American Psychoanalytic Association*, 31: 101–126.

Campbell, J. (1989) *The Improbable Machine*. New York: Simon & Schuster.

Cartwright, R. D. (1977) *Night Life*Englewood Cliffs, NJ: Prentice-Hall.

Churchland, P. M. (1988) *Matter and Consciousness*. Cambridge, MA: MIT Press.

Crick, F. H. C. & Mitchison, G. (1983) The function of dream sleep. *Nature*, 304: 111–114.

Dennett, D. (1978) *Brainstorms*. Cambridge, MA: MIT Press.

Dennett, D. (1991) *Consciousness Explained*. Boston, MA: Little, Brown.

Forrest, D. V. (1992) Artificial mind: the promise of neural networks. Paper presented at the 36th Annual Meeting of the American Academy of Psychoanalysis, May 1, 1992.

Frick, R. B. (1982) The ego and the vestibulocerebellar system: some theoretical perspectives. *Psychoanalytic Quarterly*, 51: 93–122.

Galatzer-levy, R. M. (1988) On working through: a model from artificial intelligence. *Journal of the American Psychoanalytic Association*, 36: 125–151.

Gazzaniga, M. S. (1985) *The Social Brain*. New York: Basic Books.

Hadley, J. L. (1989) The neurobiology of motivational systems. In *Psychoanalysis and Motivation* ed. J. D. Lichtenberg. Hillsdale, NJ: Analytic Press, pp. 337–342.

Hebb, D. O. (1949) *The Organization of Behavior*. New York: Wiley.

Hobson, J. A. (1988) *The Dreaming Brain*. New York: Basic Books.

Humphrey, N. (1984) *Consciousness Regained*. New York: Oxford University Press.

Jones, B. P. (1993) Repression: the evolution of a psychoanalytic concept from the 1890s to the 1990s. *Journal of the American Psychoanalytic Association*, 41: 63–93.

Kandel, E. (1983) From metapsychology to molecular biology: exploration into the nature of anxiety. *American Journal of Psychiatry*, 140: 1277–1293.

Kris, A. O. (1982) *Free Association: Method and Process*. New Haven, CT: Yale University Press.

Levin, F. M. (1991) *Mapping the Mind*. Hillsdale, NJ: Analytic Press.

Libet, B., Gleason, C. A., Wright, E. W., & Pearl, D. K. (1983) Time of conscious intention to act in relation to onset of cerebral activity (readiness potential): the unconscious initiation of a freely voluntary act. *Brain*, 106: 623–642.

Lichtenberg, J. D. (1989) *Psychoanalysis and Motivation*. Hillsdale, NJ: Analytic Press.

Litowitz, B. (1991) The new Frankensteins: models from cognitive science. Paper presented at the 16th Annual Conference of the Semiotic Society of America, College Park, MD, October 26, 1991.

Mcculloch, W. S. & Pitts, W. (1943) A logical calculus of the ideas immanent in nervous activity. *Bulletin of Mathematics and Biophysics*, 5: 115–133.

Nagel, T. (1974) What is it like to be a bat? *Philosophical Review*, 83: 435–450.

Nesse, R. M. & Lloyd, A. T. (1989) The evolution of psychodynamic mechanisms. In *The Adapted Mind: Evolutionary Psychology and the Generation of Culture*, eds J. Barkow, L. Cosmides, & J. Tooby. New York: Oxford University Press.

Olds, D. (1987) The behavioral schema: an integration of modes of learning. *Psychiatry*, 50: 112–125.

Olds, D. (1992) Consciousness: a brain-centered informational approach. *Psychoanalytic Inquiry*, 12: 419–444.

Pagels, H. (1988) *The Dreams of Reason*. New York: Simon & Schuster.

Palombo, S. R. (1992) Connectivity and condensation in dreaming. *Journal of the American Psychoanalytic Association*, 40: 1139–1159.

Reiser, M. F. (1991) *Memory in Mind and Brain*. New York: Basic Books.

Rosenblatt, A. D. & Thickstun, J. T. (1977) Modern Psychoanalytic Concepts in a General Psychology. *Psychological Issues Monograph*, 42/43. New York: International Universities Press.

Rosenblatt, F. (1962) *Principles of Neurodynamics*. New York: Spartan Books.

Rumelhart, D. D. (1990) The architecture of mind: a connectionist approach. In *Foundation of Cognitive Science*, ed. M. I. Posner. Cambridge, MA: MIT Press.

Rumelhart, D. D.Mcclelland, J. L., & PDP Research Group (1986) *Parallel Distributed Processing: Explorations in the Microstructure of Cognition*. Vols. 1 & 2 Cambridge, MA: MIT Press.

Schafer, R. (1970) An overview of Heinz Hartmann's contributions to psychoanalysis. *International Journal of Psychoanalysis*, 51: 425–446.

Shapiro, T. (1979) *Clinical Psycholinguistics*. New York: Plenum.

Skinner, B. F. (1953) *Science and Human Behavior*. New York: Free Press.

Slap, J. W. & Saykin, A. J. (1983) The schema: basic concept in a nonmeta-psychological model of the mind. *Psychoanalysis and Contemporary Thought*, 6: 305–325.

Winson, J. (1985) *Brain and Psyche: The Biology of the Unconscious*. New York: Doubleday.

Chapter 7

Dialogue with Other Sciences

Opportunities for Mutual Gain[1]

Psychoanalysis, from its very beginnings, has greatly valued what we could learn from and what we could contribute to other areas of knowledge and discovery. Creative ideas often come from such cross-fertilization, and it is inherent in the nature of science to be refreshed by discoveries from other disciplines. In the past our mutual interactions with anthropology, literature, linguistics, biography, sociology and history, as some examples, have enriched both disciplines. Currently, advances in neuroscience and cognitive sciences have aroused new interest in the exciting possibility of developing the study of mind-brain relationships and interactions. Freud himself was an early pioneer in biological interdisciplinary study, and we are reminded that he gave up this line of inquiry in part, at least, because neuroscience had not reached the point where such a project could be fruitful.

With the hope of fostering such communication the *Journal* is instituting several series of brief review articles designed to inform the psychoanalyst of the accumulating basic science knowledge in these disciplines that seem germane to our interest.

Currently, an enormous amount of new information is becoming available through techniques of molecular biology, brain imaging, genetics, computer modelling and other studies, and this may be the time to begin thinking anew of the linkages of psychology and the brain. More particularly, we may begin to ask what these new studies can contribute to psychoanalysis, as well as how the psychoanalytic understanding of mental functions may help to guide empirical studies of cognition and neural structures. Kandel (1983), some years ago, reporting on the molecular and cell biology of learning, pointed up the obvious—all mental life proceeds by alterations of brain activity, and learning represents a permanent change in the brain. Psychoanalysis, at root, is a highly specialized method of investigating and altering how and what we learn; and, we might wish to consider whether greater knowledge of brain functions will help us to a deeper understanding, and perhaps a rethinking, of some of the theories and techniques of psychoanalysis.

Freud considered the territory of psychoanalysis to be the realm of psychic conflict and unconscious thought. While Hartmann (1937) felt that in adding

DOI: 10.4324/9781003399551-8

the broad area of the 'conflict free' sphere, psychoanalysis could become an all-encompassing theory of the mind—a general psychology—most analysts today would accept that psychoanalysis is a particular branch of psychology, focused on psychic conflict, unconscious mental functioning, and aspects of development, with a special emphasis on object relations, affects and mental representations. Psychoanalysis, gathering its knowledge through its quite unique methods of study, cannot provide the explanation for all mental phenomena, but it does provide some of the essential components of a fuller understanding of the human mind.[2]

The question of the relation of mind and brain is almost as old as philosophy itself. Psychoanalysts have been deeply divided about the value of brain science or other forms of empirical study for enhancing our capacity for understanding our psyches. The argument was joined sharply in the discussion of a recent article by Peter Wolff in which, discussing the data of infant observation, he stated that 'all that is relevant for psychoanalysis must come from the couch' (1996). Among the arguments put forward against Wolff's view is that new data derived from infant observation may enrich our understanding of the cognitive capacities of the infant, the development of the self, the capacity for representing the mind of another, the vicissitudes of attachment etc., and provide psychoanalysts with new models for attempting to understand our own clinical data.

The interpretations of psychoanalysts, most analysts today would agree, are never free from the analyst's own conceptions of mental life and early development, i.e. his or her theoretical points of view. As much as we may try to listen to our patients so that we may understand the world as they experience it, we are never countertransferentially free of our deeply held beliefs about the nature of the mind. The work of contemporary neuroscientists—as well as cognitive scientists, developmental researchers etc.—should be of concern to psychoanalysts if knowledge of those fields will have an influence on our own internal mental life, i.e. our theoretical stance and our vision of the vicissitudes of human development.

In order to test whether the explosion of knowledge in neuroscience and cognitive science is significant for psychoanalysis, it is first of all necessary that we be knowledgeable about the work that is being done, and be able to translate the language of these disciplines into the domain of our concerns. Each field of knowledge, be it science or humanities, develops a specialized language that best describes the phenomena of interest to them. And, those of us who wish to find out what the neuroscientists are doing need to know how to read their literature. For productive interdisciplinary interactions it is necessary for the members of each field to be able to communicate with each other in their mutual languages. Clearly, we would welcome new knowledge that either helps to verify and enhance the understanding of some of our fundamental ideas, or challenges us to defend their validity. To the extent that psychoanalysts learn about and can participate in the work of the neighboring disciplines, we can also inform them that we are alive and well and thinking in new and creative ways that may usefully inform them. Too often, scientists with a genuine interest in complex mental functions lack access to contemporary psychoanalytic thought. It is our job to help build those bridges.

Psychoanalysis has never been an isolated endeavor. From its very beginnings it was rooted in the scientific and humanistic culture of its era, and although it now has a solid scientific and clinical base of its own, it remains the case that, like all fields of study, we cannot disentangle ourselves from the culture in which we exist. Whether it be philosophy, infant research, social psychology, brain biology, or literature, they all yield a context, which becomes part of the intellectual background in the analyst's mind, from which the analyst understands what emerges from an individual patient. Where once we were concerned about the reductionism of some forms of biology, today's biological forefront is based on hierarchical systems theory—recognizing emergent properties—and is unconcerned with trying to reduce poetic understanding to neuronal activity. A hierarchical explanatory system, including neuroscience, places psychoanalytic concepts and phenomena in a broader social, intellectual and scientific context. Listening to the patient's words remains our primary and phenomenal source of data, but our understanding of the entire patient is enlarged by the awareness of the influences of other levels of explanation. An eminent neuroscientist suggested that 'the emergence of an empirical neuropsychology of cognition based on cellular neurobiology can produce a renaissance of scientific psychoanalysis' (Kandel, 1983). We should at least understand what we are being offered, before deciding whether or not we accept it. We cannot attempt to introduce a deep knowledge of areas of neuroscience in the *Journal*, but we can provide a useful introduction.[3]

It may be helpful to provide a few samples, as an introduction to the topic. Recent research in hippocampal function provides one example of the potential benefits of an awareness of our neighbors' work. Nadel and Jacobs (1996) report the effect of stress on the hippocampus. This organ seems to be the seat of what memory researchers call 'episodic memory'—memory of autobiographical events, events marked in one's memory by a particular time and place. The hippocampus has a high density of glucocorticoid receptors. Moderate stress stimulates a slight increase in glucocorticoid production by the adrenal glands, and this may enhance our memory so that we sharply remember 'significant' events. However, under intense stress—child abuse, accidents, or wartime trauma—the adrenal output of glucocorticoid increases to high levels which inhibit the hippocampus, virtually shutting it down. Memories acquired during these times may be retained vaguely, or as general hyper-arousal states, but they lose their time and space markers. This has several implications of compelling importance to psychoanalysts. Memory of trauma may be distorted, obscured, and reduced to non-specific fear and dread, and it may be rendered timeless, never really relegated to the past, seeming always present, but because of the biology of its original registration, it cannot ever be 'restored' or 'recovered' with accuracy. As Freud described, such memories may be 'constructed', but never 'reconstructed'. Such biological information provides a basis for increased confidence in our inferences of trauma in a particular patient's past, while at the same time making us doubly suspicious of precisely 'recovered' memories under such circumstances. Further research may show in greater detail how this system works, but even this brief sketch suggests its value to the analyst in better understanding the role of constructions, and the differences between memories that are repressed, and those that were never clearly or accurately 'registered'. This biological process—based on massive amounts of glucocorticoid—helps us to a deeper comprehension of the ways ideas are at the cutting edge and not easy to fathom. However, there are some accessible and comprehensive books in this genre including Calvin (1996), Damasio (1994), Dennett (1991, 1996), Donald (1991), Humphrey (1992), and LeDoux (1996), in which our patients' memories may be deformed and even exaggerated by the underlying information processing systems when operating under situations of trauma and stress.

Memory-researchers in the past decade have carved up the realm of memory at increasingly interesting joints and have provided a glimpse into the hierarchy of systems and processes involved in memory (Squire, 1992). The major division is between *explicit* and *implicit* memory. Explicit memory roughly corresponds to memory available to consciousness, and has itself been divided into the above-mentioned *episodic* or autobiographical memory, and *semantic* memory, which is the memory for facts, history, and a fund of general knowledge. In the implicit category are forms of conditioning and associational memory, priming, and *procedural memory*.

Clyman (1991) presents a case for the importance to psychoanalysts of procedural memory. This kind of memory maintains motor schemas and procedures such as riding a bicycle or typing or even solving puzzles. It is anatomically differentiable from episodic memory—patients who have lost their hippocampus can still learn procedures, such as puzzle solving, but have no memory of having seen the puzzle before, or of having learned the procedure. This category may also include 'procedures' for dealing with people, or setting up behavior plans based on expectations from parental figures. Clyman gives an example of a neglected child who, in doll-play, tries to solve the most difficult problems himself, never thinking of having the child-doll ask the mother-doll for help. Such a 'procedure' could become a habitual pattern throughout life and be an important aspect of transference. The concept is already entering psychoanalytic thinking. For instance, Goldberger (1996) relates the development of the superego to procedural learning; the inner organization of interactions with internal and external sources of rules and punishment looks remarkably like a 'habit' learned procedurally.

Another related concept is the notion of 'schema,' applied in Piaget's developmental psychology (Piaget & Inhelder, 1969), in early computer modelling (Rumelhart, 1980), and more recently in psychoanalytic theory (Horowitz, 1988; Slap & Slap-Shelton, 1991). The term refers to habitual patterns of thought, feeling and action, and interpretations of such schemas are common in analysis. The possible relation of schemas to procedural memory is interesting to psychoanalysts, because here is a kind of process that may be unconscious, not only because of repression, but because procedures are usually learned unconsciously and remain a part of 'implicit memory'. Note that this way of explaining repetitive behaviors does not rule out the possibility that some repetitions are conflict-driven. Sometimes a schema seems to be mainly a repetition of a traumatic situation, while in other cases the pattern may be preserved in an active, stabilized conflict of motivations.

Some emotional procedures can be revealed only by their enactment and emotional experience in the transference, and by their eventual perception and interpretation by the analyst. The emergence in the transference of the deepest schemas takes time and sometimes requires the intensity achieved by multiple sessions weekly. Furthermore, there is evidence from cellular and molecular biology that certain kinds of learning require the production of new protein kinases to alter gene expression, and this occurs only after many repetitions over a prolonged period (Karasu, 1992). This may be the basis of an irreducible difference between psychoanalysis and the less intense psychotherapies, and the basis of the rationale for increasing the frequency of sessions.

One value of interdisciplinary research is that it constrains our theories and explanations to the possible, enabling us to function better as diagnosticians, and as healers. For instance, if an analysand reports a vivid memory from ten months of age we will be skeptical about the veracity of this memory, knowing that such autobiographical memories cannot be laid down at that age because —among other reasons—the hippocampus has not yet begun to function; and we will be even more curious concerning the motive for such a construction by the patient. When we are aware of the fact that the patient's narrative may be powerfully influenced by an affect disorder, we may avoid gross errors in understanding the narrative, knowing how much narratives may change under different mood states. As further examples, knowing the biology of schizophrenia or major depression will help us to avoid errors of the past, when mothers were blamed for schizophrenic children, and medication was withheld from severely suicidal patients.

Two somewhat different groups of analysts may have different interests in these interdisciplinary studies. One group includes the candidates and younger analysts, recently educated and often well equipped with the basics of brain biology, who may benefit from an update on scientific research.

Also, some senior analysts, who are interested and curious about cognitive sciences, but not about to make a major investment in learning about other sciences in depth, may want at least to acquaint themselves with some of the new scientific information, thereby increasing their appreciation of the multiple levels of sources of meaning, without having to know the basic science details. That may be all that is really needed to avoid major category errors of the past, such as interpreting the organizational difficulties of a patient with attention deficit disorder as masochistic in the traditional sense, or seeing obsessive-compulsive disorder as derived solely from anal or oedipal issues.

Now that the cognitive and neuroscientists are studying the brain at higher levels of function, and are asking questions about memory, motivation, consciousness, emotion, and symbolism, we psychoanalysts arc suddenly in the position of having an enormous amount of information to offer them. Not all psychoanalysts will be interested enough in the basic science disciplines that are involved in such study to be willing to achieve the mastery necessary for fruitful dialogue with these neighbors. But some of us have already done so and have become better informed. Psychoanalysis can only be enriched by more intimate contact with our scientific neighbors, and we hope the series of review articles that we are now beginning will help to achieve that goal.

Notes

1   Guest Editorial: David D. Olds and Arnold M. Cooper. Previously published in the *International Journal of Psychoanalysis* (1997), Vol. 78, 219–225.
2   Already, a number of psychoanalysts have made fruitful contact with neighbouring fields: developmental psychology (Stern, 1985, 1990; Emde, 1994), neurobiology (Cooper, 1985; Gabbard, 1992; Levin, 1991, Marcus, 1992; Reiser, 1991, 1996; Vaughan, 1997), neuropsychology (Solms, 1997), cognitive
    psychology (Bucci, 1997; Clyman, 1991; Shevrin, 1996), computer modelling (Galatzer-Levy, 1988; Olds, 1994; Palombo, 1992), information theory (Peterfreund, 1971; Rosenblatt & Thickstun, 1977), non-linear systerns (Galatzer-Levy, 1995), linguistics (Shapiro, 1991) and semiotics (Litowitz, 1990; Olds, 1990, 2000).
3   For those more deeply interested, we suggest reading about the concepts of the neural-network workers, such as Gerald Edelman (1992), and the connectionists such as Rumelhart & McClelland (1986) or Paul Churchland (1984).

References

Bucci, W. (1997) *Psychoanalysis and Cognitive Science: a Multiple Code Theory.* New York: Guilford Press.

Calvin, W. (1996) *The Cerebral Code.* Cambridge, MA: MIT Press.

Churchland, P. M. (1984) *Matter and Consciousness.* Cambridge, MA: MIT Press.

Clyman, R. B. (1991) The procedural organization of emotions: a contribution from cognitive science to the psychoanalytic theory of therapeutic action. *Journal of the American Psychoanalytic Association*, 39 (suppl.): 349–382.

Cooper, A. M. (1985) Will neurobiology influence psychoanalysis? *American Journal of Psychiatry*, 142: 13951402.

Cooper, A. M. (1996) *Psychoanalysis in the 21st Century: Unity in Plurality.* Keynote address, 50th anniversary of the Los Angeles Psychoanalytic Institute, 28 September 1996.

Damasio, A. (1994) *Descartes Error.* New York: Putnam.

Dennett, D. (1991) *Consciousness Explained.* Boston, MA: Little, Brown.

Dennett, D. (1996) *Kinds of Minds.* New York: Basic Books.

Donald, M. (1991) *The Origins of the Modern Mind.* Cambridge, MA: Harvard University Press.

Edelman, G. (1992) *Bright Air, Brilliant Fire.* New York: Basic Books.

Emde, R. N. (1994) Individuality, context, and the search for meaning. *Child Development*, 65: 719–737.

Gabbard, G. O. (1992) Psychodynamic psychiatry in the 'decade of the brain'. *American Journal of Psychiatry*, 149: 991–998.

Galatzer-Levy, R. M. (1995) Psychoanalysis and dynamical systems theory: prediction and self-similarity. *Journal of the American Psychoanalytic Association*, 43: 1085–1114.

Galatzer-Levy, R. M. (1988) On working through: a model from artificial intelligence. *Journal of the American Psychoanalytic Association*, 36: 125–151.

Goldberger, M. (1996) *Panel.* The self-punitive patient: analyzing unconscious self-criticism. Fall Meeting of the American Psychoanalytic Association, 21 December 1996.

Hartmann, H. (1937) *Ego Psychology and the Problem of Adaptation.* New York: International Universities Press, 1958.

Horowitz, M. J. (1988) Psychodynamic phenomena and their explanation. In M. J. Horowitz (Ed.), *Psychodynamics and Cognition.* Chicago, IL: University of Chicago Press, pp. 3–20.

Humphrey, N. (1992) *A History of the Mind.* New York: Simon & Schuster.

Kandel, E. R. (1983) From metapsychology to molecular biology: explorations into the nature of anxiety. *American Journal of Psychiatry*, 140: 1277–1293.

Karasu, T. B. (1992) The worst of times, the best of times, psychotherapy in the 1990s. *Journal of Psychotherapy, Practice & Research*, 1: 4.

LeDoux, J. (1996) *The Emotional Brain.* New York: Simon & Schuster.

Levin, F. M. (1991) *Mapping the Mind.* Hillsdale, NJ: Analytic Press.

Litowitz, B. (1990) Elements of semiotic theory relevant to psychoanalysis. In B. L. Litowitz & P. S. Epstein (Eds), *Semiotic Perspectives on Clinical Theory and Practice: Medicine, Neuropsychiatry and Psychoanalysis.* Berlin: Mouton de Gruyter, pp. 81–109.

Marcus, E. (1992) *Psychosis and Near Psychosis: Ego Function, Symbol Structure, Treatment.* New York: Springer-Verlag.

Nadel, L. & Jacobs, W. J. (1996) The role of the hippocampus in PTSD, panic and phobia. In N. Kato (Ed.), *The Hippocampus: Functions and Clinical Relevance.* Amsterdam: Elsevier Science, pp. 455–463.

Olds, D. D. (1990) Brain-centered psychology: a semiotic approach. *Psychoanalysis and Contemporary Thought*, 13: 331–363.

Olds, D. D. (1994) Connectionism and psychoanalysis. *Journal of the American Psychoanalytic Association*, 42: 581–611.

Palombo, S. R. (1992) Connectivity and condensation in dreaming. *Journal of the American Psychoanalytic Association*, 40: 1139–1159.

Peterfreund, E. (1971) Information, Systems, and Psychoanalysis: An Evolutionary Biological Approach to Psychoanalytic Theory. *Psychological Issues*, 7(1/2).

Piaget, J. & Inhelder,B. (1969) *The Psychology of the Child*. New York: Basic Books.

Reiser, M. F. (1991) *Memory in Mind and Brain*. New York: Basic Books.

Reiser, M. F. (1996) The relationship of psychoanalysis to neuroscience. In E. Nersessian & R. G. Kopf (Eds), *Textbook of Psychoanalysis*. Washington, DC: American Psychiatric Press, pp. 605–633.

Rosenblatt, A. D. & Thickstun, J. T. (1977) Modern Psychoanalytic Concepts in a General Psychology. *Psychological Issues*, 11 (2/3). New York: International Universities Press.

Rumelhart, D. E. (1980) Schemata: the building blocks of cognition. In R. Spiro et al. (Ed.), *Theoretical Issues in Reading Comprehension*. Hillsdale, NJ: Erlbaum, pp. 33–58.

Rumelhart, D. E. & McClelland, J. L. (1986) *Parallel Distributed Processing: Explorations in the Microstructure of Cognition*, Vols. 1 and 2. Cambridge, MA: MIT Press.

Schore,A. N. (1994) *Affect Regulation and the Origin of the Self*. Hillsdale, NJ: Erlbaum.

Shapiro, T. (1991) Words and feelings in psychoanalysis. *Journal of the American Psychoanalytic Association*, 39 (Suppl.): 321–348.

Shapiro, T.& Emde, R. (1995) *Research in Psychoanalysis: Process, Development, Outcome*. Madison, CT: International Universities Press.

Shevrin, H. (1996) Psychoanalytic research: experimental evidence in support of basic psychoanalytic assumptions. In E. Nersessian & R. G. Kopf (Eds), *Textbook of Psychoanalysis*. Washington, DC: American Psychiatric Press, pp. 575–603.

Slap, J. & Slap-Shelton, L. (1991) *The Schema in Clinical Psychoanalysis*. Hillsdale, NJ: Analytic Press.

Solms, M. (1997) *Introduction to Neuropsychology*. New York: International Universities Press and London: Karnac Books (forthcoming).

Squire, L. (1992) Declarative and non-declarative memory: multiple brain systems supporting learning and memory. *Journal of Cognitive Neuroscience*, 4: 232–243.

Stern, D. (1985) *The Interpersonal World of the Infant*. New York: Basic Books.

Stern, D. (1990) Joy and satisfaction in infancy. In R. A. Glick & S. Bone (Eds), *Pleasure beyond the Pleasure Principle*. New Haven, CT: Yale University Press, pp. 13–25.

Vaughan, S. (1997). *The Talking Cure: The Science behind Psychotherapy*. New York: Putnam.

Vivona, A. J. (2009) J. (2009). Leaping from mind to brain: a critique of mirror neuron explanations of countertransference. *Journal of the American Psychoanalytic Association*, 57: 551–558.

Wolff, P. H. (1996) The irrelevance of infant observations for psychoanalysis. *Journal of the American Psychoanalytic Association*.

Chapter 8

Consciousness

A Neuroscience Perspective[1]

Introduction

The majority of consciousness research is steeped in an evolutionary perspective and a fundamental assumption of 'mind-brain unity,' Single-cell organisms do not need brains, because they interface directly with their environment through chemo-tactic receptors. The brain evolved as an information processor, to bring the 'outside inside' so that the whole organism is privy to environmental stimuli. Primitive brains react reflexively. The higher vertebrate brain emerged because natural selection favors brains that respond rapidly, yet are flexible enough to adapt to changing environments.

For neuroscientists, 'mind-brain unity' refers to the way in which the brain encodes information as configurations of electrically activated neural networks. Network patterns function as a kind of Morse code that can represent the world. Networks are built up from individual neurons or groups of neurons (neuronal groups) by the intrinsic properties of nerve tissue. All nerve cells intrinsically generate electrical oscillations, independent of external and internal sensory input, and signal their excitement to neighboring cells through synaptic connections (Hobson, 1994; Llinas, 1990). Because neurons have so many synaptic connections to other neurons, even small variations of firing in local neuronal groups lead to significant variations of firing within the widely distributed neural networks that underlie complex brain functions.

Because the concept of consciousness is complex, it is studied much like the fabled elephant, in which one wise man touches the ear, another the trunk and another the leg. In parallel fashion, this article breaks the subject down into the 'what, how, where, when, why and whence' of consciousness. Following this, the theoretical work of neuroscientists Llinas, Edelman, Tononi, and Hobson is presented, since they attempt to integrate the diverse data into a coherent picture. We have chosen to discuss their theories because they address a broad range of the concepts neuroscientists struggle with, and although they disagree on a number of points, there is much overlap and much that is compatible between them.

DOI: 10.4324/9781003399551-9

Historical and Philosophical Background

'Western thought', influenced by the ideas of Plato and Descartes, has always associated the idea of consciousness with dualistic notions of the mind. There is the rational 'conscious' mind and the irrational 'unconscious' mind; the irrational usually being associated with the 'mythic', or spirits, or the Devil, which induce forbidden wishes, dreams and irrational behavior. Descartes takes the long-established split between 'divine soul' and 'mortal body,' and secularizes it to render a duality between 'mind' and 'body', which has become part of our 'common sense', and is difficult for 'Western' cultures to remove from daily thinking. This dualism assumes that there is a 'self' or 'mind' over and against a 'body'. It is inherent in 'traditional' dualism that some kind of central coordinator or inner homunculus brings all brain processes together to produce rational conscious thought (Dennett, 1991). Dualism, some might argue, also pervades the thinking of psychoanalytic theorists who separate the conscious mind from the unconscious one.

At the heart of human experience, the question of consciousness has captured the interest of prominent philosophers, who often refer to it as the 'mystery of consciousness' (Churchland, 1996; Searle, 1997). In no other area of neuroscience is the philosophical as intertwined with the scientific. Therefore, any discussion of consciousness ought to include at least mention of the major philosophical debates. One debate centers around the question of whether the brain is essentially a computational device. Within this debate there are those who believe that the brain can be likened to a computer, with the brain as the 'hardware' and the mind as the 'software'. They assert that eventually computers will be able to do all that the brain can do. This viewpoint, typified by the philosopher Dennett (1991), is often called strong AI (artificial intelligence). Dennett conceptualizes the mind as a 'virtual' machine created out of the neural networks of the brain's 'hardware', similar to the way in which computers can simulate virtual reality for pilots to learn how to fly a plane. Dennett believes that the 'mind' is independent of the 'machine' that creates it, and therefore we can learn little of the mind from the study of anatomy and physiology. The mathematician, physicist and philosopher Penrose (1994) typifies an opposing view. He argues that the human brain is not like a computer, because the mind is too complex to be reducible to the mathematics of computer programmes. He and the philosopher David Chalmers (in Searle, 1997) argue that our current science, including computer science, biology, chemistry, even physics, is insufficient to explain consciousness. They believe that eventually a revolutionary advance in the field of physics will be able to explain it.

Another major philosophical debate centers around the idea of mind-brain unity, i.e. mental phenomena are the result of the activity of neurons. On one side of the debate are those, such as Eccles (1989), who find the inherent 'reductionism' in mind-brain unity objectionable. They argue that the 'soul' and other higher human mental functions, such as self-reflection, cannot be reduced to biology and chemistry. They want to reserve some kind of phenomena beyond the physical to explain these. On the other side of this debate are philosophers, such as Searle (1997) and Churchland (1996), who consider consciousness to be an ordinary biological phenomenon comparable to growth, digestion or the secretion of bile. Consciousness is a function of the brain in the way that digestion is a function of the stomach. They strongly believe that neuroscience will eventually be able to explain consciousness completely.

Essentially all neuroscientists reject the idea of a 'mental-physical' dualism. Both Searle and Churchland maintain that eliminating dualism, however, does not mean reducing human experience, such as spiritual feelings or subjective qualities like beauty, to mere ions, molecules and synapses. But their reasons differ. Searle contends that lower-level neuronal processes lead to 'emergent properties' such as consciousness and the private subjective qualities of personal sensory experience (called 'qualia' by philosophers). An 'emergent property' is one that can be causally explained by the behavior of the elements of a system, but is not a property of any of the individual elements of the system, nor a summation of the properties of the elements. The liquidity of water is an example. The behavior of the H_2O molecule can explain the liquid state of water, but neither hydrogen nor oxygen are liquids. Churchland believes that Searle's view that physical events lead to mental events sidesteps the issue. Churchland believes that the 'physical' and 'mental' cannot be separated, and that physical properties of the brain do not simply cause mental states. She argues that electricity is not caused by the movement of electrons; it is the movement of electrons. Temperature is not caused by the mean molecular kinetic energy; it is the mean molecular kinetic energy. In a similar fashion, causation and identity of conscious states are one and the same. Churchland believes that our ability to accept that consciousness is a property of the neural processes of the human brain will come in time with greater scientific understanding. According to Olds (1998), process dualism may have a place in thinking about the brain-mind relationship. By process dualism he means that the 'semiotic' processes that convey information in life forms, distinguish the living world from the non-living, physical universe. In his model, consciousness is a source of information about brain processes.

Another important debate taken up by philosophers is called 'the binding problem'. While initially 'the binding problem' was identified in relation to perception, it now has expanded to other brain functions such as memory, consciousness and representation in general. As well described by Crick (1994), 'the binding problem' refers to the fact that modular brain areas are specialized for processing different aspects of sensory experience, such as colour, shape and spatial location, yet the brain is able to integrate signals that are separated in space and time into a whole unified experience. In object recognition, the separate modalities of touch, sight and sound are integrated into whole objects. In conversation, separate phonemes are integrated into words and into sentences and into whole conversations. In binocular vision, the two separate images from each eye are integrated into a single visual image. Thus, when we see a blue ball moving diagonally down a ramp, although the brain processes each feature in a separate modular brain region, we nevertheless 'see' the whole event, not the blue colour separate from the spherical shape, separate from the diagonal line of motion. For philosophers, and neuroscientists alike, 'the binding problem' is a central dilemma that must be explained by any neuroscience theory of consciousness.

The Nature of Consciousness: the What?

There is a growing consensus that whatever consciousness is, it is not a unitary thing, but is a class of phenomena that includes several different states, all having in common the general property of being aware (Mountcastle, 1998). Philosophers and neuroscientists emphasize that understanding 'subjectivity', the experience of being conscious, is the 'hard' problem in contrast to the 'easy' problem of describing the neurophysiology and neuroanatomy of consciousness (Chalmers, in Searle 1997). Although it is very difficult for neuroscientists to agree on an exact definition, most use consciousness in the ordinary sense of the word, meaning awareness (Hirst, 1995; Moscovitch, 1995). Consciousness is a psychological or mental phenomenon in which we are aware of perception, of memory, of thought, of action, of self, and of the very process of being conscious.

Consciousness is not an 'all or nothing' phenomenon (Hirst, 1995). There are varying degrees of consciousness; unconsciousness gradates into consciousness; and unconscious mental contents can have an effect on consciousness. Whether a stimulus becomes conscious depends, in part, on the degree of sensory analysis and on one's exact definition of unconscious versus conscious. Using a strict definition, Hirst argues that 'unconscious' applies when stimuli are processed only to a 'shallow' degree or 'low-level'. 'Low-level' analysis includes only the physical attributes of stimuli and most probably involves the primary sensory cortices. These representations are so impoverished they cannot support conscious recognition, but can still influence other mental events. Examples of 'low-level' analysis are the shape of the letters of the word 'bottle', the circles and contours of a face, and the spatial location of an object. Hirst proposes that 'primed' memory, implicit learning tasks, and 'subliminally' presented stimuli involve only 'low-level' sensory processing and therefore remain fully unconscious in the 'strict sense' (for more on memory, see Pally 1997b). These findings are consistent with the work of Shevrin, who proposes that stimuli that involve a paucity of exposure (e.g. 'subliminal' stimuli), although not consciously registered, may in fact 'prime' later thoughts and images that emerge in the clinical situation (Shevrin et al., 1996).

In a less strict definition of unconscious, the 'iffy' 'twilight' area where there is some, albeit very vague, degree of awareness, a more complex or 'deep level' of analysis is involved, most probably involving association cortices. Analysis is considered 'deep' once it involves some degree of identification of objects and their meaning. Bisiach & Berti (1995) discuss 'unconscious' in relation to anosognosia and hemineglect, syndromes that can result from cerebrovascular damage (i.e. stroke) in the right hemisphere, most often in the parietal region. Patients with anosognosia, despite significant paralysis on their left side, deny conscious awareness of their disability. In the case of hemineglect, patients report no conscious awareness of sensory information to the left side of their body. Bisiach and Berti propose that patients with anosognosia and hemineglect are 'unconscious' of disability and stimuli only in this 'less strict' sense. They do evidence that 'twilight' range of at least some level of conscious awareness on certain cognitive tests and physiological responses, such as the galvanic skin response or 'GSR' (a measure that reflects skin sweat production). Bisiach & Berti (1995) believe these syndromes suggest that the significant distinction is not between unconscious and conscious at all, but between states of 'coconsciousness'. They theorize that the apparent lack of conscious awareness in these syndromes is due to a lack of sufficient integration between dissociated 'co-states' of consciousness. Unlike psychoanalytic theory, neuroscientific paradigms of the unconscious involve 'lower-level' representations that do not involve symbolic meanings. Also, that which appears to operate unconsciously might rather be considered a dissociated state of consciousness.

Some neuroscientists consider that desynchronized encephalographic (EEG) activity correlates with conscious states (Edelman, 1989; Hobson, 1994; Llinas & Churchland, 1996). From this perspective, since both waking and REM sleep involve desynchronized EEG activity, waking and dreaming are considered to be alternate states of consciousness, that differ only in the origin of their sensori-motor inputs.

The Process of Consciousness: the How?

Consciousness is often discussed in relation to the 'a' words: awake, alert, aroused, attentive, aware, self-aware, all of which depend on activation of circuits ascending from the brainstem to the cortex. Because of their wide anatomical distribution and neurochemistry, brainstem systems are able to provide the global activation of the brain necessary for consciousness to occur. The reticular activating system drives arousal. It 'announces' to the brain regions higher up, 'stimulus coming! get ready!' The locus coeruleus, the major source of brain norepinephrine, contributes to alertness and attention. Activity in the locus coeruleus 'turns on' in the morning to wake us up from sleep. Activation of the pontine circuits is necessary for the 'consciousness' of dream sleep.

Attention is necessary for something to reach conscious awareness. Attention implies focus on something, whether an object, sensation, thought or image. While we can pay attention to, and be conscious of more than one thing at a time, there are limits. Consciousness cannot hold onto many things at a time. The ability to attend to more than one piece of sensory information depends on how hard it is to keep the two pieces of information segregated. It is easier to hold in consciousness one auditory and one visual message than either two auditory or two visual ones. It is easier to hold in consciousness a list of animal terms and a list of vegetable terms than two lists of either animal terms or vegetable terms. For events to be consciously perceived, they must be significant to the 'self'. The 'self-system' is as essential to consciousness as an intact perceptual system is to perception. One way to conceptualize consciousness is as the interaction of the 'self system' and 'non-self system' (i.e. external world). According to Damasio and Damasio (1996) the 'self system' involves both the invariant activity in neural mechanisms that represent body state, motor actions and relationships, and the changes in those representations in response to sensory stimuli. Because the right hemisphere, more than the left, is connected to somato-sensory information and the autonomic nervous system in both halves of the body, the 'self system' may be more localized in the right brain. The Damasios and others such as Edelman (1989) consider that consciousness involves very rapid shifts back and forth between 'self system' representations and the representations of sensory images.

In a related model by Gray (1995), a central 'comparator,' on a moment-to-moment basis, compares the current state of the organism's perceptual world with the predicted state derived from the 'self-system'. Most of the time the brain keeps reaffirming that nothing has changed from what would be predicted. When something does change (something moves, or something unexpected happens), the comparator notes a mismatch, and that is the instant of consciousness. This theory may have promise, from an analytic point of view. A patient lying on a couch has a rather static visual environment, especially with the eyes closed. Because the brain is always looking for change, on the couch with so little external distraction it will look for change and follow the change in the stream of thoughts and associations.

A distinction is often made between the content of consciousness and the process that produces it. We are conscious of objects, ideas, meanings, decisions and actions—but not of the brain processes themselves that produce consciousness. There is a tendency, perhaps unfortunate, to conceptualize 'process' and 'content' as a kind of 'container' and 'contained' model. Clearly this distinction is problematic since it is hard to imagine that there could be a container that did not contain anything, or a conscious content with no process. However, Lakoff and Johnson (1980) contend that although 'container models' may be conceptually flawed, we are nevertheless somewhat constrained into using them. This is because—as they argue—language and thought derive from bodily experience. For example, we conceptualize feelings as derived from within the body, such as 'the love in my heart'. A strong advocate of the container model, Baars (1996) conceptualizes a 'global workspace' in which processes such as attention and short-term memory contain the mental contents of which we are conscious at that moment.

Using the 'process-content' distinction, Solms (1997) elaborates on Freud, and theorizes that consciousness is like a sense organ perceiving inwardly, a kind of built-in monitor of other brain functions. Solms believes that the contents of consciousness are the data of the senses, the data of memory and the inward appreciation of affects. Solms concludes that the process of consciousness is the same process that produces sensation and perception, thought and affect. While they might argue with his 'process-content' distinction, Llinas and Edelman, whose work is elaborated on later in this article, would agree with Solms that consciousness requires no new neural processes. Consciousness differs only in that it results from more complex integration of the same basic processes that produce other mental phenomena.

The Anatomy of Consciousness: the Where?

A number of neurological syndromes initially led neuroscientists to the conclusion that some localized region was the 'seat' of consciousness. For a time, it was considered the cortex, since damage to the primary (striate) visual cortex leads to loss of conscious awareness of visual stimuli. However, rather fascinatingly, unlike a person with damage to the retina, or optic nerve, the 'cortically' blind person reports no conscious awareness of seeing anything, but when walking can avoid most obstacles in their path. This condition is known as 'blindsight' and may be the result of the kind of 'low-level' analysis discussed by Hirst (1995).

The syndrome known as 'split brain' arises from a cut in the corpus callosum, which divides the two hemispheres (Gazzaniga et al., 1962). Of interest in the present context are studies in which an object is presented visually to the isolated right hemisphere. When asked to name the object, it is as if the visual stimulus does not enter consciousness, because the patient will say 'I see nothing!'. At the same time, experiments show that the object is perceived and registered at some level. The patient can point to the correct object, and rate feelings about the object, such as liking it or not. In one experiment the picture of a nude man is presented to the isolated right hemisphere of a woman. She says she 'sees' nothing, but at the same time she blushes and giggles. It is assumed the person receives the images up to the level of object recognition in the right temporal 'association' cortex. But transfer into the 'linguistic' left brain is missing. Self-reflective consciousness seems to require that step.

Other syndromes at first glance might also appear to support a localized model of consciousness. A stroke in the parietal cortex of the right hemisphere leads to the unilateral hemineglect syndrome. The patient cannot even conceive of anything of interest on the left side of the body, or in the left half of their visual field. In essence the person is not conscious with regard to the left hemispace. And in the other syndrome caused by right parietal damage, anosognosia, the patient behaves as if not conscious of any paralysis of the left side, stoutly denying that anything is wrong at all.

Even recently, because of the role of the hippocampus in episodic memory, Moscovitch (1995) theorizes that it is a kind of 'centre' for consciousness. He believes that all consciously perceived information is automatically processed by the hippocampus and is later recalled as conscious explicit memory (see Pally, 1997b). He feels that consciousness is a 'feature' of explicit memory, separate from the content. When memory is retrieved, the features of perceptual content are linked with the feature of consciousness. Others disagree with Moscovitch, since the hippocampus is not essential for consciousness. A patient with hippocampal damage or Alzheimer's disease may have memory deficits, but is still considered conscious.

These syndromes make it tempting to conclude that there is a special role for 'this that or the other' brain region in consciousness. However, most neuroscientists today believe that there is no anatomical locus of consciousness, no 'Cartesian Theatre' where 'it all comes together', nor any specialized consciousness centre. Consciousness is not a localized process, but involves the integration of widely distributed modular brain regions. Except for a few types of brain damage, such as to intralaminar nuclei of the thalamus and perhaps to the brainstem, there are few brain lesions that produce a global loss of consciousness (Llinas & Churchland, 1996). Even removal of an entire hemisphere in cases of tumor leaves the patient fully conscious. Kinsbourne (1998) points out that local lesions do not eliminate consciousness. They produce only a limitation on what one can be conscious of. For example, damage to the primary visual cortex eliminates conscious vision and damage to the auditory cortex eliminates conscious hearing. Kinsbourne emphasizes that consciousness involves the integration of modular brain regions, and that the specifics of what we are conscious of is always processed in relation to the context of whatever else is happening at the same time. In other words, as he says, conscious 'awareness stands out not by what it is, but by the company it keeps' (1995, p. 1323).

Despite the fact that there is no anatomical location or 'seat of' consciousness, we do subjectively experience that the separate brain functions 'all come together', as a multi-modal integration of perceptions. The zebra always has stripes that stay on the zebra and not next to it; and the sound of its hooves comes reliably from its direction.

The Temporal Nature of Consciousness: the When?

In our subjective sense, consciousness appears to be the initiator of behaviour, the decision maker, the centre of will. The work of Libet et al. (1983) suggests otherwise, by revealing that conscious awareness occurs after the fact. Subjectively we experience that first we decide what we want to do and then we act on it. However, in fact the conscious mind is the 'last to know'. For example, the reflex withdrawal from stepping on a tack is followed by consciousness of the act. But Libet's work also demonstrates that even with a voluntary decision to act, an electrical readiness potential in pre-motor areas is detected almost half a second before conscious awareness of the decision. Computations and cogitations leading to the decision to act are initiated first; then later some of them enter the narrow stream of consciousness. Although Libet's experiments demonstrate that subjects are consciously aware of their decision to act shortly after their 'brain' has made the decision, the conscious awareness is registered so quickly that our subjective experience is that we consciously made the choice.

The Function of Consciousness: the Why?

Some argue that life's tasks could all be done without consciousness, that consciousness is only an 'epi-phenomenon' that 'just happens to accompany' thought and action, and serves no evolutionary adaptation (Gray, 1995; Chalmers, 1996). However, most neuroscientists believe that consciousness evolved as a means by which we can adaptively tailor our responses (Edelman, 1989; Tononi et al., 1992). With consciousness we selectively choose between a number of response options, as well as inhibit responses already initiated but consciously perceived to be inappropriate to the situation. As an example, we are consciously aware that the person we are talking to says something different from what we anticipated. As we respond, we can change the response already 'cued up' in pre-motor regions, even as we are speaking it. The need to tailor one's behaviour in ways that are not pre-wired reflexes requires self-monitoring of one's own behaviour as quickly as possible. The quickest we become conscious of something is about .5 seconds after the fact— 'almost but not quite' instant self-monitoring. Such selective choice and behavioural inhibition most probably involve circuits in the pre-frontal cortex (Knight & Grabowecky, 1995).

Libet's experiments, in which subjects are aware of their decision shortly after they have made it, might appear to aid the 'epi-phenomenon' argument. However, consciousness of a decision, although 'after the fact' of decision-making, is adaptive because it occurs 'before the fact' of actual action. Without consciousness, you would have to wait until you saw what action you took ... to know what action you had decided to make. This is what appears to occur in 'split-brain' patients, in which the right brain may not be consciously aware of a command to the left hemisphere to take action, for example 'walk!', until they actually get up and walk. Without conscious awareness one would stand a poor chance in a physical contest with a person who is conscious, who knows what he decided to do very quickly after his 'brain' decides, not waiting until his body has moved. Consciousness of decision-making helps 'fine-tune' behavioural responses. For example, in reaching for an object, initial attempts are often not accurate and need fine-tuning as the object is approached. Rather than 'waiting to see' what we did and then 'fine-tune it', conscious awareness of the decision to act lets us quickly know what we 'planned' to do and, when necessary, quickly modify the plan. This feedback system operates as what is called primary consciousness, the awareness of the current continuous stream of perceptual and motor events in 'real time.'

In self-reflective consciousness, the ability to reflect on mental processes including primary consciousness, human beings maintain a kind of 'virtual reality' in which we can make speculations and plans that anticipate changes in the environment. This helps us deal with very rapid and complex changes of human environments. Humphrey (1992) suggests that in the social realm, self-reflective consciousness helps us to predict our own behaviour in order to subject it to the inhibitions necessary for social life; and conscious monitoring of our own emotions helps us to gauge the intentions of others and thereby predict their behaviour.

In so far as consciousness is a form of feedback, it plays a part in a representational or semiotic system (Olds, 1990, 1992, 1995, 2000; Deacon, 1997). In this model, in self-reflective consciousness the incoming sense data are re-represented symbolically, and thereby made independent of their source. This creates a 'virtual scene'. An analogy is a video camera. If there is no tape in the camera only a fleeting image occurs, which disappears when the camera is turned off. If there is a videotape recording the input, the scene is preserved, and exists independently of the external reality. It can be replayed, but it can also be edited. Similarly, when we bring memories to consciousness as scenes or in words, this is considered to be symbolic re-representation. Because memory is reconstructed, a representation of an event can be preserved as a 'virtual' scene, but it also can be altered. Herein lies the opportunity for the error and distortion of so-called 'false memory'. But as memory is consciously retrieved and re-worked in therapy, herein also lies the opportunity for change.

The Development of Consciousness: the Whence?

It is becoming more apparent that the 'self' and consciousness arise from a dyadic, interpersonal milieu. The infant has many inborn potentials, but they flower only in intense and frequent interactions with the mother and other caretakers. The epigenetic development of mental and physical capacities require time and synchrony with body growth, central nervous system (CNS) growth and the attunement of the mother. By implication, conscious awareness of perceptual events, emotional events, social events and aspects of one's own inner life develop over time within a socio-emotional context. Some current developmental theories suggest that the 'sense of self' emerges out of the internalization of the dyadic relationship with the mother, and that the development of 'self' consciousness emerges as the infant takes the 'self in the dyad' as an object in its inner world.

Llinas: The Brain as 'Reality Emulator'

According to the theory proposed by the neuroscientist Llinas (Llinas & Pare, 1996), neural activity of the brain is intrinsically organized to represent the world. The brain has within it pre-formed 'templates' for how to respond to the general outlines of the environment it is expected to live in. Over the animal's lifetime the intrinsic activity is modified in response to the specifics of the animal's actual environment. Llinas, along with neuroscientists such as Edelman, Tononi, and Hobson, conceptualizes the brain as a 'reality emulator'. Despite the subjective experience that we sense the outside world, it is the brain's neural activity patterns that 'simulate' reality.

The theoretical proposal of Llinas and the others is that the brain operates fundamentally as a closed system. They are not suggesting that the external world has no influence on the brain. Rather, the closed system means that the brain is essentially self-activating, already has intrinsic activity that can represent the world, and that brain neural networks are active even in the absence of inputs from the outside world. The actual sensory inputs and response outputs of an individual serve only to shape and hone the specifics of that intrinsic activity.

In the closed system model, what is proposed is that certain brain capacities such as cognition, while they mature with development and learning, exist a priori in the brain at birth as a result of the vicissitudes of evolution. For example, from the very first time light hits the retina, many animals including primates automatically begin to develop a visual world (Weisel & Hubel, 1974). As a result of neural network plasticity, during development there is continuing refinement of cognitive images and meanings. As an example, at birth the infant brain can respond to all phonemes. To acquire its native language during development, neural network plasticity leads to enhanced recognition of the phonemes it hears, while the ability to recognize those 'not heard' is lost.

The closed system model emphasizes that we do not directly apprehend the outside world. What we do experience is the brain's intrinsic neural activity being modified by sensory inputs. In fact, as we can see from optical illusions such as the Kanizsa triangle (see Pally, 1997a), the nature of the perception can differ from what is present in the external stimulus. In the closed system model, the dreams that occur during REM sleep are a good example of intrinsic brain activity unmodified by the external environment. Llinas and the others like, perhaps somewhat humorously, to describe waking consciousness as a dream modified by sensory input and motor output. The closed system model may help support psychoanalytic notions of psychic reality. We do not necessarily experience what is actually 'out there'. Rather, the intrinsic design of the brain, along with other intrinsic factors such as evolutionarily determined processing biases, influence what we perceive and what we remember at any given time.

Sensori-motor Templates of the Environment

The brain evolved a special kind of connectivity within the sensori-motor system so as to enhance the animal's ability to predict changes in the environment on the basis of incoming stimuli and to formulate adaptive responses to that change (Llinas & Pare, 1996; Kinsbourne, 1998). Intrinsic activity is generated in sensory and pre-motor areas, which readies the animal for 'likely' sensory inputs and movement outputs. Llinas theorizes that certain neural circuits connecting these areas function as sensori-motor templates. What he means is that sensory perception is automatically connected to the pre-motor areas 'most likely' to be utilized in response to the sensory stimulus (Llinas & Pare, 1996). Reciprocally, motor responses automatically 'tune' sensory areas to sensory inputs most likely to result from that motor response. This enables what Llinas refers to as predictive behavioural interaction, in which a built-in 'anticipatory' system enhances the animal's ability to respond quickly to environmental situations. Llinas's idea is that as we move around the environment, we develop simple images of what we will be moving into. When an animal sees a banana, this automatically modifies pre-motor activity to implement motor programmes required for reaching for the banana; and movements to reach for the banana modify sensory activity to 'tune' the visual system to see bananas. Similarly, hearing your friend speak automatically 'cues up' the programmes for words you are 'likely' to use in response. Your response then 'tunes' your hearing for your friend's 'likely' reply. This is why we can sometimes mis-speak. When someone finishes a sentence differently from how we anticipated, we might still blurt out what was already 'cued up' by the automatic sensori-motor template connections.

This linked automatic sensori-motor connectivity helps us to understand the idea of consciousness as a feedback system. Consciousness lets you know what object you have seen, what you decided to do about it, and then by consciously seeing your movement, lets you know what action you have taken. At each step in the automatic linked sensori-motor response, conscious awareness allows us to determine whether we were correct in our prediction of what was seen, decided or done. If predictions prove inaccurate, consciousness allows us to shift out of 'automatic' into 'choice about' perception, decision, action. You notice you have mis-spoken and make the correction.

According to Llinas, and Edelman as well, as long as inputs from the environment are consistent with predictions there is no need for consciousness! When actual inputs do not match with predictions, consciousness intervenes. Because it involves a high degree of integration between brain regions, consciousness allows for rapid selective choice between alternative responses. The banana you are reaching for has an unexpected colour and texture. Consciousness enables you to recognize it as a plastic fake, not worth picking up. Unless the environment changes in a way that is not anticipated, the brain just keeps doing what it has been doing. This is why you can keep driving without being consciously aware of the road, thinking of something else, until your exit appears.

Premotor-sensory connectivity is illustrated when research subjects wear inverted lenses for extended periods of time. Initially subjects 'see' the world as upside-down (inconsistently with vestibular and proprioceptive inputs). As subjects actively walk around, sensory activity is automatically adjusted. Subjects again 'see' the world right side up (consistently with other sensory inputs). Subjects who only passively experience the world (i.e. sitting on a chair with wheels) do not adapt to the inverted lenses. Llinas concludes that behavioural interaction with the environment modifies intrinsically generated images.

Coherence and Cognitive Binding

Brain modules process the individual stimulus features of the environment (for more on perception see Pally, 1997a). Currently the most accepted hypothesis for feature 'binding' and 'discrimination' is that neural cells responding to the same 'feature' develop a synchronous firing pattern. In binding features of a cup (i.e. contours, colour, texture) all cells responding to features of the cup exhibit synchronous firing patterns. In discriminating between two auditory tones, all cells responding to each frequency exhibit synchronous patterns of firing. The inferior olive, thalamus and neocortex have intrinsic activity that, Llinas theorizes, functions as a 'pacemaker' to entrain the synchronous activity in widely distributed neural groups (Llinas, 1990; Llinas & Pare, 1996).

Llinas, as well as others, such as Crick (1994), theorize that in human beings 40 Hz oscillatory activity in the sensory cortex is particularly involved in conscious perception of stimuli. Subjects are presented with six sets of two clicks at inter-stimulus intervals from 3 to 30 milliseconds, and report whether they 'hear' one or two clicks. At intervals up to 13.7 milliseconds, only one click is consciously perceived. At intervals greater than 13.7, two clicks are consciously perceived. Magnetoencephalography (MEG) can be used to determine the presence or absence of 40 Hz activity in various cortical regions. MEG is a non-invasive technique that can localize cortical brain activity by means of surface (i.e. scalp) recordings of the underlying cerebral cortex. MEG recordings are selectively sensitive to the magnetic fields that arise from current flows in cortical neurons. MEG recordings over the auditory cortex reveal that when two clicks are presented, but only one is consciously perceived, only one peak of synchronous firing at 40 Hz is observed. When two clicks are presented, and two consciously perceived, two peaks at 40 Hz are observed.

Except for smell, sensory messages from the world reach the cortex through the thalamus and 'loop back' to the thalamus, via thalamo-cortical neural circuits. The thalamo-cortical circuits are divided into two looped systems, the specific and the intralaminar. In the specific system, sensory information retains its modality specificity, such as colour or sound frequency. In the intralaminar circuits sensory information is diffuse, meaning that the modality specificity of the sensory information is not identifiable. Both 'loops' make connections with the reticular nucleus of the thalamus. Llinas theorizes that 40 Hz oscillatory activity in thalamo-cortical circuits binds stimulus features into conscious spatio-temporal events (Llinas, 1990, 1991; Llinas & Pare, 1996). Along with Edelman and Tononi, he proposes that a 'conjunction of synchronous activity' between the specific and intralaminar loops, made possible by connections in the reticular nucleus, produces the binding necessary for consciousness. The content of consciousness is carried in the specific system and the temporal context in the intralaminar system. Together they generate a single cognitive event. Damage to specific circuits leads to deficits only in consciousness of individual sensory modalities. Damage to intralaminar circuits leads to deep disturbances in consciousness. Llinas believes that the intralaminar nucleus of the thalamus serves as a 'pacemaker' to synchronize activity at 40 Hz in modular brain regions.

Edelman and Tononi: Neural Darwinism

Edelman and co-investigator Tononi are basically in agreement with many, although not all, of Llinas's ideas. They fundamentally agree that the brain is a closed system; that sensory and motor functions are automatically linked towards adaptive responses to the environment; that the thalamocortical system is central to consciousness; that consciousness is the result of synchronization and binding together of diverse modular activity; and that there is no localized 'place' in the brain that coordinates and organizes modular activity (Edelman, 1989, 1992; Tononi et al., 1992). The theoretical work of Edelman and Tononi is derived from Edelman's Nobel Prize-winning research, in which he discovered that the immune system operates along the same principles of population variation and selection that Darwin proposed for species evolution. Edelman (1998) believes that variation and selection in populations is a fundamental aspect of biological forms. His theoretical application of Darwin's theory to development and function of the higher vertebrate brain is called 'neural Darwinism' or the theory of neuronal group selection (TNGS).

Theory of Neuronal Group Selection: Variation, Selection and Re-entry

All neuroscientists agree that the function of the brain is to generate adaptive behavioral responses to the environment. The question they all face is 'could a program of genetic instructions account for all the possible responses to environmental situations an animal is likely to encounter?' For life forms only capable of a few reflexive responses to a limited set of stimulus inputs (move towards light, withdraw from loud noises) a genetic program might be sufficient. But in the case of the higher vertebrate brain, which is capable of perceiving such a variety of stimulus situations and responding in such flexible ways, most neuroscientists assume that the material contained in the genome is not enough. In essence, Edelman developed his model as a way of explaining both that no set of genetic instructions produces our ability to respond adaptively to the world, and that while our experience is unified, there is no anatomical location where unity is accomplished.

TNGS hypothesizes that the genome programs only for the rough outlines of neurons and synapses. It goes on to speculate that the brain can develop all the necessary functional neural pathways it needs for adaptive behavioral responses, without specific genetic instructions, because of the specialized nature of its anatomy and physiology. The theory contains three basic points regarding this 'specialized nature' of the brain. The first is developmental selection. At birth, genetic programmes have laid out a general anatomical arrangement of neurons and synapses with an over-abundance of synaptic connections. An almost infinite 'variation' of ways exist for these neurons and synapses to be functionally organized into neural networks.

The second point is experiential selection. Overlapping the early post-natal period and continuing on throughout life, experience carves the functional neuronal pathways from the rough anatomical layout. The network pathways that are actually utilized during experience are selected by strengthening the synaptic connections between the neurons. Those not utilized are weakened and pruned back. By analogy, Manhattan has streets and intersections that result from a 'city plan'. The possible 'routes' people actually take to get home, to work, to school, or to play are almost infinite and result from actual experience.

The third point is the process of re-entry. Re-entry refers to the idea that the brain contains massive parallel neural connections between brain regions that enable bi-directional reciprocal electrical signaling, such that activities in different modular regions mutually influence one another. Although re-entry is Edelman's term, most other neuroscientists would agree with the idea of massive parallel bi-directional signaling. Massive re-entry connections exist between the cortex, and structures such as the thalamus, basal ganglia, hippocampus and cerebellum. The amplification of synaptic transmission made possible through re-entry permits local neural activity to influence rapidly the selection of neural pathways linking even distant brain regions.

TNGS uses re-entry as the key mechanism for explaining how there is unity of perception and behavior despite the fact that there is no 'central processor' or detailed set of instructions coordinating functionally segregated areas. Edelman and Tononi (Lumer et al., 1997) propose that the synchronization of activity made possible by re-entry enables rapid shifts in activity in large populations of neuronal groups. Re-entry functions to 'select' the particular neural pathway that underlies the perceptual and behavioral experience of the animal by linking widely distributed areas into complicated patterns, rather than by feeding all the information into some centrally coordinating region. This is why consciousness takes time. Stimuli, memory or emotions must persist for sufficient duration to enable re-entry to produce the synchronization of firing necessary to integrate widely distributed neural networks.

Complexity theory further refines the TNGS (Tononi et al., 1994). Consciousness requires the complexity inherent in the coexistence of localized segregation in conjunction with overall integration. The localized modular activity that is integrated involves not only those neuronal groups that become active in the experience, but those that are inactive as well. What this means is that to be conscious of a particular sensory event, such as the color red, is to simultaneously distinguish it as 'not yellow, not blue, even not sound and not touch'. Similarly, Kinsbourne (1995) argues that what we are consciously aware of depends on its relation to other contents of which we are not consciously aware.

The Value System

Despite enormous plasticity there are constraints on the eventual organization of the brain. What is referred to by neuroscientists as the value system, serves as a bias towards selecting those neural pathways that bring about behaviors that enhance survival. For example, as an infant develops the ability to grasp and eventually to feed itself, roughly speaking, two value constraints that are considered to operate are 'movement to midline is better than movement away from midline' and 'eating is better than not eating'. What this means is that in the early phase of the process a variety of pathways are activated, but eventually the synaptic connections are strengthened in those neural pathways that subserve the value constraints. For example, a baby begins with random hand and arm movements. It develops the ability to grasp an object held directly in front of it, as the neural pathways that become active when the baby moves its hand towards the midline are selectively strengthened over those neural pathways that are activated as the baby flings its arm outwards. In order for grasping to become refined into self-feeding, networks that subserve movements associated with successfully getting food to the mouth are 'selected' over pathways subserving shaky movements that occasionally get food to the infant's cheek. Most generally agree that value constraints are the result of cholinergic and aminergic neuromodulatory systems, since acetylcholine, dopamine, norepinephrine and serotonin neurotransmitters modulate changes in synaptic strength.

Experimental data in human beings support the idea that 'values' such as motivational salience influence neural selective mechanisms. Tachistoscopic presentation of a series of dots will not be perceived consciously if the duration of each stimulus presentation is too short. If the duration is lengthened to a few milliseconds, under normal conditions the subject will say 'I see something but I don't know what'. However, if the subject is deprived of food, they will say 'I see pieces of meat' and if deprived of water, they say 'I see droplets of water'.

The Hierarchy of Brain Functions That Leads to Consciousness

Objects in the outside world activate patterns of neural activity in the brain. According to neuroscientists, perception involves the brain's ability to recognize the patterns of neural activity not the objects themselves. These patterns result when re-entry correlates activity within multiple sensory modalities and the motivational value system. For example, a specific correlation of color, contour, and texture may lead to a neural pattern 'recognized' as apple but that is more likely to be perceived when the animal is hungry rather than satiated.

Edelman, perhaps more than other neuroscientists, emphasizes the distinction between primary consciousness and self-reflective consciousness. According to Edelman primary consciousness is the awareness of the current perceptual scene in 'real time', i.e., the 'here and now'. It is produced when re-entry connections link ongoing perception with a special kind of memory referred to as value category memory. This is the conceptual memory of what has been salient in the animal's environment, essentially the animal's experiences of 'reward' and 'adversity'. Primary consciousness provides a coherent scene that allows the animal to link complex changes in the environment, which may not be causally associated in the outside world, but which help the animal to predict danger or reward. For example, value category memory stores the information 'this tree is near where I encountered a predator last time I was at the watering hole'. Even though the tree and predator are not 'causally linked in the environment' their associations are salient, and therefore they are meaningfully linked in value category memory, and thus linked in an ongoing conscious scene.

What differentiates human beings from animals is the capacity for self-reflective consciousness (SRC). Primary consciousness exists only in 'current concrete' experience. Edelman's hypothesis is that SRC results from re-entry correlations of the 'present and concretely bound' primary consciousness with activity in symbolizing and language regions such as pre-frontal cortex, Broca's and Wernicke's regions. The pre-frontal region symbolizes experience that occurs during the social transmission of language. In this way, during verbal interactions with others, the brain generates symbolic categories such as self, non-self, actions, images, even its own internal sensations, and relates them to ongoing events of primary consciousness. Symbolic categorization frees SRC from the constraints of the immediate present. The contents of SRC can be held in mind and manipulated without resorting to interaction with concrete aspects of the external world.

Binocular Rivalry

Binocular rivalry is one of the best ways to study the neural correlates of conscious awareness, because it illustrates how sensory inputs may impinge on the brain but not be consciously perceived. Edelman and Tononi (Tononi et al., 1998) use it to defend their idea that consciousness, rather than resembling a bright spotlight illuminating a small area on a dark stage, as many (such as Baars, 1996) conceptualize it, but involves high degrees of integrated activity between many regions of the brain, even the 'silent', 'dark' ones.

Rivalry occurs when two dissimilar images are presented to the two eyes. The individual consciously sees only one image at a time, with a switch in perceptual dominance occurring every few seconds. Perceptual transitions between each view occur spontaneously without any change in the physical stimulus. You can experience this phenomenon using the Necker cube (see Pally, 1997a, p. 1025). Each eye observes a slightly different orientation of the cube. As one looks directly at the cube, the conscious perception spontaneously alternates between the two orientations. Binocular rivalry is one phenomenon used to distinguish between attentional mechanisms and conscious perception, since even though attention is directed at a constant image the subjective conscious perception fluctuates.

Neural responses associated with the physical presence of the stimulus can be distinguished from those associated with conscious awareness of the percept (Farber & Churchland, 1995) Rivalry studies in monkeys using single cell recording, and in human beings using fMRI (1), indicate that activity reflecting the physical presence of the stimulus remains constant in 'striate' visual cortices (Lumer et al., 1998). However, when the stimulus is consciously perceived, activity in 'extrastriate' visual cortex and inferotemporal cortex shows alterations that correspond to each perception. Tononi et al. (1998) investigate binocular rivalry in human beings using MEG, which measures activity simultaneously in all cortical regions. With the use of special goggles, one eye is presented with the image of a red vertical grating, and the other eye is presented with a blue horizontal grating. Both images are presented continuously, but subjects consciously perceive only one image at a time, with spontaneous alterations between the two. Brain activity for each stimulus is widely distributed throughout the cortex, whether or not the subject consciously perceives the stimulus. But the areas where activity is more intense differ according to whether the stimulus is perceived consciously or not. They conclude that this supports the idea that consciousness involves shifts in synchronous firing in large, distributed populations of neurons.

Functional magnetic resonance imaging (fMRI) can detect changes in oxygen consumption. It can be used to measure localized neuronal activity in the brain because glucose is metabolized when neurons generate electrical impulses and oxygen consumption is a reflection of glucose metabolism. Like positron emission tomography (PET), which also measures glucose metabolism, fMRI has excellent localizing ability; in addition, it has significantly better temporal resolution.

Hobson: Dreaming as a 'State' of Consciousness

The dream research of Hobson is included in this article because it assumes many of the postulates of Llinas, Edelman and Tononi and serves as an illuminating application of their theoretical models. He assumes that the brain is essentially a closed system with intrinsically generated neural activity, and the similarity in EEG activity indicates that dreaming and waking are alternate states of consciousness (Hobson, 1994; Hobson et al., 1998; Braun et al., 1998).

Hobson focuses on the three cardinal brain-mind states: waking, dreaming and non-dream sleeping. Numerous animal studies indicate that during the waking state the aminergic neuromodulatory systems (i.e. noradrenergic and serotonergic) are 'on' and the cholinergic system is dampened (Hobson et al., 1998). During REM sleep the opposite is the case, with the aminergic 'off' and the cholinergic 'on.' In other words, REM sleep is generated by the cholinergic system and waking by the aminergic system. Hobson's theory is that shifts between brain-mind states are produced by 'reciprocal interaction' of aminergic and cholinergic neuromodulatory systems. During waking, aminergic activation inhibits activity in cholinergic neurons and REM activity is suppressed. Reciprocally, during REM sleep, the aminergic system is 'turned off', releasing the cholinergic system and dream activity from suppression. What results is that waking consciousness is mediated by noradrenalin and serotonin, and dream consciousness by acetylcholine. Hobson's hypothesis is supported by a number of pharmacological studies. For example, noradrenergic agonists (clonidine) injected into the brainstem decrease

REM. Reciprocally, cholinergic agonists and cholinesterase inhibitors (carbachol) induce REM sleep.

After studying literally thousands of human subjects who are awakened during different stages of sleep and asked to report their antecedent mental activity, what Hobson (and numerous others) have found is that, while dreams do occur during non-REM sleep, those that occur during REM sleep tend to be more bizarre and more vivid. Hobson has identified highly consistent characteristics that distinguish dream cognitions from waking ones. REM dreams are filled with strange associations between objects, scenes and actions. Orientation as to time, place, person and focus of attention are continually and rapidly shifting. Recent memory is patchy. Insight is almost absent. Emotions run high and involve mainly anxiety, anger and joy. From this perspective, dreaming is similar to an organic 'delirium', but in the case of dreaming it occurs nightly, and we 'recover' each morning.

These aspects of dream cognition are presumed to reflect differential activation of various brain regions resulting from the different projections of the aminergic and cholinergic systems from the brainstem to other brain regions. The cholinergic system originates in the pontine nuclei, the noradrenergic in the locus coeruleus, and the serotonergic in the dorsal raphe. PET scans during REM, when cholinergic circuits predominate, reveal that activity is increased in extrastriate visual cortex, basal ganglia, limbic and paralimbic regions, and activity in striate (i.e. primary) visual cortex and frontal cortex is decreased. Conversely, in the waking state, PET scans reveal that the striate and frontal cortex are activated. Hobson suggests that because of the almost seizure-like electrical firing that characterizes REM sleep, pontine activation of limbic, basal ganglia and extrastriate visual areas cause dreams to contain highly disorganized, emotionally intense visuo-motor programs. Since, during REM, activity in primary sensory and frontal cortex is dampened, rational thought and sensori-motor responsivity to the external world is likewise diminished. Hobson agrees with the idea proposed by Llinas, Edelman, and Tononi that dreams are a conscious brain state unmodified by external reality. The main difference between dreaming and waking is that, during REM dreaming, cortical regions that mediate interaction with the external world (primary sensory and frontal cortex) are shut down, and information processing is driven instead by internal sources (pontine cholinergic circuits). The reason we can't orient ourselves in our dreams or remember them is that the aminergic systems that sustain orientation and memory are shut down. Hobson argues that dreams contain strange associations, not owing to unconscious dynamics, but because sensori-motor cortices are driven by highly excitable centers in the pons without the top-down control of the 'rational' and 'volitional' frontal cortex. However, they are emotionally meaningful because they include salient emotional memory contained in limbic circuits.

No conclusive answer has emerged regarding the function of either sleep in general or REM sleep in particular. Hobson believes that the most promising avenue of research implicates REM sleep as a means of consolidation of learning and memory. The aminergic neuromodulatory system that supports the acquisition of new information is shut down during REM, and therefore memory cannot be acquired. However, under the sway of the cholinergic system during REM, learning and memory consolidation occurs as synaptic strengthening forges new connections between the 'already acquired' information contained in the sensori-motor and emotional programs of dream sleep. Although there is much debate on this issue, the work of Reiser (1991) is pertinent here. Reiser notes research showing the influence of the day residue on dream content, and points out that the apparently random aspects of dreaming stimulated by the pontine-geniculate-occipital waves, actually favors themes resulting from recent activities, and leads to associations that can be psychodynamically significant.

Clinical Correlation and Conclusions

For every evolutionary advance there is a price. The symbolic thinking embedded in self-reflective consciousness affords an almost infinite flexibility in the ways human beings can conceptualize the events of their life. The price is indecision. Too many possibilities as to how to interpret events leads to confusion over what behavioral response to choose. According to a theory of Ramachandran (Ramachandran et al., 1996), coherent belief systems evolved to narrow the number of choices in order to provide consistency and coherency in determining what to think and how to behave. Ramachandran uses the condition known as anosognosia to support his theory. Anosognosia manifests in the small percentage of patients with right-sided stroke who deny their illness (Bisiach & Berti 1995; see also Pally, 1998). When asked to perform a task, such as pointing to the doctor's nose with their left hand, patients deny their disability but come up with ingenious excuses as to why they cannot perform the task: 'I would like to, but I have terrible arthritis and it hurts too badly to lift my arm'.

Anosognosia has generally been considered a defense against the painful awareness of disability. Ramachandran argues that this explanation fails because patients with left-sided stroke, an equally upsetting disability, rarely display anosognosia. He argues instead that anosognosia results from the different role played by the right and left hemisphere with respect to belief systems. The left hemisphere is the interpreter, and is primarily concerned with taking all the bewildering sensory inputs and making sense of them by ordering them into a coherent belief system. By limiting the number of ways to interpret events, the brain is not overwhelmed by all the possible explanations that could be arrived at. This protects the brain from being paralyzed by indecision as to how to act. The left hemisphere's goal is to maintain its belief system at all costs. When information inconsistent with the belief system occurs, rather than revise the belief system, the left hemisphere either denies the inconsistent information, or 'confabulates' to make it consistent. Thus, we analyze the data in our sensory environment in terms of the belief systems we have constructed.

The strategy of the right hemisphere is fundamentally different. The right hemisphere functions as an anomaly detector. When inconsistent information reaches a sufficient threshold, the right hemisphere 'decides' it is time to revise the belief system. If, however, in the case of right hemisphere stroke the anomaly detector function is impaired, the unimpaired left-sided interpreter maintains its original beliefs. Despite seeing that the left arm is paralysed, instead of revising the belief system (i.e. that the body is healthy), the left hemisphere denies the paralysis and confabulates to rationalize the motor incapacity. An experimental procedure as odd as the syndrome itself, suggests that the patient is consciously aware of the paralysis 'at some level'. Cold water is irrigated into the patient's left ear (right hemisphere). For a period of up to thirty minutes, the patient's denial clears and they acknowledge their disability. It seems as if the increased stimulation to the right hemisphere may temporarily repair the anomaly detector.

Gazzaniga (1998), who originated the concept of the left-hemisphere interpreter function, supports Ramachandran's theory of a differential cognitive role for right and left hemisphere that can lead to incorrect perceptions. In a test of memory with split-brain patients, when asked to report on an experience, the right brain reports a veridical account and the left generates many false reports. It is theorized that as a result of the left hemisphere always looking for the order and meaning of experience even when there is none, it can also include false information into its schema of what happened, if it fits with the belief. In a test of predictive capability, a subject must guess whether a light is going to appear at the top or bottom of a computer screen by pushing a button. The experimenter manipulates the situation so that 80 per cent of the time the stimulus appears on the top, but in a random sequence. It is quickly evident to all subjects that the light appears on top more often. Invariably, normal subjects adopt the strategy of trying to figure out the pattern and deeply believe that they can. However, using their strategy they are correct only 68 per cent of the time. If on the other hand, they had simply pushed the top button every time they would have been correct 80 per cent of the time! Rats, whose brain does not have the interpreter function, press only the top button and are correct more often than the normal human beings. Tests with split-brain patients reveals that the right brain appears to react in a way similar to the rat, responding most closely to what is there and not trying strategically to identify meaningful patterns.

Although the theories of Ramachandran (the right-hemisphere anomaly detector) and Gazzaniga (the left-hemisphere interpreter) are speculative, they suggest a number of clinically relevant points. Our conscious belief systems influence what we consciously perceive. The result is that conscious perceptions may not accurately reflect what occurs 'out there' in our environment. Additionally, it implies that not only do people resist knowledge of unconscious mental contents, they resist knowledge of conscious material as well, if it does not fit with their consciously held interpretations of reality. What may occur during the interpretation of transference is the engagement of the anomaly detector in the right hemisphere, alerting the individual to the need to revise their neurotic belief system.

In conclusion, primary consciousness and self-reflective consciousness evolved to enhance survival. Presumably primitive organisms do not have consciousness. They respond with 'hard-wired' inborn reflexive behaviour. Even in human beings, that which we do automatically, such as riding a bike or tying shoelaces, does not require conscious monitoring. Also, when no salient or meaningful change occurs in the environment, we do not attend consciously, as in the case of driving and not consciously paying attention. What consciousness provides is a means by which we notice changes and can flexibly choose the most adaptive response to that change. Consciousness provides a feedback system for the individual to monitor rapidly not only changes in the environment, but also their own minute-to-minute responses to those changes. We attend to and may be conscious of the most salient changes that occur.

In self-reflective consciousness, the self is taken as an object. Once the self can become an object of perception and interpersonal interactions can become internalized, one can reflect on one's own patterns of behavior, and one can represent them symbolically. A representation of any sort is more malleable than that which it represents. At the level of human self-reflective consciousness, we have 'representations of representations' that can be manipulated independently of 'concrete reality'. As a result of the flexibility inherent in consciousness we are open, on one hand, to forgetting and distortions, but on the other to the possibility of learning, growth and therapeutic change.

Note

1 Previously published by Regina Pally and David D. Olds in the *International Journal of Psychoanalysis* (1998), Vol. 79: 971–989.

References

Baars, B. (1996) *In the Theater of Consciousness: The Workspace of the Mind.* New York: Oxford University Press.

Bisiach, E. & Berti, A. (1995) Consciousness in Dyschiria. In *The Cognitive Neurosciences.* Cambridge, MA: MIT Press, pp. 1331–1340.

Braun, A. R. et al. (1998) Dissociated pattern of activity in visual cortices and their projection during human rapid eye movement sleep. *Science,* 279: 91–94.

Chalmers, D. (1996) *The Conscious Mind: In Search of a Fundamental Theory.* Oxford: Oxford University Press.

Churchland, P. S. (1996) Toward a Neurobiology of the Mind. In *The Mind-Brain Continuum*. Cambridge, MA: MIT Press, pp. 281–303.

Crick, F. (1994) *The Astonishing Hypothesis*. New York: Macmillan.

Damasio, A. R. & Damasio, H. (1996) Making images and creating subjectivity. In *The MindBrain Continuum*. Cambridge, MA: MIT Press, pp. 19–27.

Deacon, T. (1997) *The Symbolic Species*. New York: W.W. Norton.

Dennett, D. C. (1991) *Consciousness Explained*. Canada: Little Brown & Co.

Eccles, J. C. (1989) *Evolution of the Brain: Creation of the Self*. New York: Routledge.

Edelman, G. (1989) *The Remembered Present*. New York: Basic Books.

Edelman, G. (1992) *Bright Air, Brilliant Fire*. New York: Basic Books.

Edelman, G. (1998) Building a picture of the brain. *Daedalus*, 127: 37–69.

Farber, I. B. & Churchland, P. S. (1995) Consciousness and the neurosciences: philosophical and theoretical issues. In *The Cognitive Neurosciences*. Cambridge, MA: MIT Press, pp. 1295–1306.

Gazzaniga, M. S. (1998) The split brain revisited. *Scientific American*, July issue: 50–55.

Gazzaniga, M. S. et al. (1962) Some functional effects of sectioning the cerebral commisures in man. *Proceedings of the National Academy of Sciences of the USA*, 48: 1765–1769.

Gray, J. (1995) The contents of consciousness: a neuropsychological conjecture. *Behavioral & Brain Science*, 18: 659–722.

Hirst, W. (1995) Cognitive aspects of consciousness. In *The Cognitive Neurosciences*. Cambridge, MA: MIT Press, pp. 1307–1319.

Hobson, J. A. (1994) *The Chemistry of Conscious States*. Boston, MA: Little Brown & Co.

Hobson, J. A. et al. (1998) The neuropsychology of REM sleep dreaming. *Neuro Report*, 9: R1–R14.

Humphrey, N. (1992) *A History of the Mind*. London: Chatto & Windus.

Kinsbourne, M. (1995) Models of consciousness: serial or parallel in the brain? In *The Cognitive Neurosciences*. Cambridge, MA: MIT Press, pp. 1321–1329.

Kinsbourne, M. (1998) Unity and diversity in the human brain. *Daedalus*, 127: 233–256.

Knight, R. T. & Grabowecky, M. (1995) Escape from linear time: prefrontal cortex and conscious experience. In *Cognitive Neurosciences*. Cambridge, MA: MIT Press, pp. 1357–1371.

Lakoff, G. & Johnson, M. (1980) *Metaphors We Live By*. Chicago, IL: University of Chicago Press.

Libet, B. et al. (1983) Time of conscious intention to act in relation to onset of cerebral activity (readiness potential): the unconscious initiation of a freely voluntary act. *Brain*, 106: 623–642.

Llinas, R. R. (1990) Intrinsic electrical properties of mammalian neurons and CNS function. *Fidia Research Foundation Neuroscience Award Lectures*, 4: 175–194.

Llinas, R. R. & Churchland, P. S. (Eds) (1996) *The Mind-Brain Continuum*. Cambridge, MA: MIT Press.

Llinas, R. R. & Pare, D. (1996) The brain as a closed system modulated by the senses. In *The MindBrain Continuum*, ed. R. Llinas & P. Churchland. Cambridge, MA: MIT Press, pp. 1–18.

Lumer, E. D. et al. (1997) Neural dynamics in a model of the thalamocortical system. II. The role of neural synchrony tested through perturbations of spike timing. *Cerebral Cortex*, 7: 228–236.

Lumer, E. D. et al. (1998) Neural correlates of perceptual rivalry in the human brain. *Science*, 280: 1930–1934.

Moscovitch, M. (1995) Models of consciousness and memory. In *The Cognitive Neurosciences*. Cambridge, MA: MIT Press, pp. 1341–1356.

Mountcastle, V. B. (1998) Brain science at the century's ebb. *Daedalus*, 127: 1–36.

Olds, D. D. (1990) Brain centered psychology: a semiotic approach. *Psychoanalysis and Contemporary Thought*, 13: 331–363.

Olds, D. D. (1992) Consciousness: a brain-centered informational approach. *Psychoanalytic Inquiry*, 12: 419–444.

Olds, D. D. (1995) A semiotic model of mind. Presented at American Psychoanalytic Association Meeting; December 1995.

Olds, D. D. (2000) A Semiotic Model of Mind. *Journal of the American Psychoanalytic Association*, 48: 497–529.

Pally, R. (1997a) How the brain actively constructs perceptions. *International Journal of Psychoanalysis*, 78: 1021–1030.

Pally, R. (1997b) Memory: brain systems that link past, present and future. *International Journal of Psychoanalysis*, 78: 1223–1234.

Pally, R. (1998) Bilaterality: hemispheric specialisation and integration. *International Journal of Psychoanalysis*, 79: 565–578.

Penrose, R. (1994) *Shadows of the Mind*. Oxford: Oxford University Press.

Pinker, S. (1997) *How the Mind Works*. New York: W.W. Norton.

Ramachandran, V. S. (1996) Illusions of body image: what they reveal about human nature. In *The Mind-Brain Continuum*. Cambridge, MA: MIT Press, pp. 29–60.

Reiser, M. F. (1991) *Memory in Mind and Brain*. New York: Basic Books.

Searle, J. R. (1997) *The Mystery of Consciousness*. New York: New York Review of Books.

Shevrin, H. et al. (1996) *Conscious and Unconscious Process: Psychodynamic, Cognitive, and Neuropsychological Convergence*. New York: Guilford Press.

Solms, M. (1997) What is consciousness? *Journal of the American Psychoanalytical Association*, 45: 681–778.

Tononi, G. et al. (1998) Investigating neural correlates of conscious perception by frequency- tagged neuromagnetic responses. *Neurobiology*, 95: 3198–3203.

Tononi, G. et al. (1992) Reentry and the problem of integrating multiple cortical areas: simulation of dynamic integration in the visual system. *Cerebral Cortex*, 2: 310–335.

Tononi, G. et al. (1994) A measure for brain complexity: relating functional segregation and integration in the nervous system. *Proceedings of the National Academy of Science*, 91: 5033–5037.

Weiser, T. N. & Hubel, D. H. (1974) Ordered arrangement of orientation columns in monkeys lacking visual experience. *Journal of Comparative Neurology*, 158: 307–318.

Chapter 9

A Semiotic Model of Mind[1]

A theory of signs is presented to arrive at a model of mind that provides a smooth transition from inanimate matter to the thinking brain. Principles of information theory and semiotics are invoked to create a conceptual scheme that can contribute to an understanding of the "mind-body problem." The thesis is pursued that in living systems, as opposed to inorganic ones, there occurs the phenomenon of semiotic transmission of information. The result is a "dualistic-materialist" position; the dualism arises from the fact that at the beginning of life a set of processes comes into being different from those of the inorganic world. This model has implications for psychology and psychoanalysis. It allows for semiotic systems at different levels—e.g., the molecular, the neural network, the language system, and higher mental functions—to be integrated. Analytic concepts such as free association, clinical technique, feedback systems, personality structure, transference, and repetition compulsions can be understood in both biological and semiotic terms. This model interdigitates with linguistic studies already done in psychoanalysis, as well as with biological models extrinsic to the field.

Despite centuries of work by philosophers and theologians seeking to explain the difference between mind and brain, and decades of work by biologists and psychologists, the puzzle is still with us. For Freud—and for us, the psychoanalysts who have followed him—the issue has remained alive. Today, with new information arriving from neighboring sciences, the question becomes ever more pressing, for it impinges on the very nature and definition of our discipline. The problem centers on the difficulty of integrating psychoanalysis with the more strictly biological disciplines.

A version of this problem has troubled psychiatrists for years, whenever they have stopped to contemplate their use of both medication and psychotherapy. When we try to understand how a medication can effect change in a patient with a mood disorder, an anxiety disorder, or even a psychotic disorder, we run up against the problem. The medication effected a change in what traditionally has been considered a "mental" phenomenon, such as self-esteem, predictions of the future, self-confidence, a sense of alienation, or other "personality variables." These same psychological phenomena have on

DOI: 10.4324/9781003399551-10

occasion been changed by purely verbal therapies, and in fact were thought to be the main targets of such therapies. Opinion is divided regarding the superiority of one kind of treatment over the other in dealing with these areas. One frequently hears comments such as "The patient has a bipolar disorder, but he also has psychological issues," or "The patient first needs to have the affect disorder treated with medication, and then she will require analytic treatment for personality problems," or "Axis I disorders we medicate; Axis II disorders we refer for therapy." Despite the fact that it is now acceptable to say that medications have an impact on personality, and that psychotherapy modifies brain structures, the confusion persists, and we have trouble really believing such statements.

The mind-brain problem has been more intensely discussed among philosophers and physicists than among biologists. Nonetheless, in all camps there remains some version of the mind-brain split. This may be handled by an outright Cartesian dualism or by attempts to consider mind as "emergent" out of brain processes. Some try to make the problem go away by an "eliminative materialism," essentially a seamless monism.

Corollary to the mind-brain problem is the "meaning-versus-cause" problem. We commonly think that cause happens in the brain, and meaning in the mind, or between minds. We see serotonin and dopamine as having causal effects, whereas words and gestures convey meaning. There are many confusions in this realm of discourse. Causal connections are thought to be physical, whereas meanings inhabit the universe of symbols, which are thought not to be. But meanings as signs are transmitted by visible expressions or by sounds, and are received by eyes and ears tied to complex neurological systems. The meaning, however, lies not in the physical connection but in the pattern of physical connection, an immaterial concept. But is a pattern really immaterial? One could go on at length citing instances showing that causes and meanings are hopelessly entangled if we use the models currently available.

In response to this recurrent perplexity, I propose a model intended to clarify and help resolve the mind-brain dichotomy. I plan to develop a theory of signs to arrive at a model of mind that provides a smooth and continuous transition from inanimate matter to the thinking brain. In previous work (Olds 1990, 1992, 1994) I have presented simple semiotic models in initial attempts at such a mind-brain integration. Since then, I have found that a more complex semiotic system, including different kinds of signs, adds to the theory in important ways. The result is a "dualistic-materialist" model describing the transition from the inanimate to the animate, and from the primitive animate to the cerebral and the cultural.

One may well ask why we need to go so deep to deal with a problem at the "high end" of the living world. One reason is that attempts to deal with the dualist/monist argument at the mind-brain level have never really worked. Why not go to the origin of life, where the dualist process began? In the argument that follows it may seem that I am drawing on information and concepts from widely disparate fields of inquiry that cannot possibly have relevance to psychoanalysis. I hope that readers will see that these apparently distant concerns are necessary to the argument, and that in the end it is no surprise that we should have to go so far afield to answer so profound a question.

My purpose here is to continue a project of exploring the unifying, syncretic properties of semiotic theory. Peirce (1897), Sebeok (1986), Eco (1984), and Deely (1986), among others, have brought semiotics to the fore. However, these authors are not well known to analysts, and difficulties can arise from the concepts, which seem at once simple and baffling. The jargon is at times inconsistent and confusing. I myself have found it tough going to grasp these ideas, and even harder to communicate them to those not already immersed in the theory. The ideas of Bonnie Litowitz (1990), who has brought ideas from her field of linguistics to bear on psychoanalysis, provide important background for my project. Analysts have themselves done important work in a similar vein. Edelson (1975), Rosen (1977), Muller (1996), Shapiro (1991), Makari and Shapiro (1993), and others have made important efforts at integrating psychoanalysis with general linguistics. My aim corresponds to theirs in attempting to gain greater understanding of language, which forms part of the very bedrock of our discipline. With semiotic theory, however, I attempt to make more general statements about signs and sign systems as the basis for a metapsychology. I consider the sign to be a concept basic to both biology and psychology, much as the inorganic molecule is to chemistry and the atom to physics.

Precis Of the Argument

The purpose of the argument is to provide a plausible explanation of the mind-brain distinction, such that psychology and psychoanalysis have a firm foundation on a principle, operative throughout the living world, from the bottom to the top, from the molecule to the mind. The principle is that of semiosis, in which one thing can stand for another.

Semiotics is the study of signs. A sign exists in a system in which its particular properties provide a body of information carried from one part of the system to another part. Examples of sign systems include the transfer of genetic coding from DNA to protein using RNA; a neurotransmitter taking information from one neuron to another; a pheromone molecule carrying information from one mammal to another (a sign, for instance, of estrus); a rat pup's ultrasonic cry, which gets the attention of the mother; a human baby's recognition of its mother's voice; one person's greeting to another, which may convey, in addition to the ritual gesture, much affect and attitude toward the recipient; a sigh from a patient on the couch giving volumes of information about what has just been said; and indeed any word, gesture, or symbol carrying information in any human culture.

Readers often have trouble conceiving of the sign—which carries associations with the nonmaterial and "purely cultural"—as a biological, materialist building block. In most minds a sign must "stand for something to someone." But at the basic, building-block level there is no "someone," (i.e., no interpreter in the usual sense). My own inquiries in this realm began with signs at the familiar level, at the level of language, where symbols carry information from one person to another. Once I became familiar with the "standing for" relationship, I began to wonder if we could see it functioning at subhuman levels, even sub-organism levels. In other words, my use of sign relations at the molecular level is a potentially controversial extension of the semiotic concept, though I think it a justifiable extension of Peirce's theory, in accord with Sebeok's conception (1986). In short, symbols of cultural origin do require an interpreter, but we may be able to envision subsymbolic entities—icons and indices—not requiring an interpreter. I will argue that "interpretation" is simply the result of the semiotic instance. For example, a unicellular organism may encounter a nutrient gradient and therefore direct its course upstream. Beyond that behavior there is no separate act of interpretation.

I will argue that a ladder up the evolutionary hierarchy is articulated by coding relationships, in which information is transferred from DNA to RNA to proteins and, by way of proteins, to structural elements and semiotic entities such as antibodies and transmitter molecules. In the brain the same principle allows brain elements—possibly neural networks—to stand for percepts, memories, images, and other mental phenomena. The same distinction that exists between mind and brain exists between levels all the way up from molecule to mind. The hoped-for end result is to remove the fuzziness from the concept of mind, and some of the theoretical mystery from the mind-brain connection. Although we may not yet know the mechanism by which semiosis works at all levels, we can expect someday to find it. In the meantime, mental processes are in the same conceptual world as all other biological processes, including the immune system, the bone-healing system, the neurotransmitter systems, the genetic system, and the workings of enzymes and recognition proteins. Psychology, orthopedics, pharmacology, genetics, immunology, and all the other life sciences dine at the same table, that of the sign. In the first half of this paper I develop this argument in more detail. In the second half I present a few of the implications of this model for a psychoanalytically oriented theory of mind.

The Origins of Life

In the primal soup of the planet's youth, so we think, life began. There have been numerous theories as to how this came about. One held by many today is that molecules of carbon, nitrogen, hydrogen, and oxygen, mixing in the sun-drenched pools of water, were on occasion brought close enough together to chemically bond. Another theory, more recent, offers a different scenario—namely, that the "soup" was the nearly freezing water trapped beneath the huge ice sheath that covered the earth in its early history. Into this water, from hydrothermal vents in the earth, hydrogen, methane, and ammonia bubbled up, reaching concentrations adequate for the formation of larger organic molecules. Yet another theory is based on evidence that some organic-molecule precursors came with the debris raining on the earth from outer space. In all of the theories, at least those not positing divine intervention, there is a spontaneous or extraterrestrial generation of small organic molecules. Some of these molecules combined and grew to a size where they could serve as catalysts for other molecular events. In catalysis, two molecules attach themselves to the catalyst molecule in such a way that they are forced into proximity and can combine into a larger molecule. Would this large molecule then constitute life? Not really, since life requires more than a single organic molecule. Living beings must by definition be able to organize molecules so as to transform and use energy, and to reproduce themselves.

Reproduction and Evolution

Reproduction, then, is a necessary part of the life process. Evolution is secondary, and depends on there being a rapid reproductive cycle. The only way change leading to more advanced organisms can occur is for there to be chances for error and variation in the process of reproduction.

Once the complex molecule mentioned above was built, it had only two possible futures: it might simply deteriorate, or it might first reproduce itself. Certain molecules apparently did self-catalyze copies of themselves. Some precursors to the DNA molecule eventually developed in nature, and evolution could begin. It is possible that RNA played this role for millions of years before DNA (Maynard Smith and Szathmary 1995). Mutation occurs when reproduction is in process and a copying error is made. When that error—randomly caused by the destructive outside influence of a punishing environment or cosmic radiation—happens to make a slight adaptive improvement, the new organism may thrive.

Thus, if evolution is to occur, the growth of life beyond the first molecular stage, reproduction is necessary. Since a complex organism cannot be built in one step, a long sequence of reproductions must occur for the infinitesimal steps, the adaptive variants, to add up. That cumulative process has led to the amazing variety and complexity in the biosphere as we know it today. (For a rich discussion of the biology of genetic processes, see Pollack 1994; for a more complex discussion of the formation of the first molecules from auto-catalytic sets, see Kauffman 1993.) These authors present a cogent account of the requirement for the nucleic acids (RNA or DNA) and the proteins to engage in a dialogue of reproduction:

"The most fundamental distinction in biology is between nucleic acids, with their role as carriers of information, and proteins, which generate the phenotype. In existing organisms, nucleic acids and proteins mutually presume one another. The former, owing to their template activity, store the heritable information: the latter, by enzymatic activity, read and express this information. It seems that neither can function without the other."

(p. 61)

One possibility, in the earliest times, is that RNA functioned both as information carrier and as enzyme. Interestingly, once a process is established that includes reproduction and the adaptive use of error, that process is built in and remains with us. The process that got us here requires death; once the new organism is reproduced, the old one is no longer necessary. Indeed, it is adaptive in that it gives up its molecules to make new organisms. In other words, a secondary adaptive function of individual death is that it allows the recycling of molecules. Even more important, it makes room for new, more adaptive organisms.

As I hope to show later, the relationship between levels in the evolutionary succession is both causal and semiotic. Once the system of one thing standing for another emerged as molecules made copies of themselves, the potential for evolution, indeed its inevitability, also emerged.

The Law of Effect

The law underlying the process of evolution is called the Law of Effect (see Dennett, 1978, pp. 71–89). This is so simple and basic a law that it is tautological: If something works it can exist; if not, it won't. If it exists, therefore, it must have worked. The law is manifested not only in the process of evolution, but also in most forms of learning, from operant conditioning, to skiing techniques, to cultural entities such as economic systems and architectural and artistic styles. A corollary to the Law of Effect, which makes it a part of the evolutionary process, is the "selectionist" principle described by Edelman (1992) among others. In order to find if something "works" and therefore can survive, it must be "tried." An instance of the adaptation must exist before it can be selected for. Thus, a random mutation occurs and leads to a phenotype change; this, if it promotes survival, will then be selected for.

Semiotics

At some point in the beginning of the life process there came a time when molecules could make copies of themselves. These were the earliest versions of RNA or DNA molecules. When a molecule copies itself, it transmits its patterned structure to another molecule. That pattern is its information content, existing in the form of electrochemical properties and geometrical shapes that describe the molecule and function as a code. The gene codon links with a certain amino acid because of its physical structure. Similarly, the antibody recognizes the antigen by physical attributes, in a key-lock fitting. The same is true of recognition proteins in one-celled animals, of neurotransmitters at their receptor sites, and of enzymes with the molecules they cause to interact. It is by means of information from the genes that the most complex organisms are built; with the higher animals, the same principle of information transfer leads to quantum jumps in complexity.

The use of structures as codes brings us to consider the sign, and the development of the theories of semiotics. Semiotics has a surprisingly long pedigree, with certain concepts of current value originating in the Middle Ages. In fact, semiotic notions have formed a kind of parallel philosophy, often considered heretical, in opposition to the establishment thought of Aquinas, Descartes, and Kant. John Deely (1986) has provided an account of the development of semiotic thinking in the early Middle Ages. The definition of sign, which persists, comes from Augustine's De Doctrina Christiana: "A sign is something which, on being perceived, brings something other than itself into awareness" (Deely 1986, p. 12). The most complete development of the idea came in the seventeenth century, with the Portuguese scholar John Poinsot (1632). The essence of this way of thinking is that signs may be objects—rocks, flags, words, or even ideas—but they are signs only insofar as they signify something else. Thus, an important distinction from mainstream philosophy was this: according to more familiar figures, (e.g., Locke and Descartes), the mind directly apprehends ideas (for Descartes, in the suprapineal gland-mind. Poinsot and others, however, believed that the mind apprehends not ideas but entities, which signify ideas. In current jargon, the brain event, say the firing of certain cells, brings to mind a tree or a concept; one has no direct awareness of the brain event.

One thing we must note is that information is coeval with reproduction. Informational structures initially developed to no other effect than to reproduce themselves. In other words, when a molecule was randomly assembled and later disintegrated, no semiotic system evolved, as there was no receiver of the information. *However, when a molecule with the right shape came to catalyze the formation of another molecule, we would have had a kind of semiotic system, in that its shape uniquely determined the product.* But if the new molecule did nothing and went nowhere, this sign did not enter the evolutionary stream.

Information Begins with Semiosis

I have been using the term "information" without defining it. Information is a quantitative term that refers to the carrying capacity of semiotic systems. At the most basic theoretical level, as described by Claude Shannon (1949), information is structure; in terms of the Second Law of Thermodynamics, it can be viewed as "negative entropy." Information is the production of order out of disorder, certainty out of possibility.

Thus, like physical structures, informational structures reduce randomness. The house is less random, more improbable, than the pile of lumber;

similarly, the gene is more structured than a soup of nucleic acids, a sentence more structured than a bunch of letters. Strictly speaking, information is not the structure itself; information is a measure of the reduction of improbability in any given message. A potential information system has more than one possible configuration: for example, a binary system can be on or off; an alphabet, having many more elements, has many more configurations.

The amount of information a system can carry with each alternative configuration depends on the total number of possible configurations in the system. Each time a configuration is displayed, it rules out all the other possible configurations; in information jargon, it reduces improbability. For example, more information results from the throw of a twelve-sided die than from the throw of a six-sided one; in the former toss, eleven possibilities are ruled out, while in the latter only five are eliminated. Another way of saying this is that in the twelve-sided die there are more possibilities, so that the probability of each one's occurrence is smaller; the throw of the die then reduces a greater amount of uncertainty. Information is the property of a system, not of a given message. Information is not to be equated with meaning, because it does not tell you what the message means, but only how expectable that particular configuration of elements in the system is.

Information theory deals with two major issues. The first is the amount of information that can be carried by a given system, such as a die, an alphabet, a language, or a genetic code. The second is the maintenance of a message structure against the pull of entropy. During World War II Shannon was concerned with the transmission of information (e.g., radio messages), and with the fact that message structures tend to degrade (e.g., because of static electricity, obstructions, and distance), just as any structure will if not maintained. Genes are maintained by the strict rules of replication and cellular methods for gene repair, as well as by the nonsurvival of mutants. Linguistic messages are maintained by many forms of redundancy, so that in human speech, for instance, we can usually understand the message, even when we hear only half the words spoken. Even so, illustrating the fragility of language as an information carrier, in the game of "Telephone," in which a message is whispered from one to another in a circle of people, it is remarkable how rapidly the message alters to the point of being unrecognizable.

The nucleic acid system is an admirable information/semiotic system. It contains four different nucleotides, which may be strung in an infinite number of strings, providing a genetic language with an efficiency paralleling that of human language. The four nucleotides are adenine, guanine, thymine, and cytosine. (RNA works the same way, using the same nucleotides, except that for RNA another nucleotide, uridine, is used instead of thymine). When the molecule makes copies, a complementarity rule ensures faithful reproduction. Adenine attaches to thymine, and guanine to cytosine. A DNA molecule in copying itself produces a complement, not a copy; if the complement copies again, that complement will be identical to the original molecule. Similarly, when RNA molecules are constructed, nucleotides are lined up on the DNA molecule in the same complementary fashion.

The way this information is used to build a protein is as follows. Although RNA is a long chain of nucleotides, the information unit is the codon, which is a triplet of nucleotides; every three nucleotides in the long chain is an informational unit, a "word" in the genetic language. There are sixty-four ways to combine four nucleotides in a series of three. Each of these ways encodes an amino acid. The protein chain is lined up as the amino acids attach to the RNA triplets and then become attached in the chain.

Pollack (1994) credits Erwin Schrödinger with a predictive notion, formulated in 1944, about the basic molecule of life, the idea of an aperiodic crystal. Schrödinger (1944) thought that when such a basic molecule was discovered it "would be both very stable and contain much information, despite the contrary quality of these two attributes.... The paradox was this: the gene had to have crystalline stability but it could not take the form of a crystal's purely periodic, informationally barren repeat. DNA—the base-paired double helix—completely removes the sting of the paradox from Schrödinger's prediction. DNA is, precisely, an aperiodic crystal" (Pollack 1994, p. 28). Watson and Crick worked out the DNA structure in the early 1950s, dramatically verifying Schrödinger's prediction.

Dualism Versus Monism

The system I am describing has a dualistic aspect. My approach to the monism-dualism discussion is somewhat different from the usual arguments. Churchland (1986) provides an excellent review of the arguments on both sides. Churchland spells out the arguments for and against various kinds of dualism. Her sympathies lie with eliminative materialism, a reductionistic, monistic view that there is but one kind of substance. She persuasively resolves many of the issues that divide her view from both substance dualism and property dualism. Cartesian substance dualism posits a physical substance interacting mysteriously with a mental universe of non-matter. That view has few adherents among philosophers these days. More accepted is the notion of property dualism, according to which there is no way to finally reduce the difference between subjective feelings, such as the sense of self derived from introspection, and the "objective" view of a person from the external point of view of a hypothetical observer. Even if we correlate a person's statement, "I am me and I am feeling happy," with a particular localization on an fMRI readout, we will never capture the subjective experience expressed. Churchland tries to resolve the problem by saying the brain event and the mental event are the same event, period. In the same way, light is the same as electromagnetic radiation; it is not caused by radiation, it is radiation. In general, I agree with her arguments against substance and property dualism and would accept that their differences are derived from the way one poses the arguments. But I would like to try out the notion that a semiotic model is useful in explaining a multilevel dualism in living processes.

In the semiotic model the essential dividing line is not at the brain-mind level of functioning. Instead, there are many dividing lines, in what might be called a process dualism, a possible variant of property dualism. When we focus our attention on sign systems rather than mental function alone, we see that the first dualistic boundary is at the point where life begins. As described above, life begins with the semiotic principle, which requires the presence of systems in which signs function. Thus, a different process comes into being.

The first step in this process must go something like this: a molecule of a certain size develops, containing carbon, hydrogen, oxygen, and possibly nitrogen. Certain molecules of this sort, with or without the aid of other catalytic molecules, can serve as a template to align complementary molecules, essentially making copies of themselves. At that instant those processes that we call life—reproduction, semiosis, information, and evolution—have their simultaneous beginning. In the process, oxygen is consumed, not only as a structural atom but also as a source of energy, the energy that binds the atoms in the new molecule from the free state to a structure-bound state. That process is one in which a previously random distribution of atoms becomes constrained into a structure. This is the conveyance of information, and it follows the mode of information processing, which, in binding the random atoms, reduces probability to the structures of the molecules. At the same moment, a system begins to exist—that is, the system of the molecule and its complementary molecule. It includes 1) the template molecule; 2) the substrate; and 3) the complement molecule. The complement is formed by information from the template in a process that goes up the entropic gradient: it reduces entropy and increases information. In the system the complement is a sign of the template; it is contingent upon it and takes its information from it. At this point a system has been born—a simple one, but one that is the basis of all life.

The crucial aspect of the semiotic model is that everything that makes a sign a sign comes from outside the sign. Thus, something becomes a sign only because of the system in which it participates. This principle is often forgotten, a lapse that leads to the unnecessary attribution of an uncanny or nonmaterial quality to signs.

This first prototype is the model for the DNA molecule, which carries the code for all currently living organisms. It functions as I have just described, by arranging for a complementary molecule to line up in parallel to it and carry its information. In cell fission and replication, that complementary molecule is another DNA. But during the normal day-to-day processes of the somatic cells of an organism, the process is one of spinning off messenger RNA molecules that carry information in their structures, outside the nucleus into the cytoplasm, where they impart their information in the building of proteins through the assembly of chains of amino acids. Here we have a mediated sign system in which the RNA is the carrier of information from the DNA to the protein. The system, then, is one that includes the DNA as the transmitter, and information is conveyed to the RNA by virtue of a set of rules. In a subsequent step, another semiotic event occurs when the RNA, using another set of rules, conveys its information to a protein molecule. This occurs in an endless chain. The protein then carries information. Its structure allows it to provide the information (expressed in its shape and properties) or to act as either a structural element or as an enzyme or other biologically functioning entity. As we see, structure and information are almost identical here. For it is the structure that is the information; the structure provides the unique "lock" that other molecules fit into like "keys" when they enter into biochemical processes.

This system is key to there being a semiotic process at all. It helps provide an answer to the question, "Why do we need anything beyond simple causality? The lugs in a key-lock system work by pushing or pulling, just like billiard balls; so what's so special?" As I have mentioned, it is the system in which it exists that makes something a sign. The point is that this kind of system does not exist in the prevital universe. One could counterargue, "But what about the laws of nature? The planets go around the sun in a preordained path, guided by the well-known physical forces; why isn't that the same kind of system?" There are two answers to that. One is that the semiotic system itself operates according to the basic physical laws, but the actual structures of the living systems were set up long after the universe was formed in accordance with those laws. Second, these system laws govern a particular act of structuring that is reproducible. In contrast to living organisms, inanimate nature has no systems for reproducing structures. Hence it is a radical departure in the physical universe when such systems begin; it is so radical that it initiates the simultaneous emergence of several major processes.

In the argument presented here, the brain-mind level, where we are used to thinking in terms of dualism, is simply a derivative of the basic dualism that appears when signs and life begin. At every level in the biological hierarchy, from molecule to mind, the same semiotic relationship obtains. In the brain we conceive of storage events, possibly neural circuits or "nets" that stand for percepts. There may in addition be events that stand for integrations of percepts into object representations, and in human beings yet other circuits that stand for object representations, abstract concepts, and cultural entities. Then there are the many output phenomena of the brain: thoughts, feelings, symbols, language, art, buildings, techniques, crafts, etc. Each of these represents a sign system in which signs stand for the person in a way to be communicated to the world.

Peirce's Trichotomy of Signs

My earlier semiotic model, based on Poinsot and Saussure, says simply that a sign is something that stands for something else. In the work of the American philosopher Charles Sanders Peirce, a more complex model of semiosis is to be found, one that proves quite useful in a hierarchical understanding of psychology. Peirce's model is often referred to as a "triadic" system, because it contains several trichotomies. In an overarching trichotomy, he recognizes not only the signifier and signified of Saussure, but in addition, and this is crucial, a system in which these function, a set of rules that he calls a "Third." In another trichotomy, Peirce saw that there are three distinct kinds of signs, or different ways in which one thing can stand for another. This distinction is extremely useful in elucidating the function of language and other forms of communication. Peirce elaborated his system to include ten (and ultimately sixty-four) different kinds of signs, but the distinctions he makes become so fine and complex as not to be useful for the present endeavor. The three basic types, based on the different relations signs can have to their objects, are icon, index, and symbol.

An icon stands for its object by virtue of being similar to it. An icon can be a diagram, a map, or a more fully representational picture. An index stands for its object by contiguity, by a physical, spatial, or temporal connection to the object, or even by a causal connection to it. Examples are a pointing gesture, an arrow, or a noise by which I locate the noisemaker. There are two basic things an organism needs to know about an object in itself as object—what it is and where it is in space and time. Icons tend to be about "what"; indices about "where" and "when." We also need to know the object's affective valence to the self—we might say the "why." As I will discuss later on, this third major characteristic is necessarily subjective, and is related to the sense of self. Affects make use of both indices and icons.

Then there is the symbol. This represents its object by social convention. The other two signs can be used in informational exchanges by unicellular creatures, but symbols require a human social community. Symbols include words, tokens, flags, and almost all the items in a culture. A symbol is more complex than the other two sign types; Icons and indices can represent their objects in a one-to-one relationship. A symbol has varying degrees of relationship with its referent, but its most important relationship is with all the other symbols in the language, or in the culture. In other words, the symbol "bottle" (the word) can refer to an object in the world that we call its referent, an object Webster defines as "a rigid or semi-rigid container typically made of glass, having a comparatively narrow neck or mouth and usually no handle." But the symbol's relation to the palpable object is in a sense trivial, in comparison to its relation to all those words used in the previous sentence to make the object's composition and function clear.

It must be remembered that there are few, if any signs of a pure type. An index often has iconic properties of similarity. A birdcall, as an index, says, "I am over here." But it is the iconic "shape" or temporal pattern of the call, the complement to the other bird's receiver, by which it is recognized and stimulates a response. An icon may often have indexical properties. A road sign with a cartoon drawing of a gasoline pump is an icon, but its presence before a highway exit indicates "You can get fuel here at this exit." At the level of symbols things become much more complex. A symbol may have iconic and/or indexical properties. On a dashboard, a cartoon of an oilcan may flash on, serving as an icon, but also functioning as an index calling attention to it, and thereby referring to a symbolic phrase meaning "low oil pressure." In another example, the word "I" is a symbol, but also necessarily an index of the speaker; the English word, being a single letter, is also an icon for the "individual." A word may have onomatopoeic (iconic) aspects in its sounding, as with the name of Jonathan Swift's horse-people, the Houyhnhnms.

Parenthetically, it must be said that there is an irony in the fact that the discipline of semiotics, which deals with the very basics of communication, has some of the most ambiguous jargon to be found anywhere. For present purposes though, we can say that in most usages, "icon" implies similarity; we might say an icon is a sign constrained by the physical identifying properties of the object, its properties, which tell us what the object is. "Index" implies some kind of directive pointing function or causal connection; it is a sign constrained by the location, the where of the object, or the relationship between objects. "Symbol" is used here, in Peirce's sense, as a specialized term implying arbitrary, culturally determined reference, and is therefore not constrained by the nature or location of the object. In other usages, however, "symbol" may refer to all forms of sign.

If we begin at the molecular level and move upward, we see that we are always dealing with information exchange. The mode of neurotransmitters is the use of complementary electrochemical-spatial properties—a kind of physical shape—which is an iconic mode. When these iconic transfers have been made, and an autonomic or affective response has been engendered, this response functions as both an iconic and an indexical sign to the person, who feels excited, depressed, angry, etc. Some widely distributed neurotransmitters such as dopamine, norepinephrine, and serotonin are thought to produce physiological aspects of basic states of emotion. The process involves establishing an autonomic set, a complex of bodily and emotional feelings. These feelings come packaged with signs of their presence for communication to others; each emotional state has a facial and body pattern that acts as a form of mimetic communication.[2]

What, Where, And Why in The Brain

Let us consider the "what, where, and why," which we have discussed from a semiotic point of view, in terms of basic brain anatomy, taking the visual system as an example. Reflected light conveys color, shape, and other visual phenomena to the retina, which transfers data via the lateral geniculate ganglion of the thalamus to the occipital, or primary visual, cortex. It is thought that the primary sense data are perceived separately, by cells designated to pick up simple sensory stimuli. The secondary visual cortex assembles the data into objects. This assembly is accomplished in two ways. One is the putting together of information to recognize what (or who) an object is.

This secondary cortex is found in the temporal lobes. Another assembly locates the object in space and possibly time. This occurs in the parietal lobes. The object is also viewed in its affective valence, as good, bad, or otherwise, for the welfare of the self. Contributions to this come from the limbic system. LeDoux (1996) has described two emotion systems: one, "quick and dirty," that takes a loose iconic approach—anything that looks at all like a snake leads to reflex avoidance—and uses a short circuit through the thalamus and amygdala; the other allows for more considered value decisions, made at slower speed and using the cortex. Higher-level cogitations about the object, such as how to use it, what its significance is, how it relates to the self, what its associations are, are handled in the prefrontal cortical areas. At the same time, language can be brought to bear on it, and it can be handled within the symbolic order.

These gross, and grossly oversimplified, divisions of brain anatomy suggest that what, where, and why are natural kinds, and that the different requirements for answering each question are fulfilled in different brain regions. It is now known that the regions are not so clear-cut, and that almost any brain function has distributed aspects, but it still seems to be that these semiotic aspects are handled by different systems.

In semiotic terms we can say that in each major cortical area there are neural-nets or cell assemblies that are signs in the sense used here. The sign in the temporal lobe will code for the shape and other essentials to recognize the object; this representation we would call primarily iconic. The parietal version may take some of the same sense data, but will use them to represent the spatial relationships of objects with respect to the self. This picture of the field will be iconic, in that it is like a diagram of the viewed world, but it has an indexical quality, in that its purpose is to indicate where things are. In fact, its status as icon or index depends on the location of the self vis-à-vis the scene. If the self is observing the scene from without, the scene is displayed as an icon. If, however, the self is a participant, it is embedded in the scene and will use indexicals to locate other entities in the scene. In fact, fMRI studies show that the cells that come into play when preparing the muscles and limbs to reach for an object are mostly in the parietal area. The distinction may also be made in describing dreams: in one dream the dreamer is completely participant (relationships are indexical), while in another the dream scene may be viewed from outside or above (iconic). To fill out this view of memory a little further, the hippocampal region seems to be the seat of episodic memory, the autobiographical memory for events. These must include data from both temporal-lobe "what" information and parietal-lobe "where" data. The current view is that the hippocampus labels the what and where with a "when," a "time and date stamp" necessary for there to be an organized event memory.

The limbic version signifies affective valence. It has generalized effects on the body as a whole. For the one-celled creature the precursors to affect are the simple detectors for pH, sugar, or light, directly connected to the motor system, that signal the organism to move toward a good environment or away from a bad one. As we go up the evolutionary ladder, we get more differentiated affects that represent many other affective characteristics (e.g., anger, sadness, joy). These are represented by physiological changes in the body, including changes in body posture and facial expression, that communicate the affect to others, as well as, via feedback loops, to the self.

The Physical Nature of Signs

One factor to keep in mind is that the nature of each kind of sign determines the kinds of information it can convey (Olds, 1992). For instance, a letter "H" could be made of brass; it could then be part of a brass nameplate; if heavy enough, it could be used as a weapon; or, if there was a lock that it fit, it could be used as a key. The same letter composed of lines of sand on a table could not have these uses. A more telling example is the nature of spoken verbal signs, as opposed to sign language (Sacks, 1989). Both are symbolic, and both are digitalized, giving them great flexibility and informational efficiency. But they have different physical properties, and these may have influenced which mode of utterance won the evolutionary race to be the human mode of natural speech. Sign language is very effective and practical in daylight, and has the virtue of being silent and therefore not indexically alerting to predators. It may also work over longer distances than audible speech, or in a windstorm. Hence the use of flashing light and semaphore systems between ships at sea. Spoken language, however, has the advantage that it does not require line-of-sight and can therefore go around corners; it is particularly useful in the dark. Possibly most important is that the oral/aural mode leaves the hands and eyes free to do other things.

Forms of nonverbal communication other than sign language demonstrate further that different modes have different properties. The predominant forms of affect communication are the prosodic and gestural modes. We convey how we feel by tone of voice, facial expression, and bodily posture.

The distinct nature of the three semiotic modes forces differences as well. An icon, particularly a neurologically instantiated one, is constrained by the nature of its referent; storage is in the form of a prototype, built from multiple instances. With categories—say "caretaker," "mother," or "authority figure"—the iconic representation emerges from experience. An experience quite distant from the prototype—e.g., a person who has learned that authority implies violence and constant criticism encounters a benign authority figure—will not immediately alter the prototype. Instead, the prototype will "assimilate" the newcomer and render it as a negative transference object. However, repeated instances of the new paradigm may eventually accumulate to change the prototype—an important aspect of analytic therapies.

In contrast, because of its nonessential connection to its objects, the symbolic order provides for greater flexibility. A verbal-symbolic representation of the prototype "authority figure" can be changed instantly, simply by adding the word not: "Oh, I see, authority figures are not all mean and critical." However, as we know all too well, that bit of insight will not immediately change the transferential behavior in relation to the iconic representation. The noncongruence of these two kinds of signs—icon and symbol—is the bread and butter of psychoanalysis. A major virtue of the symbolic is that it is so flexible, so freely used by the imagination for counterfactual simulations and trial actions. This process may produce insight, without change in the indexical and iconic orders. But in the verbal, analytically oriented therapies it can lead the way toward change at these other levels.

How this works—how verbal-symbolic insight leads to permanent change in the entire person—is still not clear and will be a major aspect of future research (see Olds in press). One important factor may be the notion of trial action. For instance, someone might have a maxim of life, or theory of behavior, such as the dictum "If I have any success, I will be severely punished." The person may go through life without challenging this dictum, which will be enacted unconsciously, and feel safe in the assurance that the theory is validated: success has assiduously been avoided, and—sure enough—punishment of the sort unconsciously feared has never occurred. Without therapy, the person may never even think of challenging the theory. The evolutionary principle is that if it isn't tried, we'll never know if it works—a corollary to the Law of Effect. Similarly with the neurotic's theories of life. The trial actions afforded by language and the capacity to imagine hypothetical alternatives allows us not only to entertain these alternatives but to consider their possible results. Herein lies the utility of Winnicott's notion of play as applied to analysis. New alternatives can be tried, and the results, when contrary to expectation, may lead to change at the iconic and indexical levels. Thus, the verbal can lead the way to change, though it does not usually produce it instantaneously.

Recapitulation So Far

I have presented a semiotic model that I hope will be useful in thinking about some of the basic concepts in biology and psychology. The most important points I think are as follows:

1. The sign can be seen as a basic unit in biology and psychology, parallel to the inorganic molecule in chemistry and the atom in physics. Basic does not mean irreducible. Each of these basic units has constituent parts; molecules, organic or inorganic, are constituted of atoms and atoms consist of subatomic particles.

2. In nonlinguistic sign systems the units, be they molecules, neural networks, or mimetic signs, are made up of elements, particular combinations of which make up particular signs. With language, the most recently evolved semiotic system, we have a "double articulation" in which units of one level become the building blocks of the next; phonemes are combined into words, and words into sentences.

3. The semiotic approach allows us to use a single concept—that of the sign—to discuss DNA, proteins, neurotransmitters, medications, thoughts, words, and concepts.

4. The model is substance monistic (it posits but one kind of matter) but process dualistic (semiosis involves a process not found in inorganic nature).

5. Basic to life are semiosis and evolution. Once molecules can make copies of themselves, evolution—via variation and selection—become possible and inevitable.

6. C. S. Peirce's semiotic model allows us to relate different kinds of signs to important natural kinds: the what (the icon represents the object by being similar to it) and the where (the index represents the object by denoting its location and relationships). We can extend the theory to include the autonomic and mimetic sign system, which denotes the affective valence of a percept. The symbol, the basis of language and cultural artifact, represents by convention and has no intrinsic, necessary relation to the object. Convention produces essential connections to an object, or class of objects, and to the other symbols in the language.

7. We live in a hybrid culture, what Peirce calls a "sea of signs." Every sign we use has all three aspects—iconic, indexical, and symbolic—but in each case we may discern a "primary" function (e.g., pointing as index), while the other two functions are present but secondary.

The Semiotic Model's Relation to Psychoanalytic Theory

If we accept this semiotic model of life processes, we can use it to examine some of the higher, more complex processes with which we are familiar. I will take a brief look at several phenomena of interest to psychoanalysts in terms of the model and indicate potential avenues for further exploration. I will discuss transference, free association, linguistics and multiple-code systems, hemisphere specialization, enactment, and development psychology.

Transference

The analytic relationship is shaped by the transference, the perceived resemblance of the analyst to an early figure. This would seem to be iconic. The standing-for, in connectionist terms, is a partial similarity that is enlarged to make a match (Palombo, 1992). That match, having been made, has positive and negative aspects. In therapy one may make use of the positive aspects to develop a therapeutic alliance. But another goal of therapy—particularly analysis, where it is a long-term goal—is to un make the match, to render clear the differences; becoming aware of these differences in turn renders the patient's interpersonal relations more reality-based and less shaped by transference. The analyst helps the patient to this awareness by imposing the symbolic on the system. With words—clarifications, interpretations, enactments—the analyst helps the patient make distinctions. Drawing attention to apparent similarities allows the patient to become aware of the differences. To see that two things are similar is part of pattern recognition, but this may occur in the absence of pattern discrimination. Transference is akin to the lack of discrimination shown when people are less able to individualize members of another race than they are members of their own; both are instances of a failure to discriminate within a pattern recognition. In the transference mode, all authority figures are alike, all maternal figures are alike, etc. In analysis we interpret current feelings in terms of reactions to past figures. We also enact a role ultimately inconsistent with the transference icon.

Free Association

To encourage the development of underlying mental patterns in psychoanalysis, we try to allow the analysand to follow trains of thought with minimal constraints from the requirements of practical reality. In theory, the discourse will be more guided by internal goals and directions, thereby allowing the emergence of themes based on unconscious processes. One way in which associations are linked is via tropes of language, particularly metaphor and metonymy, which Lacan described as the mainstays of the language of the unconscious. Here Peirce and Lacan converge: iconicity and metaphor both represent by similarity, index and metonymy by contiguity and physical, causal connection. Another major relationship between Peirce and Lacan is in the trichotomy of modes. Muller (1996) has noted that Lacan's is yet another "triadic" system and has pointed to the similarities between Peirce's icon, index, and symbol and Lacan's real, imaginary, and symbolic.

Deacon (1997) points out that an icon, or a similarity, may result from a failure to distinguish. Recognizing difference may be more difficult than recognizing similarity. For instance, a young child in saying "doggie" may refer to the entire animal kingdom; only with time and experience are differentiations made. Similarly, unfamiliar objects and members of another race may be iconized and less differentiated. This may be particularly relevant to transference, because some transference paradigms are set up in children who have not learned many discriminations, and a few icons are overinclusive. Failures to differentiate are often more prevalent at times of stress and altered states of consciousness.

Multiple-Code and Linguistics Models

The idea that information comes in a variety of forms with essentially different vehicles is not unique to semiotics. In general linguistics the notions of a
different relationship between symbol and referent go back at least to Saussure. More recently, psychoanalytic theorists have focused on these vehicles.
Shapiro (1991; Makari & Shapiro, 1993) has differentiated the syntagmatic
(which approximates the symbolic) from the paralinguistic—prosodic elements of tone of voice and facial expression (possibly something like the
iconic) and both of these from the kinetic—aspects of speech and expression
involving the motor elements and rhythms of communication (thus showing
aspects of the indexical). These vehicles form a unique combination in any
patient, and provide a multitrack source of information in the analytic
process.

Another approach, Bucci's "multiple-code" system (1997), has elements
similar to those of the semiotic approach, particularly where this system
works at the top of the semiotic hierarchy and explicates the psychological
level. For Bucci, too, the human communication and information-processing
system is divided into three modes: the subsymbolic, the nonverbal symbolic,
and the verbal symbolic. In this model, subsymbolic representations are built
up in a connectionist mode—a prototype built from repeated instances—
such as I have described for the iconic sign mode. Bucci's subsymbolic mode
probably includes both the iconic and the indexical, and she divides the
symbolic into the verbal and the nonverbal. She and her colleagues, using
this tripartite model in analyzing psychoanalytic transcripts, have conducted
considerable research in this promising and potentially very important area.

These models have a similar purpose—namely, to provide clarification of
different semiotic levels—and it is possible that a juxtaposition of the models
will be heuristically valuable.

Hemisphere Specialization

What we have been saying about the different kinds of signs may be useful in
thinking about hemisphere specialization. Evidence has been accumulating
regarding the different kinds of information handled by the two hemispheres.
The left hemisphere has evolved to specialize in language, the primary symbolic form of human semiotics. This is most likely the most evolutionarily
advanced function. The right hemisphere handles many kinds of nonsymbolic signs, spatial images, gestalts, and affectively toned items. Closer to the
brain function of other primates, it can communicate exquisitely, but not
usually with language (Joseph, 1982; Levin, 1991). The evolutionary changes
that brought the left hemisphere into the symbolic order led to a process by
which icons and indices could become symbols. Language evolved using
sound forms developing into verbal symbols and syntactic structures. This

required a kind of linear processing, unlike much right hemisphere activity, but much like motor behavior, which occurs in one-dimensional trains of activity. Speech, itself a motor activity, must occur in a linear fashion. One cannot speak two sentences at once, any more than one can walk in two directions or at two different speeds at once. Before speech were gesture and mimetic communication; these too must be linear, like all motor activities.

This is an important point illuminated by Donald (1991). In his view, the high-level motor process and praxis harnessed by early hominids in the use of tools required a new level of experience-derived skills, or procedural memories. These skills, perfected using the motor (left) hemisphere, allowed for complex learned behaviors on quite a different plane than the more hardwired behaviors, in other species, of courtship, nest building, or food gathering. The ability to learn complex procedures, along with the expanded voice apparatus of later hominids, provided the background for learning the elaborate, fine-tuned sequencing of mimetic and spoken language.

The ability of the right hemisphere to represent and integrate internal objects and object relations, particularly in nonverbal media, has been receiving increased attention (Pally, 1998, forthcoming; Schore, 1997; Watt, 1990). The right brain is seen to be harboring a rich set of representations of objects, relationships, and affective connections. Joseph (1982) has proposed that the right hemisphere matures earlier than the left, and in the process establishes stronger connections with the limbic affect systems. The left brain connects to the motor system and consequently, in humans, to the speech system. Watt (1990) describes the phenomenon of internalization as nonverbal representations with affective significance, predominantly right hemisphere oriented. In his view, an important effect of psychoanalysis is the translation of the experience of the nonverbal internal objects into language. With the semiotic model we can push this idea further. The kinds of representations that are nonverbal are iconic and indexical signs.

The complex signs standing for internal objects are to some extent constrained by the objects. In other words, they represent some of the qualities of the objects, in that they are similar in visual imagery and affect tone to the originals. Indeed, if we use the connectionist idea of prototype formation, we can see the internal object as a prototype resulting from a summation of many experiences. An example may be Stern's point (1985) that an infant, shown a number of faces, will show evidence of strongest "recognition" of a mathematical average of the images, an image it has never seen before. Thus, we have a kind of prototype icon built up from many experiences of certain objects.

The psychoanalyst encounters a patient who has an object icon, produced by thousands of experiences of the object, and such an icon is naturally rather resistant to change. Verbal insight may help in making clear some things about the experience behind the icon. But it is increasingly apparent that one result of analysis is the change in the prototype itself. Here we invoke the possibility of corrective emotional experience, in which the new behavior of the analyst must be repeated many times, and become part of the expectable environment, if it is to affect the model built up by earlier experience.

Enactment

A question must be raised regarding the semiotic nature of enactment. In recent psychoanalytic theory this has become an important concept, one with roots both in the psychoanalytic notion of repetition compulsion and schema formation (Slap & Slap-Shelton, 1991) and in cognitive science and its elucidation of different types of memory. The concept of procedural memory refers to memory for processes such as motor activities like skiing or driving, and is contrasted with episodic and semantic memories involving the explicit conscious storage of experience and facts. Procedural memory (Clyman, 1991) underlies enactments of all kinds, including the acting out of repetitive schemas in the transference, schemas learned in childhood or in later traumatic situations.

What kind of a sign is an enactment? The answer is complex, but we can see that in some ways the behavior pattern of a transference enactment is iconic vis-à-vis the experiences leading to the particular kind of transference. The word pattern suggests an icon, in this case one that unfolds over time, and this pattern is constrained by the nature of the original experience. But there are also indexical aspects, especially in transferences infused by insecurity and separation anxiety. Thus, experiences involving intimacy, proximity, and distance will be highly charged, and will lead to repetitive patterns of response. There are also symbolic aspects; the analyst as authority figure may be represented in a dream by a policeman, the uniform being the socially derived symbol of authority. In analysis, repetitive behaviors in the transference, unconscious to the patient, become recognizable signs to the analyst.

In a larger sense, a person's behavior may be organized by encompassing "narrative structures." These have been discussed by, among others, Bruner (1990), Dahl (1988), and Luborsky and Crits-Cristoph (1988). These structures may represent the archetypal stories and myths that organize the fantasy life and behavior of a person's entire life. They have iconic, indexical, and symbolic aspects.

Developmental Psychology

There are two major streams in infant research that would seem to map onto the semiotic categories. One is the notion of attunement, brought to our attention by Stern (1985, 1989), the richly varied and constantly responsive activity of mother and infant in which each mirrors the other, in rhythm, sounds, and tactile stimuli. In Muller's words (1996), "In early infancy iconic relations are enacted. The mother's smiling gaze brings about its replica in the infant; the infant's smiling gaze, in turn, produces a mirroring response in the mother" (p. 59). This behavioral paradigm may be the ultimate in communicating "whatness"; through it the mother becomes known to the infant, and the infant becomes known to itself through that mirroring.

The other stream is that of attachment and its complex evolution (Bowlby 1988; Ainsworth and Bowlby 1991; Goldberg, Muir, & Kerr, 1995). Attachment signals would seem to be primarily indices; they indicate where the infant is, and they elicit proximity and caretaking responses in those nearby. In releasing behaviors, they are like mating or aggressive gestures—evolutionarily derived signals.

Primatologists who work with attachment theory have described an increasing complexity of attachment behaviors through the evolution of primates. The five behaviors—sucking, crying, clinging, following, and smiling—designated as attachment behaviors by Bowlby, Ainsworth, and others have important semiotic aspects. All have physical causal aspects in bringing the infant closer to the mother. At the same time, they have semiotic aspects; they act as signs that release instinctual behaviors in the caretaker. Chimpanzees and humans have all five of the behaviors described by Bowlby, Old World monkeys (such as the rhesus) have four (they do not smile), and the more primitive New World monkeys have three (their following behavior is nonspecific). Suomi (1995) writes that attachment behavior is a form of imprinting, an elaboration of a form of learning present in some birds and more primitive mammals. The evolution of the complexity of attachment behavior repertoires coincides with an increase in semiotic capacity in these evolving species.

Both of these paradigms begin very early, possibly within days of birth, and they precede the functioning at the symbolic level (Beebe & Lachmann, 1988). When the symbolic level is attained, late in the first year, it adds to and integrates with the other two. It is likely that the iconic and indexical feed the symbolic in crucial and profound ways as yet not fully understood. The work of Lakoff & Johnson (1980) suggests that these issues are the basis of the metaphors that form language—another fruitful area to explore.

One piece of research that suggests the usefulness of semiotic categories in understanding psychoanalytic process is that of Spence, Mayes, and Dahl (1994). They examine the well-known case of Mrs. C. (Teller & Dahl 1986) and try to correlate the occurrence of indexicals—pronouns referring to the two participants (I/you, you/me, etc.)—with the tendency of the analyst to intervene. They found a significant correlation between closely spaced indexicals—for example, the words you and me with few words in between them and any intervention, including an interpretation or any other verbal response. They understood this as the analyst unconsciously responding to the increasing use of the pronouns, which use suggests that the patient is talking about the analytic pair and their relationship; the analyst can be predicted to respond in some way. They see a mutual influence in the dyad, possibly a reexperiencing, of the mother-infant mutual interactiveness described by infant researchers. Not only that, but the apparent responsiveness of the analyst to closely spaced indexicals seems to increase toward the end of the analysis. They interpret this as an increasing attunement as the analysis progresses, with a positive feedback system established in which the patient, feeling understood, speaks more freely about the analytic relationship and the transference, and in which the analyst takes the cue and responds more effectively, which continues a benign cycle.

Summary And Conclusions

I have attempted here to present a model of mind based on sign systems. It draws together the systems of Saussure and Peirce to argue that the sign can be seen as the basic unit of living, as opposed to non-living, systems.

This model helps us relate some major mental phenomena of interest to psychologists and psychoanalysts. Neural networks carry information about things and persons, which are iconic. They may be carried by connectionist-like systems as prototypes derived from repeated experiences; as such they represent a set of experiences abstracted, and leading to transferential expectations of persons in the current world, including the analyst. Other networks, or associated systems of networks, carry indexical information regarding the relations between objects and between the self and objects. These too may result in transferences based on these relations and on behavioral associations with objects. Finally, symbols carry information via language and other cultural entities.

A central point of all this is that this model gives a unified framework in which to fit our clinical theories and research paradigms. The notion that everything a therapist does has semiotic implications at one level or another may help unify our sense of what we do. And as a basis for asking research questions, it should provide heuristic models as sources of questions about the effects of therapies at various levels. A practical implication of the classification of signs lies in the different levels of semiotic freedom. The index and icon, being closely "adherent" to their referents, are very slow to change. Analysts have found that the flexibility inherent in symbolism has provided an aid to changing behavior and personality patterns. Use of the symbolic to achieve distance and gain perspective on the subsymbolic provides a powerful source of freedom not available to subsymbolic organisms.

The philosophical value of this argument is that we have a satisfactory dualistic model of living process, in which the sign is the atomic entity. From the point of view of psychology and psychoanalysis, the model shows us a set of differing modes of representation that illuminates the ways the mind works at various levels and gives us some insight into the multilevel effects of psychotherapy and psychopharmacology. It also renders a continuous hierarchy within the living world, identifying some basic entities that function at all levels. Some of the same laws operate in semiosis at the molecular level as up the line to the mental and linguistic levels.

One possible use of semiotics in relation to psychoanalytic theory is that it helps us resolve certain antinomies within the theory, particularly between biological reductionism and hermeneutics. These apparently incompatible models in fact refer to the same organism, the human being, and they do so via a common underlying principle, the semiotic. Because of this we can see that all biological processes have a semiotic aspect, and so do all hermeneutic phenomena.

This brings us back to the questions at the beginning of the paper. How do we reconcile a biological and pharmacological view of mental function with the psychoanalytic? We have had the experience of a medication altering the most subtle of personality functions, as well as the experience of psychoanalysis modifying affective and cognitive pathology usually considered biological.

One way to look at this is to see the basic neurotransmitter systems as semiotic. The broadcast transmitters such as dopamine and serotonin are general information systems affecting activation levels in distributed areas of the brain. They are molecular signs in a vast hierarchy or community of neurons. This same community has inputs at different levels, all of which can lead to immediate behavioral responses, as well as long-term changes. The sign systems interact so that the pharmaceutical agent, the verbal intervention, the behavioral modeling, and the transference enactment all feed into an interactive system. This kind of thinking could help relieve the current malaise in psychiatry and reverse the impoverishment of training programs that omit any consideration of psychodynamics. This model provides a rationale for more fully rounded psychiatric education.

The semiotic approach may be particularly appropriate now because it parallels our growing awareness of the role of community; of the self as arising from the dyad; and of the importance of an intersubjective stance in understanding psychology. The connection, it might be said, is only analogical: as it takes two to develop a self, so it takes, two, the sender and the receiver, to have a sign. But there is more to it than that. The semiotic system of icons and indices requires two parties and a third, the system in which they function, just as the realm of the symbolic is created socially, in Peirce's terms, in a triad: sender, receiver, and the culture (the Third) in which they function. A symbol is nothing without a community. Indeed, there must be a community for there to be a symbol at all, and a *sign* of any kind enhances the community—from the mother-infant dyad to the whole social, symbolic world.

The semiotic model is particularly timely from a scientific point of view. In the world of cognitive science, researchers are being confronted with the need to explain higher levels of brain-mind function. In this realm traditional reductionism is at its worst in providing explanatory models. Psychoanalytic concepts are gaining respectability for their ability to embrace the necessary levels of complexity at the phenomenological and psychological levels. Semiotic paradigms too are finding a place; as I have argued, they can synergize with psychoanalytic concepts. It may not be too bold to predict that the underpinnings of the theory of mind that we will find most useful for a new psychoanalytic model will include, as conceptual contexts for our research, semiotic theories and the theories of complexity (non-linear dynamics, chaos theories, connectionist paradigms). It seems a pleasant irony that "the decade of the brain" has been so successful, and has brought cognitive science to such a concern with higher mental functions, that it may emerge as the "decade of the mind."

Notes

1 Originally published in the *Journal of the American Psychoanalytic Association* (2000), Vol. 48: 497–529.
2 Four works that explicate Peirce's model and apply it to evolution and human development in greater detail are Deacon (1997), Hoffmeyer (1997), Litowitz (1990), and Muller (1996).

References

Ainsworth, M. D. S. & Bowlby, J. (1991) *An ethological approach to personality development*. American Psychologist, 46: 333–341.
Beebe, B. & Lachmann, F. M. (1988) *The Contribution of Mother–Infant Mutual Influence to the Origins of Self- and Object Representations*. Psychoanalytic Psychology, 5: 305–337.
Bowlby, J. (1988) *A Secure Base: Parent-Child Attachment and Healthy Human Development*. New York: Basic Books.
Bruner, J. (1990) *Acts of Meaning*. Cambridge, MA: Harvard University Press.
Bucci, W. (1997) *Psychoanalysis and Cognitive Science: A Multiple Code Theory*. New York: Guilford Press.
Churchland, P. S. (1986) *Neurophilosophy: Toward a Unified Theory of the Mind/ Brain*. Cambridge, MA: MIT Press.
Clyman, R. B. (1991) The Procedural Organization of Emotions: A Contribution from Cognitive Science To The Psychoanalytic Theory Of Therapeutic Action. *Journal of the American Psychoanalytic Association*, 39: 349–382.
Dahl, H. (1988) Frames of mind. In *Psychoanalytic Research Strategies*, ed. H. Dahl, H. Kächele, & H. Thomä. New York: Springer-Verlag, pp. 51–66.
Deacon, T. (1997) *The Symbolic Species: The Co-evolution of Language and the Brain*. New York: W.W. Norton.
Deely, J. (1986) The coalescence of semiotic consciousness. In *Frontiers in Semiotics*, eds J. Deely, B. Williams, & F. E. Kruse. Bloomington, IN: Indiana University Press, pp. 5–34.

Dennett, D. (1978) *Brainstorms: Philosophical Essays on Mind and Psychology*. Cambridge, MA: MIT Press.

Dennett, D. (1991) *Consciousness Explained*. Boston, MA: Little, Brown.

Donald, M. (1991) *The Origins of the Modern Mind*. Cambridge: Harvard University Press.

Eco, U. (1984) *Semiotics and the Philosophy of Language*. Bloomington: Indiana University Press.

Edelman, G. (1992) *Bright Air, Brilliant Fire*. New York: Basic Books.

Edelson, M. (1975) *Language and Interpretation in Psychoanalysis*. New Haven: Yale University Press.

Goldberg, S., Muir, R., & Kerr, J., Eds (1995) *Attachment Theory: Social, Developmental, and Clinical Perspectives*. Hillsdale, NJ: Analytic Press.

Hoffmeyer, J. (1997) *Signs of Meaning in the Universe*. Bloomington: Indiana University Press.

Joseph, R. (1982) The neuropsychology of development: Hemispheric laterality, limbic language, and the origin of thought. *Journal of Clinical Psychology*, 38 (suppl.): 4–33.

Kauffman, S. (1993) *The Origins of Order: Self-organization and Selection in Evolution*. Oxford: Oxford University Press.

Lakoff, G. & Johnson, M. (1980) *Metaphors We Live By*. Chicago: University of Chicago Press.

Ledoux, J. (1996) *The Emotional Brain*. New York: Simon & Schuster.

Levin, F.M. (1991) *Mapping the Mind*. Hillsdale, NJ: Analytic Press.

Litowitz, B. (1990) Elements of semiotic theory relevant to psychoanalysis. In *Semiotic Perspectives on Clinical Theory and Practice: Medicine, Neuropsychiatry and Psychoanalysis*, ed. B. L. Litowitz & P. S. Epstein. Berlin: Mouton de Gruyter.

Litowitz, B. & Litowitz, N. (1983) Development of verbal self-expression. In *The Future of Psychoanalysis*, ed. A. Goldberg. New York: International Universities Press, pp. 397–427.

Luborsky, L. & Crits-Cristoph, P. (1988) The assessment of transference by the CCRT method. In *Psychoanalytic Research Strategies*, ed. H. Dahl, H. Kächele, & H. Thomä. New York: Springer-Verlag, pp. 51–66.

Makari, G. & Shapiro, T. (1993) On Psychoanalytic Listening: Language and Unconscious Communication. *Journal of the American Psychoanalytic Association*, 41: 991–1020.

Maynard Smith, J. & Szathmary, E. (1995) *The Major Transitions in Evolution*. New York: Freeman.

Muller, J. P. (1996) *Beyond the Psychoanalytic Dyad*. New York: Routledge.

Olds, D. (1990) Brain-centered psychology: A semiotic approach. *Psychoanalysis and Contemporary Thought*, 3: 331–363.

Olds, D. (1992) The physicality of the sign. *Semiotics*, 9: 166–173.

Olds, D. D. (1994) Connectionism and Psychoanalysis. *Journal of the American Psychoanalytic Association*, 42: 581–611.

Olds, D. (2003) Affect as a Sign System. *Neuropychoanalysis*, 5: 81–95.

Pally, R. (1998) Bilaterality: Hemispheric Specialization and Integration. *International Journal of Psychoanalysis*, 79: 565–578.

Pally, R. (forthcoming) A primary role for nonverbal communication in psychoanalysis. Psychoanalytic Inquiry.

Palombo, S. R. (1992) Connectivity and Condensation in Dreaming. *Journal of the American Psychoanalytic Association*, 40: 1139–1159.

Peirce, C. S. (1897) Logic as semiotic: The theory of signs. In *Semiotics: An Introductory Anthology*, ed. R .E. Innis. Bloomington, IN: Indiana University Press, 1985, pp. 1–23.

Peterfreund, E. (1971) Information, Systems, and Psychoanalysis: An Evolutionary Biological Approach to Psychoanalytic Theory. *Psychological Issues* Monograph 25/26. New York: International Universities Press.

Poinsot, J. (1632) *Tractatus de Signis: The Semiotic of John Poinsot*, transl. J. Deely. Berkeley, CA: University of California Press, 1985.

Pollack, R. (1994) *Signs of Life*. New York: Houghton Mifflin.

Rosen, V. (1977) *Style, Character and Language*. New York: Aronson.

Rosenblatt, A. D. & Thickstun, J. T. (1977) *Modern Psychoanalytic Concepts in a General Psychology*. Psychological Issues Monograph 42/43. New York: International Universities Press.

Sacks, O. (1989) *Seeing Voices: A Journey into the World of the Deaf*. Berkeley, CA: University of California Press.

Schore, A. N. (1994) *Affect Regulation and the Origin of the Self: The Neurobiology of Emotional Development*. Hillsdale, NJ: Erlbaum.

Schore, A. N. (1997) Early organization of the non-linear right brain: A development of a predisposition to psychiatric disorders. *Development and Psychopathology*, 9: 595–630.

Schrödinger, E. (1944) *What Is Life?* Cambridge: Cambridge University Press.

Sebeok, T. A. (1986) The doctrine of signs. In *Frontiers in Semiotics*, ed. J. Deely, B. Williams, & F .E. Kruse. Bloomington, IN: Indiana University Press, pp. 35–42.

Shannon, C. (1949) *The Mathematical Theory of Communication*. Urbana, IL: University of Illinois Press.

Shapiro, T. (1991) Words And Feelings In The Psychoanalytic Dialogue. *Journal of the American Psychoanalytic Association*, 39: 321–348.

Slap, J. & Slap-Shelton, L. (1991) *The Schema in Clinical Psychoanalysis*. Hillsdale, NJ: Analytic Press.

Spence, D. P., Mayes, L. C., & Dahl, H. (1994) Monitoring the Analytic Surface. *Journal of the American Psychoanalytic Association*, 42: 43–64.

Stern, D. (1985) *The Interpersonal World of the Infant*. New York: Basic Books.

Stern, D. (1989) The representation of relational patterns: Developmental considerations. In *Relationship Disturbances in Early Childhood*, ed. A. Sameroff & R. Emde. New York: Basic Books, pp. 52–69.

Suomi, S. J. (1995) Attachment theory in non-human primates. In *Attachment Theory: Social, Developmental, and Clinical Perspectives*, ed. S. Goldberg, R. Muir, & J. Kerr. Hillsdale, NJ: Analytic Press.

Teller, V. & Dahl, H. (1986) The Microstructure of Free Association. *Journal of the American Psychoanalytic Association*, 34: 763–798.

Watt, D. F. (1990) Higher Cortical Functions and the Ego. *Psychoanalytic Psychology*, 7: 487–527.

Chapter 10

Affect as a Sign System[1]

Introduction

After long decades of being ignored by cognitive and neural sciences, the phenomenon of affect has recently become the object of intense study. Exciting work has been published in the past few years, attempting to bring affect studies up to par with those of cognition, motivation, behavior, and memory. Further research will no doubt help bring some of these theories into an integrated picture.

In this paper I will try to illuminate the concept of affect by viewing it from the perspective of biological semiotic systems. Semiotics, the study of signs, addresses the *communication* system itself, and by so doing we learn about the phenomena that are communicated. An analogy might be to the study of linguistics as way to help understand narrative. My general purpose is to see if bringing a different *point of view* to bear on affect will explicate the subject in a novel way. I will explore ideas that might clarify certain controversies in current theorizing, with the hope that as a heuristic model it may open up other questions and generate other hypotheses.

The basic model here is one of information processing. Signs carry information, and they do so by the "standing-for relationship." That relationship "brings to mind" a thing, a thought, an idea; or we may say it draws attention to, and brings to consciousness. In addition to the basic semiotic model describing the standing-for relationship, Charles Sanders Peirce, a nineteenth century American philosopher, developed a more nuanced, trichotomous model of semiotic that denotes three major categories of sign, the index, the icon, and the symbol. These categories help understand the different *ways* in which one thing can stand for another.

In this paper, I will briefly explicate the semiotic model as an alternative, heuristic point of view, capable of providing a different perspective on affect theory. I will then try to relate it to current biological models of affect. Finally, I will bring in the tripartite semiotic model, focussing on the functions of the different types of signs with respect to affect. I will use the model as a way to explore four issues relevant to psychoanalysis: 1) The question of

DOI: 10.4324/9781003399551-11

the time course of an affect; 2) The issue of drives and affects; 3) The three manifestations of affect and their dissociation; and 4) The different functions of the three types of signs with respect to affect.

The Semiotic Model

Let me first summarize the semiotic model that I have used elsewhere in trying to understand the informational function of the brain. I have previously explicated semiotic models in some detail (Olds, 1990, 2000, 2002). Semiotics, in the thinking of de Saussure, Peirce, and the Indiana semiotician, Thomas Sebeok, is the study of signs. The notion of a sign goes back at least to the Stoic philosophers, but the articulation most often cited is St. Augustine's *De Doctrina Christiana*. Saint Augustine's definition of a sign is still probably the best one around: "A sign is something that, on being perceived, brings something other than itself into awareness."

What is the need to use semiotics for this purpose? In the previous paper I used the model to look at life processes including the mind-brain relationship from a different perspective. There have been contributions from psychoanalysis and the cognitive sciences to this relationship. The cognitive sciences have been forging ahead in recent decades to a vast explanatory theory of mind and brain. In the process both these disciplines have begun to consult with each other about mind-brain function at the highest functional levels. We begin to see the possibility of a unified theory of mind and brain. But there are some unanswered questions remaining because of 1) complexity in certain areas where simple linear models do not work; and 2) the necessary dualism in a world where there are irreducible dichotomies such as those between the animate and the inanimate, and the mind and the brain. The semiotic model approaches the second of these questions, while complexity theories such as connectionist, neural-network, and non-linear systems theories address the first.

In the previous paper I outlined the way the model helps explain the dualism inherent in the crucial difference between the living as opposed to the inanimate world. The foundation of the theory is that, in living beings, things can *stand for* other things in a system. This phenomenon can help in modeling the processes of reproduction and genetic transfer, protein synthesis, neurotransmitter function, and brain function with respect to mental processes including thought, affect, memory, language and culture. The semiotic model is based on the notion of information transfer. Within a system, information can be conveyed by a sign, which stands for information in one part of the system, and transfers it to another part of the system. The advantage of the model is that we have a bridging concept, the *sign*, which has the capacity to represent, at different levels in the biological hierarchy. At each level the mode of representing may be quite different, but there is the common feature that one thing stands for another.

Essential Concepts

In discussing semiotics there are several terms that can lead to misunderstandings and disagreements requiring volumes of argument. Particularly troublesome are "information" and "meaning." I will give brief accounts of them, hoping to pursue my argument without getting sidetracked into the many confusions about their use.

Information is basically a pattern or sequence; in the present context, a sign can convey that pattern to another part of a system. Thus, RNA carries the code of the DNA, and the pattern leads to the construction of a protein. Or Morse code carries a pattern of sounds that code for letters and can be read out as words. It is often the case that the process goes from one medium to another, as with the sounds in code standing for letters in language. But this is not always so; when DNA replicates, it produces another identical DNA.

Meaning may be even more difficult. For the present argument, we might say that the meaning includes the information carried by a sign, but it is more inclusive. A peacock's display is a sign of sexual readiness, and will lead to mating. The meaning of the sign may relate more to broader issues of context and subjectivity. The meaning for the peahen may be different than for a human observer. As we develop the idea of affect as a sign, we will see that meaning may be variable depending on subjectivity and context. In this paper I will avoid the word because of the many confusions that it can cause.

The present paper will expand on the semiotics of *affect* with the same goal mentioned above: to provide a different perspective on affect, a theoretical viewpoint that may fill in some gaps in current theory. If the semiotic model is valid and useful it will not contradict other viewpoints including the neurobiological; it should provide a meaningful augmentation.

The Semiotic Model as a Point of View

One thing to make clear in presenting the semiotic model is that it is a *point of view*. It could be considered to be on the level of the metapsychological points of view. In his theoretical work, Freud (1915) described the metapsychological points of view, the "dynamic, topographical and economic aspects." (p. 181) Subsequent writers (Hartmann et al., 1946 and Rapaport & Gill, 1959) have added two others, the *genetic* and the *adaptive* points of view. These viewpoints allow explanation from deep, underlying principles, these principles not susceptible to translation into each other. For instance, the topographical point of view describes the mind insofar as it is internally structured with differentiated global functionings, whereas the economic point of view describes the effects of the flow and counterflow of energy; these are not incompatible but they are different. In the current environment, it may be useful to add the *neurobiological* point of view (Olds, 1990) and now the *semiotic* point of view. This aspectual approach allows for a model to be heuristic without forcing it to antagonize or refute other models. The heuristic value of each is that phenomena at a certain level of conceptualization may be considered as a system providing information and possible hypothesis generation within its domain.

The semiotic point of view would be one which, to paraphrase Rapaport, would *include propositions concerning the workings of signs in the transfer of information.* From this viewpoint, we follow the flow of information; we attend to patterns and structures that are transformed as information travels in living organisms.

An example might be the following: First a model in a rat, then a more psychoanalytic model in a human. A rat sees food and is hungry for it; it has learned that when it crosses the barrier between it and the food it gets a shock. *Dynamic*: the vector forces are such that the need to avoid the shock is greater than that to get to the food, and the rat does not move. Later when the hunger vector has increased the balance could shift and the rat would brave the shock and get the food. The *genetic* viewpoint would be that the rat is constitutionally wired to learn the association of certain behaviors and painful shock, and it has been subjected to such learning. The *neurobiological* viewpoint would explain this via learning paradigms in which neural networks in causal chains would lead to first the inhibition and then the action. The *semiotic* point of view would have a rat receiving two different signs, one a sign representing the body's need for food and another representing an evaluation of the situation in which a behavior is associated with shock, namely fear. There is an approach-avoidance dilemma produced by two opposing evaluations. As the hunger increases, the evaluation begins to place the importance of getting the food higher than that of avoiding the shock.

In the human example we might see in psychoanalytic terms the following: a person is ambitious for success but feels afraid that success will lead to punishment or retaliation. *Dynamic*: the vector forces are such that the need to avoid the punishment is greater than that to advance in his career; the result is an inconsistent or self-sabotaging performance that leads nowhere. The *genetic* point of view would relate inborn constitution and childhood experience leading to a constellation of attempts at success marred by recurrent self-sabotage. The *neurobiological* viewpoint would explain this via learning paradigms in which neural networks in causal chains would lead first to adaptive action and then to inhibition and self-interference. The *semiotic* point of view would have the man receiving two opposing evaluative signs, one that success is good and leads to increased self-esteem, and the other that success precedes disaster or punishment, in fact is a sign of disaster, and therefore must be avoided. There may be fantasies of being killed, beaten, or humiliated, which act as *signs* that success is dangerous. With the dynamic viewpoint, we emphasize the force vector aspects, with the genetic we emphasize constitutional and historical aspects, with the neurobiological we emphasize the neuronal structures, with the semiotic we attend to the sign systems. They all end up contributing to an understanding of one and the same phenomenon.

The heuristic value of this is that it leads us to inquire about the mind-brain connection, and mind/brain products such as affect, as being in this category of *standing-for* relationships. It should lead research investigators to look for ways in which mental phenomena behave as semiotic entities. In the present enterprise, I am turning this particular lens onto the phenomenon of affect with the hope of revealing something about affect in its communicative and meaning-producing aspect. As we shall see, it leads us to think more about the semiotic aspect of affect rather than the direct physiological effect of affect, without in any way undermining theories of neurobiology or physiology.

As organisms proceed up the evolutionary ladder, affects become more complex. There are central aspects, which may be mediated by neurons, but we have even more need to consider the system as a semiotic one in which the responses indicate value judgments, with physiological, expressive, sub-jective and motor aspects. The physiological-neurological package, con-sidered from this point of view, is part of a sign system. In mammals, the system is very complex and our theories, and even our descriptions of affects, are still unsettled. In fact, there is disagreement about the definitions of "emotion," "affect" and "feeling." Major researchers in the field have differ-ent tallies of what are the basic emotions. For instance, Ekman has 17 basic emotions, while Panksepp has three categories of emotion-like phenomena in one of which reside the four "blue ribbon basic emotions"—*seeking, fear, separation panic, and rage.*

The Roots of Affect in Unmediated Approach-Avoidance

With this simplified description of semiotics in mind, my thesis is that the affects make up a semiotic system, one that has evolved since the first one-celled animals. In those simple creatures we believe that affect constituted a simple positive-negative sign system. Even in this simple state, one can see that the affect system is an evaluation device, and in semiotic parlance it uses signs which stand for the evaluation; this evaluation leads to approach or withdrawal. For instance, a one-celled organism would approach increasing nutrient concentration, but avoid heat or too much acidity.

As an example of one of the more simple and primitive approach-avoid-ance systems, Hofer (1997) describes a bacterium that, when it encounters a nutrient gradient, its flagellae move in synchrony, directing it upstream toward increasing concentration. When there is no such obvious stream to follow, the flagellae go out of phase and the organism simply rotates in place, not going anywhere. In higher organisms there are many reflex systems that operate this way; the motor response is an automatic result of the perception.

In multicellular creatures with more complex perceptual systems, chemoreceptors persist as early forms of smell and taste, and other systems such as the visual, auditory and sensory systems evolve. With these, in organisms such as fish and reptiles, simple stimuli, such as a color or a shape, may still be hard-wired to certain responses. For instance, a frog may reflexly attack and swallow any dark small fly-sized object as if it were a fly; and it will avoid any looming object.

Eventually other objects will be recognized as conspecifics or non-specifics, rivals, or adversaries, or food. At this level comes object recognition, where qualia must be assembled to form object representations. Already the criteria for approach and avoidance have become more complex. At this level of organism—the level of fish and reptiles—we may suggest that approach may be for the purpose of conglomeration as in schools of fish, or for mating; it may also be for the purpose of fighting, and defense of territory, or for that of eating, devouring prey. Avoidance now may be for self-protection, escaping from a predator or a more powerful rival, or it may be for genetically evolved requirements for space and population distribution. But clearly, at this evolutionary level, we have more than a simple model of approachavoidance or pleasure-unpleasure. We have to have different evaluations as part of the adaptive response. A fish defending territory will not try to eat the object, and termination will occur when the object backs away; but if the object is food, the fish will pursue and devour, but only when hungry. Here the nature of the object perceived triggers the response, which has a behavioral and often a display aspect. The display may be different for feeding, fighting and sex. We can postulate that at this level, all there is to the affect is the display and the behavior; we have no idea what the subjective aspect may be. We believe from observing and experimenting that there is little freedom of response, that there is no mentalizing and evaluating between the perception and the response. We think of the response as "reflex," or "unmediated."

Mediated Affect Systems

As we work up the evolutionary ladder, the dichotomy persists—the distinction between the useful or pleasurable, on one hand, and painful, damaging or dangerous on the other. At the same time the complexity increases, so that 1) There are more differentiated affects; and 2) There are much more complicated chains of mediation, clusters of signs between input and output, between stimulus and response. With lower mammals, such as rats, things are already more complicated; there are the positive evaluations, including those towards certain pleasures, or necessities, of eating, mating, exploring and playing, as well as the negative ones of fear, rage and depression. All five senses are used to recognize and evaluate current environment and experience. There is always the basic polarity between the positive and negative;

and this polarity means affects are sometimes in opposition as in the laboratory rat or the success-phobic man mentioned above.

At the approach-avoidance level of affect, we have a basic circuit—the connection between the percept and the action is automatic. At more complex levels, however, there are inner (central) responses to the percept, which themselves are signs of what to do next. These signs evoke autonomic arousals within the organism, which are the analogs to the behavior of the simple organism. In other words, instead of automatically moving, the organism gets an internal message, manifested as the activation of arousal or inhibitory systems. That activation itself becomes a sign as it is interpreted by the organism. Owing to this intermediary system an organism has a second chance; its behavior is less tightly determined, and it can decide if it really wants to follow the indication of the arousal system. With more corticalization, as in primates and humans, that subjective response becomes more elaborate, and mediated in the social milieu. In higher animals, there is the physiological response including a tendency or urge to act, but the act may be inhibited as the urge conflicts with a competing urge. One might be angry and wish to challenge the silverback, but also be afraid to do it, and hold back. Or one might be frightened to give a public speech, but in certain conditions one might do it anyway. The fear seems to be an appropriate response to the situation, but one might over-ride it for other purposes.

The Brainstem Centers of Affect

The work of Damasio, Panksepp, and others suggests that there is at the base of the evaluation system an integration of affect and arousal. The roots of affect depend on brainstem nuclei, including the *periaquaductal gray* and the *parabrachial nucleus*. These areas make up the lowest point in what is being called the ERTAS system, or Extended Reticulo-thalamic Activating System. An elaboration of this system is beyond the limits of this paper, but it seems that at this point there is an initial division into positive and negative evaluations, leading both to activation and arousal, and also to approach or avoidance. Thus, at this level the mechanism of affect and the mechanism of arousal may be essentially indistinguishable. Arousal begins with a value judgment, and levels of arousal determine levels of affect. The sign system involved has a distinguishable circuit for each of the major affects (Panksepp, 1998). Each circuit is distributed through the neuraxis and includes these brainstem areas, in addition to specific areas in the limbic system such as nuclei in the amygdala, hypothalamus and cingulate cortex. Each of them is essentially a sign system using complexes of neurotransmitters to conduct information about value to the cortex and motor systems; these guide motivation, thought, and behavior.

Recent work by Damasio et al. (2000) supports the idea that each affect activates a cluster of brain areas:

"structures that regulate the organism's current state, by executing specific actions via the musculoskeletal, ranging from facial and postural expressions to complex behaviors, and by producing chemical and neural responses aimed at the internal milieu, viscera and telencephalic neural circuits."

(p. 1049)

In their experiment they induced subjects to recall certain memories which evoked four basic emotions—happiness, sadness, anger, and fear. They performed PET scans on the subjects as they were experiencing the emotion and compared it to a situation where they were in a "neutral" emotional state. They conclude that "these varied patterns provide distinctive 'perceptual landscapes' of the organism's internal state and that the differences among those landscapes constitute the critical reason why each emotion feels different" (p. 1051). An example of such a pattern for happiness is "the positive peak in the right posterior cingulate, the negative peak in the anterior third of the left cingulate, the positive peak in the left insula, and the positive peak in the right SII" (secondary sensory cortex). For the present argument this suggests a correlation between the subjective awareness of a certain emotion and the unique, reproducible cluster of brain activations. It is not clear if these activations are part of the mechanism of becoming aware, or *perceiving* the emotional state of the body, or are they being measured in the act of *producing* the emotional state, or both. But the point is that this complex of neurological phenomena, correlates with the affect and represents the evaluation, in this case of the memory being evoked for the experimental purpose.

An Evaluative Quale?

Each affect is a sign system, and the sign is made up of a set of neurological responses. This may be parallel to that for a complex visual sign, which includes *qualia*, or sensed qualities, of shape, location, color, texture, size, etc, each of which requires a modular brain system. Or it may be like taste, which is a blend of four different taste qualities, from four different systems. An affect may be a similar complex of responses, including arousal mechanisms, autonomic changes, motor responses of approach and avoidance, as well as physiologic responses to expected pleasure or harm. Could the affect sign be a quale, functioning like any other sensed quality of an object? Panksepp (2000b) suggests something very similar in his notion of "equale" referring to an *evolutionary quale*.

The kind of sign we are dealing with is unusual. It isn't a simple token or object that "stands for" something. It is a complex set of physiological responses standing for an *evaluation*. Thus, there is no "object" that it stands for, only a value, an abstraction. The affect starts with the awareness of a state of affairs, via perception, but also the connection of the perception with one's history, sense of self, and current contexts. So it may be that there are different entry points for an affective experience, e.g., the stimulus, the perception, the natural reflex response, the learning history, and higher-level evaluation generated by the cortex. If someone accidentally steps on my toe, I'll react with immediate withdrawal, and quick anger. As the experience is worked over by way of higher cortical centers, and I hear the person's apologies and obvious contrition, I will see it was not a deliberate attack, it was an accident, unintentional. The pain may remain but the anger may dissipate because of the top-down (cortical) modulation.

Let us try to correlate certain trains of perception, again focussing on the visual system. As described in a previous paper (Olds, 2000) the brain has evolved to provide different sign systems for certain interpretive clusterings of sensations according to certain functional categories, denoting the *identity,* the *location* and the *value* of the percept. The identity is iconic in that it depicts the visual characteristics needed to identify or recognize the object; this is done mainly in the temporal cortex. The location is the indexical relationship, conveying information about where the object is in relation to the self. The value is a third functional category, the evaluation of the object, using the affect system. A simplified version of the process would be this: A light stimulus enters the eye and a "retinotopic" icon of the object is formed. Optic neurons carry this image to the thalamus and then to the occipital cortex.[2] Experiments have shown that the image maps onto the cortex in an iconic way. (A stimulus such as an "X" sign will generate a neural firing pattern in V1—in the primary visual cortex—that has the shape of an "X.") As the activation spreads to secondary cortices, the stimulus can be compared to memory traces and, in the *temporal* cortex, identified as what it is. As it spreads to the *parietal* cortex, its image is much less detailed, and the information is generated as to the distance and direction from the self. Third, as it goes to the systems generating affect, it will be interpreted in terms of its value to the self.

Thus, the semiotic approach suggests that the brain uses three major systems to process these practically different aspects of an object. The affect may be attached faster than we can be aware of but still it is temporally secondary to the other two; it is not just another quale like the color or shape. The affect represents the object's value, and is not an inherent property of the object. In most cases affects are attributed as a result of experiential learning, usually in the form of classical conditioning. The attribution has a history in previous experience. In simple neurological terms it takes time to put together an image and an object in the visual system, and then even more time to communicate with another set of brain systems to recreate the association to the affect. We might call the affect a "secondary quale."

The affect, being an appraisal, necessarily follows the perception; there must be something to appraise. However, because of the fast, early limbic circuit, and the relatively slow pace of consciousness, the percept and affect usually appear to be simultaneous.[3] For this third step the brain has to choose which affect to connect with the stimulus. This has been learned by prior experience: mother's approaching footsteps evoke an expectation that relief is immanent. Mother's more rapid staccato footsteps may mean "watch out."

But how did the percept and affect get connected in the first place? There seem to be pre-wired connections for certain sensations indicating wetness, cold, hunger, separation, etc. with certain affect responses. In other words, how does an infant know that a pinprick is "painful" and a light caress "pleasurable?" Those connections must be prestructured. Many percept-affect connections are learned in the well-known behavioral paradigm. In this, the stimulus may be paired in time with a set of sensations, and thereby the association is made. But, also, it is generally accepted that some stimuli are pre-wired to affective response. Some species seem to have innate avoidance responses to snakes and looming objects. A chick will fall silent when any shadow passes overhead, despite no prior experience of shadows. Mouse pups with no previous experience of cats, in the middle of "rough and tumble play," will stop playing the instant some cat fur is placed in the cage (Panksepp, 1998).

The expression of affect, the signs of emotion to be conveyed to others, precedes language by a long time. And much of mammalian evolution has included an increasing complexity of affects and of their expression. The driving force for this complexity seems to have been the degree of sociality that a species develops. Going a long way back in evolution are the expressions of mating-readiness, and of aggression in the establishment of social dominance hierarchies. These may have evolved in social animals such as monkeys and primates, leading to "social" emotions such as shame or triumph. With pre-linguistic hominids, the expression via gesture, facial expression, and tones of voice became highly elaborated. As language developed in archaic Homo sapiens, we think that affects became nameable like everything else.

The Semiotic Categories of Affect

For the present argument, we must try to clarify just what kind of a sign an affect is. It is an extremely complex sign, and we may use Peirce's categories to define some subtypes of signs.

Loosely following Peirce's classification, we may consider three major types of signs, each having different properties useful for conveying particular kinds of information within and among living organisms. To briefly review these categories of signs, we can take for example the much-used object, the writing pen. If there is a pen lying on the table, there are three main ways you can bring it to mind: you can point to it, thus locating it in space and drawing attention to it—in Peirce's terminology, this is an "index;" you can draw a recognizable picture of it, otherwise known as an "icon;" or you can name it or "symbolize" it. A crucial distinction among these three ways is that the non-symbolic signs (indices and icons) are in some way *constrained* by their objects; if you use an index to represent the pen you have to point at the pen, you cannot just point anywhere you please. And if you use an icon, a drawing or a diagram, it must resemble the pen; otherwise, you won't recognize it. However, with a *symbol*, there is no necessary connection to the object; just about any set of phonemes can be used to represent anything, the ones you choose will depend on what language you are speaking. This so-called "semiotic freedom" gives the symbol incredible power, which has made it one of the major engines of human evolution.

Affects as Signs

How do we classify an affect as a sign? An affect has aspects of all three kinds of signs:

Indexical: location is important in determining what affect will be elicited. First of all, the phenomena of approach and avoidance are the clearest examples of the index that there are. *Proximity* and *distance* are among the fundamental categories relevant to survival. Basic issues of pleasure and unpleasure indicate whether one should approach or avoid. In addition, indexical values determine many specific responses. A coiled rattler three feet away will provoke one affect and response; the same snake 30 feet away will occasion a different reaction. An affect display may include indexical aspects such as *withdrawal* gestures and postures or gestures of *drawing near* and embracing. And within the body the subjective aspect of emotion may include a location, the "heart" or the "guts." The metaphors often associated with affect have indexical aspects; my mood is up or down, I'm feeling "distant," or "inside myself." In infancy, but also throughout life, the *whereness* of important objects is highly affectively salient. For an infant the where-abouts of the mother is of constant concern, proximity being possibly the most important factor in the survival of an infant of any species.

Iconic: an affect may have natural constraints including that the affect be appropriate to the situation. Increased heart and breathing rate are appropriate to situations of danger, where fighting or fleeing may be necessary. Ekman's (1994) research has supported the notion that some affect displays are uniform across cultures. Thus, we can say that the sign of affect is *constrained* by the affect; this suggests it is non-symbolic, better characterized as an icon. But if it is an icon, how does it resemble anything? We can say that the physiology of each affect relates in a non-accidental way with the situation causing it. For instance, the emergency emotions of fear and anger include sympathetic arousal and a body prepared for action. This is iconic in the sense that it is appropriate for fighting or fleeing. Sadness or joy arouses different physiological responses. It is likely that the iconic aspect of affect plays a large part in the "attunement" experience between mothers and infants. In that interaction there is much passing back and forth of affective displays, including both "categorical" emotions, the ones we have been speaking of, and the "vitality" affects, representing changes in intensity, tension and energy. Infant-research tapes have shown iconicity in the cross-modal expressions of rhythm, for instance when a mother's vocal rhythm matches the infant's banging of a rattle.

To pursue the iconicity issue further, we must say that it is important that I recognize the affect that you have. Empathy, imitation, other forms of internalization produce an iconic likeness of your affect in me. This may occur by several routes, as yet not fully understood. If we think of the iconic representation of the visual image that arises in the visual cortex, is there an analogy in the world of affect? As mentioned above we learn to associate an affect with a percept (say loud noises with fear) and we communicate our affects to others. The communication function is of major importance. By the analogy of vision, my perception of your affect may have an iconic representation in me; this would have to mean it would induce in me at least a mild version of your affect. (If you are sad I'll be sad; if you are angry I'll know it by having "trace anger;" then I will be angry or afraid of you, depending on the context.) There are intriguing possibilities for research. One such possibility is the phenomenon of "mirror cells." Experiments with the motor system in monkeys has shown that, when a monkey makes a motor act such as putting food in its mouth certain motor cells can be recorded. Then when the monkey sees the experimenter making the same motion of arm and hand, the same cells fire *in the monkey*. This direct mirroring of the others actions in one's own brain may be important in imitation and the learning of skills, possibly in all mammals. It may be that such mirroring allows for internal simulation of another's affect. As far as I know, research in the mirror cells in the receptive areas or the affective-motor areas of the brain has not been done.

Symbolic: affects are expressed non-verbally and verbally. The verbal expression is obviously symbolic by our definition of language. At first consideration the non-verbal affect expression, via body posture, gesture and facial display, is not culturally determined and therefor does not fit the definition of symbol. However, it may be *evolutionarily* determined, in a way that is not dissimilar to the cultural mode. Affect displays have evolved over the millennia. It may not be clear how each affect evolved its repertoire of physiological responses, and there may be some manifestations that now seem arbitrary, although they may have once been constrained by adaptive purpose. For instance, it makes sense that the expression of shame might include a sagging posture, derived as it may be from the dominance-submission systems in primate evolution, or that rage might be indicated by aggressive expressions of baring teeth and making frightening noises, iconic for a fighting posture. But it may be somewhat accidental that the brow furrows with worry or the eyebrows go up with surprise. This could be similar to the evolution of birdsong; each species has the inherited apparatus to produce a series of notes that is unique to the species, a kind of language whereby members of the species can communicate and be recognized. But there is no inherent constraint producing any particular series of notes. As with all forms of communication there must be a shared understanding of the meaning of the sign, so that the singing bird and listening bird have evolved to make use of the same song.[4]

An interesting sidelight here is that affective expressions have to some extent been preserved through the evolution of species. A dog and a human can easily detect anger or fear in the each other. This is different in bird-song and other displays related to mating. A dog will respond appropriately when a peacock gets angry, but will be quite indifferent to the peacock's mating display.

Also because of the vagaries of both disposition and learning there is some indeterminacy in the particular relation between an affect and its inducer. One person might evaluate a mouse running across the floor as cute or amusing, while another might react with terror. But the particular affect is expressed to the self and to others in pretty uniform ways.

It is striking that the iconic and indexical aspects of affect expressions have themselves generated much symbolism. As Lakoff and Johnson (1980) have pointed out, much of our language derives from metaphors derived from body feelings appropriate to affects: "hot under the collar" relating to anger, "down in the dumps" relating to low mood or sadness. In other words, the signs of the physiology and display of affect are translated into the symbols of linguistic emotion expression. This is interesting in that the symbolism here is directed by the iconic and indexical aspects of the non-verbal aspects of affects.[5]

A Difference That Makes a Difference?

One might wonder how this redescription via semiotic theory could make any difference other than the philosophical issue of the difference between non-life and life, or the generally interesting notion that we live in a sea of signs.[6]

There are several issues we might open up to semiotic examination to see if the model is of some heuristic value: 1) The issue of the time course of an affect; 2) The issue of drives and affects; 3) The three functions of affect and their dissociation; and 4) The different functions of the three types of signs with respect to affect.

The Time Course of Affect

There has been considerable struggle between at least two models of the time course of an affect. One is a traditional perception-first model. In this the subject first senses and identifies an object, then attaches an affect, and then has a physiological and motor response. Affects have been associated with objects through previous conditioning; and subsequently when one comes upon something dangerous or previously associated with harm or pain, one sees it, recognizes it and then responds with *fear* and jumps away. An alternative is the classical James-Lange model of affect proposed in the late nineteenth century. In this model the generation of affect is pre-conscious, mediated by somatic, physiological reactions. In the classic statement of the theory, one knows one is afraid when one realizes one is running away. The physiologic response of fear, anger or pleasure is made instantly and pre-consciously, and one learns of one's emotion by becoming aware of such a response. Although the semiotic model cannot prove either of these alternatives, it might help resolve the controversy. If we take LeDoux's model of fear in which there is a "short circuit" whereby a percept is immediately routed to subcortical structures—in the case of fear, to the amygdala—and a long circuit by way of the cortex. The short circuit is very fast but imprecise visually so that anything that looks like a snake triggers an immediate reflex jumping away. This circuit would correspond to the interpretation-first view of affect. When the cortex is used to evaluate the stimulus and conclude that the object is only a curved stick, this aspect would correspond to the James-Lange view because it is at this level that we become conscious of the experience, it's most salient and possibly first-arriving feature being the fact that I am jumping away. Each of the two steps represents a semiotic system, one for rough and ready survival, one for more deliberate judgment. It is probably even more complicated than that. Panksepp proposes a more elaborate model where there are multiple levels in the neurological and mental response, with two-way feedback in *concurrent* complex processes (1998, pp. 35–45). The semiotic analysis finds a contradiction in the model that suggests we attach the affect before knowing what the object is. Signs do not flow backward; by this I mean that a sign exists in time *after* the thing, phenomenon, or event that it stands for. The sign of evaluation must have something to evaluate, and therefore must *follow* it. The LeDoux short circuit provides the answer to the apparent paradox.

Drives and Affects

The place of drives and affects in psychoanalytic theory has had a tumultuous course. In the neuroscientific realm there may be similar uncertainty, although it seems to be a less passionately debated issue there. Damasio seems to conflate drives and affects as in the same category—homeostatic regulatory mechanisms. Panksepp does not discuss drives much in his *Affective Neuroscience*. But interestingly, in his tri-level listing of affects his level 1. seems to be really about drive like phenomena—the hungers, etc.

A paper that addresses this issue squarely is Shevrin's (1997). He points out that psychoanalytic theory has, in its flight from libido theory, taken a sharp turn toward "affect-first theory." He reviews Lichtenberg's and Kernberg's models as ones in which drives are downgraded, and almost discarded. For Lichtenberg the things considered in the past to be drives are now limited to signals, which derive all their force from associated affects. The informational model has taken over, so that even the "drives" are informational signals that initiate affective processes that lead to action. Where there seems to be no escaping the energy aspect, there are terms like "affective cathexis" which slip energy back in without much notice. Could semiotics help us here?

Let us go back to the earlier mentioned hard-wired affects represented by approach-avoidance, say toward nutrients or away from looming objects. I described them as "unmediated" affect systems, reflex and with no central intermediate phases. Or with a hunger, one gets hungry and eats. One can do that without much affect. In Freud's model the affect of unpleasure was associated with the increasing drive, say hunger, and pleasure with the satisfaction and reduction of the excitatory pressure. Thus, drive and affect were intimately related. But it may be that a drive is more about the state of the body and its homeostasis, and an affect is more about the state of the world, of the environment confronting the organism. Shevrin points out that the semantics differentiate drive from affect. You can *frustrate* or *gratify* a drive, or a "craving", but not an affect. You can *experience, express* or *suppress* a feeling but not a drive. You can *want* (drive) something without *liking* (affect) it, and you can like something without wanting it. Drives have force and affects have evaluative content. Pleasure and unpleasure are the basic affect vectors; satisfaction or frustration are basic drive vectors. Of course, there is frequent overlap; one can become angry or sad when a hunger or craving is unsatisfied. A feeling of happiness can lead to increase in sexual or creative drive. Anxiety can lead to reducing of both those drives. Shevrin describes a craving in very young children as diffuse and nonspecific. The baby is dysphoric, it cries, the mother tries to satisfy it with the small repertoire of ministrations—feeding, burping, changing, rocking or cuddling. Later the drives become more differentiated as desires; the baby, and soon the mother, through signs, "know" the baby is hungry, or wet or tired, etc.

From our point of view, we could suggest that the difference is in the nature of the sign. For a drive we have a kind of unmediated urge; the sign—conscious or otherwise—is not a value, it is directly a hunger, a wanting. The sign is a physiological sign, a sign of homeostatic imbalance. It can be conscious as with hunger, or non-conscious as with electrolyte imbalance. The body normally automatically rights the imbalance without a lot of affect. Blood sugar goes down to a certain threshold, that is a sign to various brain areas leading to physiological responses and feelings, light-headedness, stomach feelings, etc. As Panksepp points out, we have evolved so that we have this experience long before we are near starvation; there is a healthy lead-time built in so that hunger begins well before there is an emergency. The subjective sign is the representative of the drive, it is a physiological set similar to that for an affect, but it is not an evaluation as such. A value may be added, but not inevitably; if I'm hungry, I could be angry or anxious that I don't know where my next meal is coming from, or I could be pleased because I want to have a good appetite for the excellent restaurant I'm heading for.

This may help in understanding Panksepp's categories of affects. In his description there are three categories. Category 1 includes "low level emotive responses that are almost reflexive, such as startle, disgust, and the various hungers..." Category 2 are the "blue ribbon grade-A emotions." These are "expectancy" or "seeking," "rage," "fear," and "separation-distress." Category 3 are more subtle, socially determined affects, usually studied in humans. Category 1 tends to the drive and craving model. Categories 2 and 3 phenomena are more evaluative as described above and less drive-like. They are more informational and less energetic, the obverse of the situation with drives.

In summary, the difference lies in the nature of the sign. With a drive the sign is the physiological imbalance itself, and the correction is normally done automatically, with or without awareness. With an affect there is a secondary evaluative sign. It is less peremptory and possibly more complex and with more mediating steps than the drive. We might say simplistically that an affect has, or is, an extra sign that a drive does not have. A secondary feature we can note here is that an affect, value sign, is usually a quale attached to a percept or a remembered image. In other words, the affect sign is about the world and the organism within the world; an affect turns outward. A drive arises from within; the sign is of a state of homeostatic disequilibrium. Another difference may be that affects are less about current states and imbalances than are drives, but are more predictive, they are evaluations, which lead to predictions as to the organism's welfare given the current circumstances. Thus, the signs that represent the drive represent the imbalance itself—with hunger: the stomach pangs, the fatigue, the light-headedness. With affect, the signs represent the evaluation, not any particular drive-related metabolic imbalance. Another way of describing the difference is this: a drive is a semiotic system representing a departure from homeostasis necessary for survival of the organism. An affect creates a departure from homeostasis that acts as a sign to motivate the organism with respect to its environment according to values. The affect seems to have more of a top-down aspect, more room for a high-level evaluation of the state of affairs, which then enhances or reduces the immediate physiological response.

Three Aspects of Affect and Their Possible Dissociations

We can abstract three major manifestations of the affect system. One is the *physiological response* involving multiple brain centers and the autonomic nervous system indicated in research such as Damasio et al.'s experiment. A second is the *display* aspect, and the third is the *subjective* aspect. Psychoanalysts have long been aware that these three are often dissociated, possibly the most common and striking feature of our patients' presentations. In a sense each aspect can be put out of commission, temporarily or long-term. One may have the physiological and the display aspects but be unaware. One may for instance be red in the face, with knuckle white fists, and show the cardiovascular phenomena attributable to the anger response, and still say, "Who me, angry? No way!" This dissociation may be quite habitual in some people, a facet of the "repressor style" to which I'll return later.

One may have both the subjective and the physiological aspects, but not the display, as in a dissembler or "poker faced" negotiator. Here the display aspect can be sharply reduced, but such a person may fail a lie detector test, which measures the physiology. Or alternatively one may fake display, as in feigned anger in order to intimidate, or feigned friendliness to a hated rival.

Or one may have only the physiology but no display and no subjective awareness. Examples of this may be the "alexithymic" and possibly the "avoidant" child to whom I will also return later. It seems that of the three we have *very little* control over the physiologic response (with the possible exceptions of certain trance states and Yogic practices), *some* conscious and unconscious control over the display, and *much* unconscious control, mostly by way of defense mechanisms, over the awareness.

Krause (2000) points out that affect research beginning with Freud has underestimated the importance of the expressive aspect of affect. One could argue that the expressive purpose of affect is particularly important as mammals became more social. It could be that the ability to dissociate display from basic physiological response had its own evolutionary trajectory. Just as the anger and the fear clusters may have evolved as separate systems, the expressive aspects could have evolved as separate systems as well. The ability to dissemble and fake affect expressions seems to be a high-level function, well known to humans and possibly present in chimpanzees. Also, some species may find some flexibility in affect expression to be advantageous. A lion preparing to struggle with a rival in a power dispute will use a dramatic threatening display. The same animal about to attack a wildebeest, may have a similar physiological cluster of excitations, but it can well do without the display. If these two aspects—physiology and display—have evolved separately and differentially in different species, they could more easily be seen to develop separately, and at times idiosyncratically, in humans. Krause points out that certain kinds of psychopathology exhibit mixes of incompatible affect displays, such as anger and pleasure, or anxiety and pleasure. Then there are ethnic differences, such that affect display in general is more or less acceptable and uninhibited, and other areas where expression of certain affects may be curtailed. For instance, in one culture the display of contempt might be important in preserving social hierarchy, while in another culture contempt would have little value and would be considered bad manners unacceptable in a leader.

For the present discussion the most obvious semiotic dimension of affect is the outward expression. Yet the physiology and the display have an inward semiotic aspect, so that the subjective awareness of affect includes both an awareness of the physiology of preparedness and of proprioceptive sensations resulting from the display. Curiously, we can use each manifestation as a sign to generate the other two. I can think *sadly* as in Damasio's experiment and generate the physiology and expression; I can have the physiology stimulated by drugs or electrodes, or I can imitate the expression as in some of Ekman's (1994) work, and the other two phenomena follow.

This phenomenon of dissociation may be an example of the heuristic value of the semiotic approach. We sometimes speak of "carving nature at the joints." Semiotics may show us some of the joints, in this case the knife is dissociation, which suggests that an affect is made up of three semiotic systems that have co-evolved. In fact, this affect-system dissociation is the bread and butter of psychoanalysis. It has not been as much studied by neural scientists, as have other aspects of affect.

An extraordinary experiment by Heller (Heller & Haynal, 1997) may be an example of the kind of dissociation I've described. In an attempt to understand "the semiology of suicide" they observed videotapes of the facial expressions of a psychiatrist interviewing patients within three days of a suicide attempt. Following the interview, the patient and doctor filled in questionnaires aimed at evaluating the emotional quality of the interaction. The doctor wrote down his diagnosis and his *prediction* of the patient's making another suicide attempt. The interview was structured, with a set series of questions. Video tapes were made of the doctor's face and the patient's. Only after doing these things did the doctor consult the patient's previous record. The first interviews included 59 suicide attempters. A year later they found that ten of the patients had made another suicide attempt, none fatal. The video tapes were coded using a facial expression coding system devised by Ekman and Freisen (1978). In brief, the doctor predicted the risk of another attempt, using his conscious impression with an accuracy of 29 per cent; however, the coding of the doctor's face during one minute of tape allowed the investigators to predict with 81 per cent accuracy. One major difference was that the doctor *frowned* more and was more emotionally expressive and active with the future re-attempters than with a matched sample of patients who did not make another attempt.

This experiment was done with one doctor interviewing 59 patients. Although there are many reasons to question the results—the small n, the unique personality of the doctor, even the possibility that his frowning had a negative therapeutic effect. But the fact that his facial expression pattern was a more accurate indicator of his reaction to the patient's presentation than his own conscious evaluation is striking. He revealed an iconicity with the patient that even he did not realize. This is a nice example of dissociation between the display aspect and the subjective aspect. It would be interesting to have had the doctor wired for physiological measures.

The Symbol in Relation to the Other Types Of Signs

Let's take another look at the role of the symbol. Affects themselves, both in their internal and external expressions, are inborn and universal, and therefore in general would not be considered symbolic. As mentioned above however, in humans, the furrowed brow and the raised eyebrows may not be physiological requirements related to the affects involved. As with birdsongs and the barks and whines of mammals, the mutual evolution of signs, and receivers of those signs, produced a communication system. However, in human language symbols can be used to represent affects, thus standing for affects in a more arbitrary way. With human language, there may be some influence from iconic and indexical aspects as mentioned above. But the fact that a symbol is chosen arbitrarily and is different in each language makes its relationship to its referent always more distant and provisional. Symbols can be verbal (language), or non-verbal, for instance a gesture, a national flag, or an advertising logo.

This distance and provisional nature provide the symbol with the properties of flexibility and the power to help in adaptation in a complex social world. Boysen et al. (1996) describe an experiment with chimpanzees, that makes a dramatic point. If you present one hungry chimp with two plates of food, one much bigger than the other, it will always choose the larger by pointing to it. If you ask the animal to choose one, which will go to another chimp, potentially giving the other one the smaller portion, the subject chimp will not be able to make the self-serving choice. When asked to select by pointing to the food plate to be given to the other animal, it will always point to the larger and then be quite angry when this goes to the other. Children before age two have the same problem; they cannot point to the smaller—to be given away—in order to end up receiving the larger. However, in the world of primate research, there are now some chimps that have learned to count and use numbers as symbols. When the same experiment is done with such a chimp, for instance with one treat in the small portion, and four in the large one, and you ask, "Which one do you want to be given away, '1' or '4'?", it can soon learn to sign "1" and then triumphantly enjoy the big portion. In other words, when the animal has to use an index, namely point to the desired dish, it doesn't have the kind of flexibility needed. When symbols are applied, it can somehow play the game at a different level.

This experiment is enlightening with respect to symbol systems. They provide a separate world, the world of the symbolic, manipulated in the brain. Symbols, in this case numbers, have such a loose connection to their referents that they can be manipulated with great freedom, a freedom Lacan refers to as "glissance," a kind of sliding or slippage. Symbols relate more intensely to *other symbols* than to the objects in the world.

Now it appears that the symbolization of affects can be beneficial. Research suggests that affects of which one is unaware, and/or unsymbolized, are less in our control. We have a less flexible way of dealing with them, and we are unable to learn whether they are appropriate or not. A repressed person finds himself in transferential situations with an authority figure, finds himself behaving in damaging ways and has no awareness of why. Like the chimp who is unable to make the adaptive choice with respect to the two plates of food, the transference reaction is out of the person's control. Teaching the chimp to use symbols apparently allows for an adaptive flexibility. Teaching an analytic patient to symbolize affects may allow for similar adaptability.

If we look at this possibility in semiotic terms, we can imagine the following. Semiotic theory leads us to focus on the repetition compulsion as fundamental to much repetitive behavior, some, but not all of which, is maladaptive and out of a person's control. The repetition structures transference responses and many behavioral complexes we term characterologic. A repetition is by definition *iconic*. A structure of experience is repeated as a habit, also called a procedure, or procedural learning. For instance, in a patient who has intense conflicts in dealing with authority figures, the person has generalized an affective response derived in early experience with a parent or caretaker, to all those in a position of power or influence over the self. The ensuing response to such a person, involving fear and withdrawal, compulsive rebelliousness, anger and resentment, or passive-aggressive negativity, will result from the affects habitually associated with the authority figure. The affect has become an implicit quale in this situation, and the person has little choice beyond his habitual response. The iconicity implies that the experience is a *package* deemed similar, there is no freedom to parse out aspects of the experience that would break down the conviction of similarity.

In a transference reaction the affective icon is linked to a category of person. When we introduce the symbolic, by talking about a patient's experiences with authority figures, we can introduce some flexibility into the transferential system. When we do this, each element of the complex can be separated out and can be named and dealt with discretely by its name. The affect involved can be named, and the parts that might differentiate the current object from the transferential object can be named. This naming allows the individual elements to be peeled away from the affect. One might have the freedom to conclude, "Yes indeed my boss is harsh and critical, but he is not the same person as my father, and the various meanings of his behavior are different for a grown man than for a little boy." That is of course not the end of it. The working through requires many repetitions and re-experiencings of this insight that has been shared through naming—in the analytic situation. But the naming and the differentiating at the symbolic level, allied with the new patterns experienced in relation to the analyst, seem to allow for change. The symbolic order takes events and things into a virtual world, mediated by the human cortex and the social world. The virtual world can be manipulated by trial actions, imagined events and people, by re-arrangements of reality. The hard-wired affective connection, leading to phobia, inhibition, compulsion, perversion or repetition-compulsion becomes an object in the symbolic world, and the connection can be seen to be provisional. Other possibilities emerge, and one can work through to change. Affects too can become objects when they become named and become the referents of symbols. Thus, the person who can symbolize has this great advantage: feelings can be named and thus opened to question.

Lest we focus too much on the negative aspects of the iconic repetition, we must remember that the positive transference is also iconic. We enter the therapeutic relationship with hope for the repetition of the positive aspects of our childhood and the beneficent role of our caretakers. The iconic aspects we use profoundly, and for those for whom there was little good in their childhood, there may be little positive transference to count on. And we know that the separations and reunions of the present, the analyst's vacations and returns, are among the most dramatic and important repetitions that we encounter; they are iconic experiences, which generate iconic responses. Again, verbalization helps in managing these responses. It may take years to be able to verbalize what is good in the relationship, what one misses by absence and gains by presence. That too involves the symbolization of what was indexical and iconic.

There is much recent work showing more of the power of symbolization, particularly of language. Eagle (1998) reviews the growing literature showing the disadvantages of the "repressive style" and the advantages of verbal expression—the lifting of thing presentations to word presentations. He quotes Freud from 1937, saying "It sometimes turns out that the ego has paid too high a price for the services the defense mechanisms render it. The dynamic expenditure necessary for maintaining them, and the restrictions of the ego which they almost invariably entail, prove a heavy burden on the psychical economy." There are numerous lines of research on people with a repressive style, a general style that avoids consciousness of negative affects and the thoughts or memories that could trigger such affects. They may have the advantage of a more sanguine conscious mood; but they more often have a decreased immune response under stress, heightened systolic blood pressure and increased cortisol levels; they may also have heightened susceptibility to somatic conditions including ulcers, allergies, and other medical problems. Jensen found that repressor cancer patients generally had a more positive affect; but their medical history at follow up was much worse than for non-repressors. A related example is the "avoidant" child described in the literature on attachment; although unaware of and unexpressive of an emotional reaction, the toddler is manifesting many of the autonomic arousal signs appropriate to separation anxiety. Does this child become a "repressor?"

On the other side of this coin there are shown to be advantages to making use of the symbolic realm. Pennebaker and colleagues have shown that students suffering from various kinds of trauma, who are asked to write about the trauma, make fewer visits to the student health service, and have shown improved immune function. In another example Esterling et al. (1990) have shown that writing about traumatic events seems to modulate latent Epstein-Barr virus activity.

Summary and Review

To review the arguments:

1   The semiotic model provides a *point of view* of biology and brain function that allows for a smooth crossing of the mind-brain barrier; in fact, there *is* no mind-brain barrier. From this viewpoint, brain phenomena and mind phenomena are all semiotic; they are all forms of information processes at different levels of conception.

2   The model works particularly well when the functions of interest are themselves basically informational systems, such as the central nervous system and its many communicative manifestations—for instance neuropeptide systems, hormone systems, and the neural-network systems, that generate perception, memory, affect and consciousness—as well as interpersonal systems including gesture, language, and social structure.

3   We have encountered three trichotomies. There are three major categories of signs, the icon, the index and the symbol. There are three major systems for distinguishing percepts, namely identity, location and evaluation (affect), with major brain systems devoted to these distinctions. And, the affect system itself has three major manifestations including a physiological response, an expressive display, and a subjective awareness.

4   We have noted the importance of the dissociation of these different manifestations of affect, and we may suspect that such dissociation plays a part in some psychopathology; and, the undoing of such dissociations may play a part in psychotherapy.

5   When we consider different types of signs—icon, index, and symbol—we see that each type plays a part in affect systems. An understanding of the functions of the different types may be heuristic in suggesting paths of research. And, this understanding can shed some light on questions about the time course of affect, the nature of drives and affects, dissociations of the manifestations of affect, and the functions of the different kinds of signs in affect systems.

6 6. In summary, I suggest that the point of view espoused by the semiotic model has heuristic value in the scientific study of affect, at different levels of discourse.

Notes

1 Originally Published in *Neuropsychoanalysis* (2003), Vol. 5: 81–95.
2 This description relates to the corticalized brains of higher primates, particularly the human. For a reptile with very little cortex the thalamus does the work. This is LeDoux's rapid circuit, in which response is automatic and minimally mediated.
3 In fact, in laboratory experiments with word presentation, there is a delay in conscious recognition of conflict laden words such as "cancer" or "swastika," suggesting that even with symbols there is an initial quick appraisal prior to awareness (Anscombe, 1986). In such instances, it may be that the sound pattern itself has a pre-symbolic effect, like a scream or a dog's growl, via LeDoux's rapid circuit, stimulating anxiety before its symbolic reference is appreciated. This would be interesting to research.
4 Could some of the expressive aspects of affect that are not necessary parts of the physiologic arousal, such as the raised eyebrows or the sneer, be co-evolved in a more accidental way, and as mentioned above behave like symbols?
5 Here is an example of the fact that there are almost no signs that are "pure." And many symbols have some iconic and indexical aspects, which we can see especially when we follow their etymology in a language. For instance, the word "sanguine" associates a ruddy countenance with optimism and good humor, an iconic aspect (A. Chiozza, personal communication.)
6 Two other important bodies of work address similar issues and may be complementary to the present essay. One is that of Bucci (1997), who has derived the concepts of sub-symbolic, non-verbal symbolic, and symbolic forms of communication. Another is that of Lane and Schwartz (1987, 1990), who have developed a hierarchy of expressions of affect, which has an epigenetic unfolding similar to that of Piaget in his series of cognitive stages.

References

Anscombe, R. (1986) The ego and the will. *Psychoanalysis and Contemporary Thought*, 9: 437–463.
Boysen, S., Bernston, G., Hannon, M., & Cacioppo, J. (1996) Quantity based inference and symbolic representation in chimpanzees (Pan troglodytes). *Journal of Experimental Psychology and Animal Behavior Processes*, 22: 76–86.
Bucci, W. (1997) *Psychoanalysis and Cognitive Science: a Multiple Code Theory*. New York: Guilford Press.
Clyman, R. B. (1991) The procedural organization of emotions: a contribution from cognitive science to the psychoanalytic theory of therapeutic action. *Journal of the American Psychoanalytic Association*, 39 (suppl.): 349–382.
Crick, F. (1994) *The Astonishing Hypothesis: The Scientific Search for the Soul*. New York: Scribners.
Crick, F. & Koch, C. (2000) The unconscious homunculus. *Neuropsychoanalysis*, 2: 3–11.

Damasio, A. (1999) *The Feeling of What Happens*. New York: Harcourt Brace.

Damasio, A., Grabowski, T. J., Bechara, A, Damasio, H., Ponto, L. L. B., Parvisi, J, & Hichwa, R. D. (2000) Subcortical and cortical brain activity during the feeling of self generated emotions. *Nature Neuroscience*, 3: 1049–1056.

Deacon, T. (1997) *The Symbolic Species*. New York: W.W. Norton.

Dennett, D. (1991) *Consciousness Explained*. London: Penguin.

Eagle, M. (1998) Freud's Legacy: Defenses, somatic symptoms and neurophysiology. In G. Guttmann & I. Scholz-Strasser, Eds, *Freud and the Neurosciences: From Brain Research to the Unconscious*. Vienna: Osterreichischen Akademie der Wissenschaften.

Ekman, P. (1994) All emotions are basic. In P. Ekman & R. J. Davidson, Eds, *The Nature of Emotion: Fundamental Questions*. New York, Oxford: Oxford University Press, pp. 15–19.

Ekman, P. & Freisen, W. V. (1978) *Facial Action Coding System*. Palo Alto, CA: Consulting Psychologists Press.

Esterling, B. A., Antoni, M. H., Kumar, M., & Schneiderman, N. (1990) Emotional repression, stress disclosure responses, and Epstein-Barr capsid viral antigen titres. *Psychosomatic Medicine*, 52: 397–410.

Freud, S. (1915) The Unconscious. *Standard Edition*, 14: London: Hogarth Press, 1962.

Heller, M. & Haynal, V. (1997) The doctor's face: a mirror of his patient's suicidal projects. In J. Guimon (Ed.), *The Body in Psychotherapy*. Basel: Karger, pp. 46–51.

Hofer, M. (1997). An evolutionary perspective on anxiety. In S. P.Roose & R. A. Glick, Eds, *Anxiety as Symptom and Signal*. Hillsdale, NJ: Analytic Press.

Humphrey, N. K. (1984) *Consciousness Regained*. New York, Oxford: Oxford University Press.

Lakoff, G. & Johnson, M. (1980) *Metaphors We Live By*. Chicago, IL: University of Chicago Press.

Lane, R. D. & Schwartz, G. E. (1987) Levels of emotional awareness: A cognitive developmental theory and its application to psychopathology. *American Journal of Psychiatry*.

Lane, R. D., Schwartz, G. E., Walker, P. A., et al. (1990) The Levels of Emotional Awareness Scale: A cognitive-developmental measure of emotion. *Journal of Personal Assessment*, 55: 124–134.

Lane, R. D., Sechrest, L., Reidel, R., Weldon, V., Kaszniak, A., & Schwartz, G. E. (1996) *Psychosomatic Medicine*, 58: 203–210.

LeDoux, J. (1996) *The Emotional Brain*. New York, Simon & Schuster.

Olds, D. D. (1990) Brain centered psychology. *Psychoanalysis. and Contemporary Thought*, 13: 331–363.

Olds, D. D. (2000) A Semiotic Model of Mind. *Journal of the American Psychoanalytic Association*, 48: 497–529.

Panksepp, J. (1994) The basics of basic emotion. In P. Ekman & R. J. Davidson, Eds, *The Nature of Emotion: Fundamental Questions*. New York: Oxford, pp. 20–24.

Panksepp, J. (1998) *Affective Neuroscience*. New York, Oxford: Oxford University Press.

Panksepp, J. (2000) Commentary on the unconscious homunculus. *Neuropsychoanalysis*, 2: 24–32.

Peirce, C. S. (1897) *Logic as Semiotic: The Theory of Signs; reprinted in Semiotics: An Introductory Anthology*, Ed. R. E. Innis. Bloomington, IN: Indiana University Press, 1985.

Shevrin, H. (1997) Psychoanalysis as the patient: high in feeling, low in energy. *Journal of the American Psychoanalytic Association*, 45 (3): 841–864.

Solms, M. (1997) What is consciousness? *Journal of the American Psychoanalytic Association*, 45: 681–703.

Chapter 11

Nonlinear Systems Theory and Psychoanalysis

Symposium in Honor of Emmanuel Ghent

Introduction

This issue of Psychoanalytic Dialogues is assembled as a tribute to Emanuel Ghent, a beloved analyst and teacher who died on March 31, 2003. Mannie was one of the founders of the Relational Track at the NYU Postdoctoral Program, and he was a training analyst at the William Alanson White Institute. He had a long-standing interest in the frontiers of psychoanalytic thinking and devoted much attention to dynamic systems theory. He studied the work of Gerald Edelman and wrote an important paper (Ghent, 2002) amalgamating Edelman's theories, dynamic systems models, and current psychoanalytic concepts. It is therefore appropriate that a section of this issue includes three essays by thinkers in the realm of dynamic systems.

Readers of this section have a treat in store. The three papers in it give a clear and readable introduction to what many feel is an intimidating conceptual paradigm. The need for such a paradigm has emerged in recent decades as it has become clear that we have not had an intellectual instrument to help us understand the complex biological and psychological world in which we live. Dynamic systems theory is one that helps to fill in this deficit in our understanding.

For those with little previous exposure to systems models, the papers will provide an interesting and friendly introduction. For those who are more familiar with this thinking, each paper will clarify and embellish what they know. And each provides different examples of the beauty of the models. Craig Piers presents the scientific and visual patterns of chaos and fractals, Esther Thelen shows the basic applications to motor learning and physical movements, and Stephen Seligman provides applications to clinical experience and psychological development.

Here's what emerges in the theory. Biological and psychological models have long had a linear format. This format emphasizes what Aristotle called the efficient cause, a preceding event in a physical causal chain. In theory, if we know all the efficient causes at any given time, we should be able to predict events into the indefinite future. In psychoanalytic models of the past century, a similar model held sway. Psychic determinism was a foundation for the

DOI: 10.4324/9781003399551-12

understanding of mental life; therefore, future events should be predictable if we know all the variables. Major factors included drive, defense, and constitution, as well as the vicissitudes of sexual stages, resolution of the Oedipus complex, and so on. Given this battery of causal factors, we could look back into the history of the adult analysand and give a causal psychodynamic explanation of the person's present state. The sense that we could retrospectively explain things produced an impression that mental processes were determined and potentially predictable. The fact that our backward-looking explanations explained everything, and were unfalsifiable, enhanced our illusion of predictability, at least until the attacks by epistemologists such as Gruenbaum.

We have more recently been confronted with the fact that although some things are predictable - in most cases, a girl will become a woman, a certain gene structure will produce Down's syndrome, and a loss will engender sadness - the fine structure of the future is in principle not predictable beyond certain levels of probability. Identical twins may share many tastes and dislikes, but not all, and we cannot predict which. It has turned out that prospective prediction is impossible, not only because we do not happen to know all the variables contributing to behavior, but because we can't know all the variables. Important to the model is the interactive nature of the world. X speaks to Y, and Y responds with a 99.9% predictable response, but after X and Y have been in dialogue for 100 interactions, the .1% error rate blossoms into uncertainty. This conclusion has opened us to the new paradigm, and it has shown the need for at least a descriptive model that can contain the causal structure of nature and the fact that complexity can lead to unpredictability. When we look at it this way, the surprising thing is that there is any predictability at all. This is the value of chaotic systems and attractors; they give partial predictability within certain limits.

There is an apparent paradox. We now think that we cannot know all the factors between Time A and Time B, say, in the development of an organism. But even so, the model has increased our awareness of the richness of detail between A and B. We get an appreciation that some of those details may generate surprising swings in growth, such that a child from an abusive, impoverished home may do well, whereas a privileged child may do poorly. The concept that in complex systems, there is an extreme sensitivity to initial conditions means that we can never reproduce perfectly all of the variables. We don't give up determinism, but the model takes the sting out of the reduction to physical variables that has seemed to many thinkers to go beyond freedom and dignity and into a mechanical clockwork model. The idea that the current state is the product of all previous history of both the self and the entire environment leads to a more interactive self, interacting with the world and other people. The three papers that follow flesh out the implications of this concept in different and complementary ways. Piers gives us a rich, mathematically based description of the dynamic systems model. Although many find equations intimidating, it is worth a try to follow his elegant presentation showing how a system becomes chaotic in the dynamic sense. The paper gives a solid introduction to this theoretical underpinning of dynamic systems. The author has a twofold ambition: first, to present the mathematical models, and second, to show how they may fit clinical psychological phenomena, such as character rigidity and preservation of the self in the face of internal multiplicity and defensive dissociation. Some may wish to see this as purely metaphorical, an analogy to psychological structures; and some may accept it as a model that directly describes them. In either case, it provides an illuminating and mind-expanding view.

Esther Thelen's contribution is a concise explanation of how dynamic systems theory can illuminate processes of development, in humans as well as in other animals. Her classic experiments showing the continuity in the maturation of a child's motor skills have become part of the foundation of the theory. Her work has been a convincing counter to traditional linear theories of development; her experiments have dealt with the apparent discontinuity in an infant's spontaneous early leg movements, which are precursors to walking. A classical statement of the theory from her paper is this:

> How a child behaves depends not only on the immediate current situation, but also on his or her continuous short- and longer-term history of acting, the social situation, and the biological constraints he or she was born with. Every action has within it the traces of previous behavior. The child's behavior, in turn, sculpts his or her environment, creating new opportunities and constraints.

Seligman's paper is the most directly clinical one. He shares with us clinical reports and vignettes that cross the difficult terrain between theory and practice. Although most of the technical implications of the complexity theories have not been worked out, he gives some clear examples of the direction in which the theory is taking us. There is a shift away from an emphasis on single or even repeated events and traumas as unique causes of current states, and a move toward the nature of current process, even though we may find it useful to know about early trauma as a contributor to the personality. Here the emphasis is on the rigidity of structure and how this rigidity interferes with both current functioning and the ability to grow and mature. Dynamic systems theory requires, and also permits, a different mode of thinking. Seligman contrasts the "either-or" mode of linear reductionism with the "both-and" mode of complex thinking. The latter is most useful to psychoanalysis, which has already been adopting this way of thinking over recent decades as analysts have become aware of the complex vicissitudes of development and of human interactions. He implies that we have been adapting to this mode-but implicitly-as we have taken on a more dialogic, intersubjective approach to our analytic work. The dynamic systems model has given us a theory to help us understand what we have intuitively come to.

Where will dynamic systems theory take us? It is a body of theory evolving over the past half century. Early theories such as von Bertalanffy's general systems theory began to confront the problems inherent in linear causal thinking, and to deal with multilevel causal trains. It even gave voice to the idea of equifinality, an idea somewhat like Aristotle's final cause. This allows us to include "top-down causation" in our explanatory reasoning, in that fantasies may contribute to decision making, or adaptation may contribute to evolutionary development. A more recent theoretical model has been that of connectionism, or neural network theory. This is a parallel processing model in which multiple causal chains contribute to complex end results, mostly applied to neuronal systems and computer simulations of brain functions. It has provided useful models to explain how perceptual systems can identify and classify objects or how a language learner masters syntax. The current dynamic systems model is similar to the earlier ones, but it has added the mathematical models of chaos, attractor systems, and fractals, all necessary concepts in dealing with truly complex systems.

From our vantage point today, it appears that dynamic systems theory is destined to play an important role in the future of psychoanalytic theory. But whose future? Dynamic systems theory meshes particularly well with the relational, interpersonal models and may collaborate productively with the increasing information coming from the biological sciences. But will it be limited to "American psychoanalysis," described by Mitchell and Harris (2004) as moving into the extra- and interpersonal spaces emphasizing the dyad and focusing less on the individual interior? Could it be useful to the British and Continental and South American schools, in which one-person psychology is still prevalent? I see no reason why the theory could not be applied in more traditional analytic psychologies. The brain works on dynamic principles, and the biological substrates of affects and cognition develop according to dynamic models of ontogeny. But it is hard to predict if dynamic systems theory will be seen as interesting and useful to other schools of psychoanalysis.

In the meantime, the models are proving to be incredibly important in the evolution of the analytic theories based on ego psychology and object relations, and especially to the newly emerging theories that make use of input from the biological and brain sciences.

References

Ghent, E. (2002) Wish, need, drive: Motive in the light of dynamic systems theory and Edelman's selectionist theory. *Psychoanalytic Dialogues*, 12: 763–808.

Mitchell, S. A. & Harris, A. (2004) What's American about American psychoanalysis? *Psychoanalytic Dialogues*, 14: 165–191.

Chapter 12

Identification

Psychoanalytic and Biological Perspectives[1]

Introduction

Now that psychoanalysis and cognitive science are beginning to speak to each other, there is a strong wish to find ideas and concepts that will bridge between the two worlds, and allow for conversation and mutual exploration and research. Since psychoanalysis has been traveling its isolated path, increasingly distant from the behavioral and mind sciences, several historical trends in the evolution of psychological constructs have emerged: One is that the same *term* has been used in both realms but in different ways. Examples might be *memory*, not carefully defined or explored in psychoanalysis, but increasingly differentiated into diverse types in cognitive psychology. Or, the concept of the *unconscious*: analysts tend to refer to the *dynamic unconscious*, while other sciences may study the *cognitive unconscious*, unaware of implications of conflict and repression.

Another trend is that a *concept* has developed in one field and not in another. Phenomena such as *conditioning, procedural memory* and *priming* have been the objects of intense research elsewhere, but are only now creeping into the analyst's vocabulary. In the other direction the same is true in that some of our concepts, such as *transference* and *internalization,* are unfamiliar, and uninteresting, to non-psychoanalysts. Currently bridges between the two areas are being built. On the one hand, books such as Pally (2000) and Solms and Turnbull (2002) have presented cognitive science concepts to psychoanalysts. On the other, a great deal of research has been done of interest to both sides, for instance the burgeoning infant-observation research, the developments in attachment theories, and the psychological research into psychoanalytic concepts, such as that of Shevrin and his colleagues (e.g. Shevrin et al., 1996).

A third project, which is only beginning, is that of taking major *psychoanalytic concepts* and connecting them to the outside scientific world, so that on one hand they may be better explained and defined scientifically, and on the other, that they be made intelligible and brought into the dialogue with cognitive scientists.

DOI: 10.4324/9781003399551-13

In this paper I hope to make a preliminary attempt to perform a piece of this third task with the concept of *identification*. First, I will briefly review some of the psychoanalytic views on this phenomenon as a subtype of the more general concept, internalization. I will try looking at some of the information coming from other disciplines that might elaborate our understanding of our concept. In doing this I will be mindful of the fact that when one discusses higher forms of mental function such as the self, internalization, memory, empathy, and consciousness, it is hard to separate one and omit discussion of the others. Each term explains much about the other terms, but it would be a very large book that would try to deal with them all. For example, identification plays a major part in the development of the ego, the self, and object relations. Identification, as well as introjection, is important in the establishment of moral values, the superego. Empathy and identification are closely entwined. These neighboring entities will be mentioned but not fully explored.

In a nutshell my argument is this. We analysts have elaborated several concepts under the rubric of internalization, based on many years of experience with our patients. We have described the phenomena more fully and richly than any other discipline. We may now be in a position to add information about the evolutionary and biological roots of these phenomena. I will argue that the evolution of primates led to a high level of imitative ability in parallel with cortical expansion, which allowed for new forms of memory. The neurobiologist's discovery of the mirror neuron revealed a property of brain by which it perceives by virtually enacting others' actions. In infant development a dyadic interchange takes place involving imitations and attunements, so that the infant takes on many characteristics of the parent in the process of internalizing behavior, affects, and communicative skills including language. We can speculate that there has been an evolution leading to human identification that would involve 1) the evolution of multiple memory systems, in particular procedural memory; 2) mirror neurons developing in mammals; 3) imitation evolving in mammals and increasing in importance in primates; 4) the prolonged plasticity of human childhood allowing for imitation and attunement; and 5) most recently the advance of mentalism or theory of mind possibly exclusively in humans. The evolutionary push to imitation and internalization may have social roots beyond the value to the individual, particularly in the transfer of culture.

Although I will briefly review some of the psychoanalytic ideas on the subject, mainly in order to introduce the concept, the aim of the paper is to bring in views from other sciences that might enrich our understanding of the phenomenon. There are many different biological disciplines, and their fields of interest often overlap. I will choose from among them a few that have produced information on the topics I want to use in the discussion. I will first draw from cognitive psychology some information on the different types of memory, as well as some data and opinion about types of learning, particularly *instruction, practice* and *conditioning*. In order to discuss another term important in the discussion, *imitation*, I will turn to the animal behaviorists who have been working intensely with primates as well as other animals to understand imitation, and to differentiate it from other forms of learning. In bringing in information about imitation and attunement, now in human infants, I will look to some of the infant observation literature. I will briefly question what is the influence of genetics on the transmission of characteristics we often associate with identification, by introducing some information from genetic research. Finally, I will consult the neurobiologists who have advanced the idea of the *mirror neuron*. Although I am looking at several sciences in a brief and selective way, I hope to gather some findings that may come together to enlarge our view of the concept under discussion.

Most psychoanalytic discussions in this area, begin with the larger concept of internalization, and discuss identification within that context (i.e. Schafer, 1968; Meissner, 1971). In order to make the topic manageable I will introduce identification under the larger rubric, but then will focus the discussion on identification alone.

Identification and Internalization

In psychoanalytic thinking, the term internalization has a long and rich history. From Freud's use of the terms identification, introjection and incorporation to current use of these concepts, there has been a focus on the apparent fact that representations of objects and object relations, are stored in the mind, and that they exist not only as percepts or stored images, but that they alter the person and structure the personality. For analysts the concept of internalization has a robust and almost unquestioned validity and usefulness in clinical work. When we see a person acting, often unconsciously, just like mother or father, we have no hesitation in referring to identification with, or internalization of the parent. However, in many areas of the world of cognitive science, the term internalization seems to have very little use. I have asked a couple of memory researchers about the term and they had never heard of it, and when it is explained to them, they find it mildly interesting but of no particular relevance to them. I have found this fact curious and disturbing. My point is that here is a useful and meaningful concept that analysts have been working with for about a century, and that the brain researchers have not taken into account and have not considered worthy of research. If we are to bring our concept into the wider world, it will be helpful if we can relate it to the language and research of the brain sciences. We may learn something about our concept and find it more scientifically validated, and the brain scientists may see our concept as potentially worthy of further investigation in their particular disciplines.

Let us focus in closer on our use of the concept of internalization. Schafer (1968) has given a classic and still useful set of definitions for most of the terms surrounding the concept. He describes a basic triad. *Incorporation* involves a kind of fantasy of taking in the object in a way that resembles eating it. The fantasy is of taking in the whole object, which one may then identify with. *Introjection* is the taking in of the object as a kind of fantasy and retaining that object in a virtual inner space such that one can have a dialogue with it. This may more accurately be described as internalizing the object *relationship,* in the form of a virtual dyad. In the relationship mental space, the introject remains other; it may be a source of self-criticism, self-admiration, advice, warning, generally feeling like an internalized parent. Thus, introjection is one of the central mechanisms for the internalization of moral values. *Identification* is the modification of the self to resemble the other; with identification the object does not remain as an inner other.

The history of the concepts has been much more complex than the above suggests. There have been other definitions of the terms. For instance, Loewald (1973) saw identification as an early phenomenon, pre-individuation, so that the infant and parent are one. Subsequently the forms of internalization may be defensive in nature as attempts to repair the awareness of the loss of an object. Loewald and others have seen internalization as a taking in of regulatory mechanisms, which are at first provided to the infant from parents, and which later serve as internal regulators in an autonomous individual. Important to him is that identification is a primitive pre-differentiation state, which may persist into adulthood. In analysis, a patient may start out in that state or regress to it.

For Loewald, internalization was a developmental end result, in which the self separates intrapsychically from the object to form an autonomous self. "In internalization it is a matter of transforming these relations into an internal, intrapsychic depersonalized relationship, thus increasing and enriching psychic structure: the identity with the object is renounced." (p. 15) Etchegoyen (1985), in his comprehensive review, speaks of primary and secondary identification, the former being a pre-differentiation phenomenon, the other being a taking-in of the other after the other has become a separate object.

Schafer himself radically reviewed the concepts in his paper, "Internalization: Process or Fantasy?" (1972). In his attempt to clarify analytic concepts using Action Language, he imposed a behaviorist scheme on our vocabulary, attempting to root out the many reifications of abstract concepts that infest our language. The various forms of internalization came under this knife in the attempt to get rid of the somewhat mystical or ghostly aspects we give to "introjects" and "identifications." He concluded that the only real entity that could be salvaged was the fact that people do *fantasize* that they have incorporated another person, or that they are speaking to an internalized other. Although analysts still seem to use internalization concepts in this reified way, and sprinkle the terms liberally in their case reports, Schafer's attempt was useful in at least pushing us to try to clarify these complex concepts.

When we look at how the term is used, we see there are two major sub-types. One might call incorporation and introjection "ingestive" or "interiorizing;" they involve the idea of taking another personal object inside some kind of space. This differs from identification, which has to do more with imitation, taking on the characteristics of the other. We might say that one is a fantasy of taking in the body of the other, while the other is taking on the form or the identity of the other.

Identification

Now to bring the focus onto the phenomenon of identification. This term also has many meanings, some of them confusing and mutually contradictory. Many analysts see identification as the process of changing the self to resemble the other, consciously or non-consciously. This may be for a child identifying with parents, for friends or spouses identifying with each other, or patients identifying with analysts.

Identification also can be thought of as a process and as a result (Hartman & Loewenstein, 1962). The *process* implies the verb "to identify," and that itself has two meanings. One involves imitation, conscious and unconscious, as well as more practical aspects of learning procedures and patterns of behavior that resemble the other. One may identify also with the goals and values of the other, and take one's life in the direction of achieving those goals. A second meaning of the term is as an influence on perception; it is apprehension of the other as similar to oneself. Analysts sometimes use the term in the sense of thinking of oneself as like the other, often inappropriately so, as in "pathological identification," or "over-identification"—thinking one is more like the other, or that the other is more like one, than one really is.

There are also important differences with respect to the nature of the *object* identified with. We think of identifying with beloved objects, certainly common in childhood and with lovers, mentors, leaders, and friends throughout life. In this vein there may be identification with an idealized object in generating a "wished for self-image (Milrod, 1982). There is also identification with the lost object, described by Freud, Bowlby and many others. This is usually seen as a defensive measure, a way of—in fantasy and imitative action—trying to reverse the loss. This seems to be a necessary step in the process of mourning. A third is identification with the aggressor. Anna Freud and others saw this in children of the holocaust. A classic paper by Emch (1944) posits that in some cases, where one or both parents are "unknowable," because of chaotic, violent, or unpredictable behavior, or prolonged absence, the child may imitate the most salient behaviors with the unconscious aim of providing some predictability in the child's troubled life. Coates and Moore (1997) have written about this in abused children where the imitation and identification with the terrifying opposite-sex parent is so intense that it can lead to extreme identification resulting in gender identity change.

Now let us turn to other disciplines and see how some of their findings may help illuminate our topic.

The View from Cognitive Psychology and Memory Research

The branch of mind science that deals with mental phenomenology, derived from the clinical examination and psychometric testing of patients is usually referred to as cognitive psychology or neuro-psychology. This discipline took some of the first great steps towards the association of behavioral pathology and lesions of the brain. In so doing much of the brain was mapped out during the 19th and 20th centuries. With respect to neuro-psychological investigation and memory there is the classical example of the case of HM, in which the patient underwent surgery for the bilateral removal of his hip-pocampus and later revealed a severe amnesia (Scoville & Milner, 1957). This led researchers to the association of the hippocampus and *episodic memory* for recent events, and the separation of this function from the learning of skills and habits, now referred to as *procedural memory*. Solms and Kaplan-Solms (2001) have recently made a major contribution in this tradition in relating brain anatomy to higher mental functions of particular interest to psychoanalysis. Until recently this *clinico-pathological method* relied on autopsy studies to confirm the anatomical correlations with pathology. In recent years much of that work can be done using imaging technology.

The procedural subtype of memory may be an important aspect of the identification process, because it is habits and skills and behavior patterns that we imitate in taking on the characteristics of the other.

Procedural Memory

Procedural memory has come forward in recent years as one of the types that may be particularly relevant to psychoanalysis. Clyman (1991), in a by now classic paper, has described a kind of emotional procedural memory, that represents the emotional schemas developed in childhood, and which becomes a building block of transference in later life. This has shown promise of being a kind of bridge between memory research and the basic concepts of psychoanalysis. How are procedures learned?

We might consider that procedures are learned from several sources, which have been studied by neuro-psychology; let us look at some of the more important ones: *instruction, practice, conditioning and imitation.*

Instruction. Instruction may be a uniquely human phenomenon since most definitions of instruction involve language. This part of the process may itself be conscious, since it is partly verbal and often the result of a deliberate conscious wish to learn. Primatologists have studied chimpanzees to find evidence of actual instruction in the sense of the adult actively teaching an infant, and have found very little. A mother may facilitate the learning of nut-cracking by doing it in the presence of the infant, but there seems to be nothing like the human activity of deliberately showing and helping to learn. This fact goes along with the notion that, as far as we know, chimpanzees do not develop a theory mind as it is conceived by students of human development. In human teaching, the steps of a procedure may be spoken aloud and may be memorized in words. These words can guide behavior into channels where only practice will make perfect.

Practice. An important way to learn a procedure for humans is to start with the instructions and keep trying until one goes beyond them to a "feeling" that one has mastered it. This feeling of mastery, derived from getting the piano piece or the golf stroke just right, lies in the behavioral realm and is usually beyond words. As in the case of instruction, non-humans don't seem to explicitly use practice to improve a skill, although they do "try and try again," and such repetition may improve performance.

Less familiar to us as sources of procedural learning are *conditioning,* and *imitation.* The first is the *primary source of learning* in most animals. As we will discuss later, imitation has emerged as very important in higher primates. And as recent work has shown they are not always easy to distinguish from each other, with some workers holding that conditioning is the only form of learning in non-human species.

Conditioning

I use this term to refer to the forms of learning that are "consequence contingent"—forms that rely on reward and punishment. Classical behavioral theory distinguished two major types of conditioning. One, made famous by Pavlov, is *respondent* or *classical* conditioning. In this form, two stimuli are paired such as food and a bell. Pavlov found that after some experience with dogs with such a pairing, the dog responded to the bell as well as to the food, with an expectant salivary response and other indications of expecting something to eat. The other form is operant conditioning in which the animal is "rewarded" by doing certain things. In the classical experiment a rat would tend to push a lever after finding by accident that after it pushed the lever, food would appear. Operant learning is thought to be important in much procedural learning.

The literature on imitation and conditioning is often confused because what looks like imitation in one person's definition is actually conditioning in another's. The difference between the two is quite important. Conditioning may be the earliest form of learning, available even to paramecia; imitation seems to be a recent achievement, some would say available only to humans. If we turn to the animal behaviorists, we can gain more insight into this phenomenon.

The View from Animal Behavior Research

Another discipline that has contributed information relevant to our subject is the group of sciences of animal behavior, including evolutionary biology, physical anthropology, and primatology. From them a great deal has been learned about imitation.

Imitation

Byrne's (Byrne & Russon, 1998) rigorous definition of imitation is the *learning of novel behaviors by way of observation*, in a process that can be differentiated from the complex set of other behavioral learning modes. Imitation itself is a complex phenomenon as yet not well understood. The process of copying would seem to be straightforward. In fact, we may see an imitation-like phenomenon in newborn infants, who stick out their tongues in apparent imitation of another person (Meltzoff, 1990). Children seem to learn much of what they do by this method, most obviously language. Smith (2001) points out that the phenomenon is not limited to children. His description of the way residents in the class he was teaching began to shuffle in their gait and tend to smoke pipes, in imitation of their charismatic mentor, is a striking example in adults.

Aping In Apes

Franz de Waal who runs the Yerkes Primate Center in Atlanta, has made intensive study of the higher cognitive abilities of apes. His recent book title, *The Ape and the Sushi Master* (2001), refers to the lore that an apprentice sushi master spends many years doing scullery work in the Master's kitchen before being allowed even to touch a knife. After all these years he is ceremoniously given a knife and is an expert, simply because he has been watching the master at work.

Curiously, de Waal (2001) uses the term "identification," but in not quite the same way as do analysts. In his usage, the term relates to the intense bond between one primate and another, or a non-human primate and a human. His concern is the nature and in fact the actuality of *culture* in monkeys and primates. Much of culture is passed on through generations by various forms of learning by imitation. He denotes this phenomenon using the acronym, BIOL – Bonding and Identification-based Observational Learning. He points out that in the past people have described apes as *merely* imitating, as though this is an inconsequential capacity. We now view it as a high-level function. He says:

"Think about it: how does one get from watching another individual's actions to performing the same actions for the same purpose? Imitation requires that visual input is converted into motor output, telling the body to re-enact what the eyes saw."

(de Waal, 2001; p. 219)

There are countless examples of complex imitation by primates, especially primates raised by humans. The imitation often has no obvious reward. Russon (1996, p. 166) describes an orangutan imitating the entire process of brushing teeth, using a toothbrush to mimic this human activity. Another example is represented in a photograph taken by Robert Yerkes in 1923; in the picture we see a young bonobo, Prince Chim, sitting with a book in hand looking convincingly as though he is reading intently (de Waal, 2001). Some imitations, such as those which yield food from cracked nuts, or from a refrigerator, yield obvious rewards. But many, such as the "teeth-brushing" and the "reading" yield no apparent immediate benefits.

De Waal's view is that in primates a *primary drive to imitate* is at work, its reward being the sense of conformity in a group. In a relatively strict view of imitation, it is learning new behavior. It is not just stringing together known behaviors—by copying a model, a parent or a peer, *the goal being secondary in importance to the act of copying itself.* Implied in this is an emotional bond between the mentor and pupil, such that the pupil wishes to imitate the mentor in order to be like that person, or to enhance the bond with that person.

De Waal's version of the evolutionary development leading to human culture holds that early monkeys and later primates evolved imitative skills, which have led to (non in-born) cultural advances. Examples are the learning to wash sand-covered potatoes in Japanese macaques, and the cracking of very hard nuts by chimpanzees.

When primates are raised by humans their mimicry abilities are given full reign because now, they have much more complex beings to copy. Thus, human-raised chimpanzees and bonobos have shown advances in communication and language skill that are astounding. There are now two interpretations of this phenomenon. Tomasello (1999) who has raised chimpanzees and written about the differences between them and humans with respect to intentionality and theory of mind, views the imitative capacity as one that is engendered by being raised in human company. In other words, a new capacity has emerged in the new environment. De Waal (2001) disagrees and feels that imitation begins with early primates and occurs in the wild, and expands when they are raised by humans because, in their earliest most plastic phase, they form intense attachments to humans. This motivates them to use their already extant imitative ability to mimic human culture up to their physical and neurological potential capacities.

What has become clear is that this *plastic* phase really is plastic, and allows for impressive environmental influence. Apes raised in the wild do show a culture learned from their fellows. But put them with humans, and they take impressive further steps in cognitive and cultural abilities. The "poster boy" of this enterprise is Kanzi, a male bonobo raised and taught by Sue Savage-Rumbaugh at Georgia State University (Savage-Rumbaugh & Lewis, 1994; Shanker & King, 2002). The surprising thing about this story was that Savage-Rumbaugh had for some time been trying to teach an adult female, Kanzi's adoptive mother, to learn and use linguistic symbols. The mother did very poorly, and the teaching was finally brought to an end. Only then was it discovered that the infant Kanzi, who had been present during all the lessons, suddenly demonstrated that he had learned most of what was being taught. Now Kanzi may be the world's leading ape linguist.

Minding in Humans

Michael Tomasello (1999) has written an important book based on research in both primates and human children, describing a great deal of work showing the similarities and differences in cognitive abilities and social skills at the two evolutionary levels. His central argument is that in the first year of life the human infant develops a unique cognitive ability, namely an ability to sense the intentionality of another person, to sense that the other person has goals and a causal will like one's own. In his view, this revolution, occurring at about nine months of age, does not happen in any other primate.

The key observation with children in the end of the first year is that they find the need to *share* experience. They point to objects to draw them to another's attention, they hold things up for show, they bring others to an object to see it, and they demonstrate actions to show others. This inherently social capacity, lays the groundwork for much of the evolution the human is heir to. One important ability is the understanding of causality, which Tomasello attributes to the extension of the sense of the other's intentionality to explain forces and causes in the inanimate world. This would be expected to enhance the ability to make and use tools and develop technology.

The nine-month-old's appreciation of another's intentionality is part of a series in the ontology of interpersonal understanding. He describes three levels. The first is in young infants: understanding others as "animate beings," appreciating behavior and even goal-like direction of motion. This capacity is present in all primates and many other mammals. The second is the appreciation of intentionality in the nine-month-old. The third occurs at about four years of age when others are understood as "mental agents." With this third stage the child not only understands the other as having an interior self and will, but also begins to understand what the other may know or be thinking.

With respect to imitation, there is something that should be mentioned about evolutionary "advance." Deacon (1997) has made the point that in order to learn to symbolize, hominid species may have had to *lose* some of their talent for operant learning. Trial and error learning is a high art among other primates. He feels that in order to move beyond the immediate reward system, and into symbols, we had to become worse at operant learning; we had to be able to distance ourselves from immediate contingency or consequences of behavior in order to let the symbolic world take shape. This is a hard concept to grasp. But an experiment by Tomasello (1999) and colleagues may show an apposite point, in that all human capacities may not be simply bigger and better. In an experiment comparing the learning of certain tasks by chimpanzees and young children, tasks that *required operant learning more than imitation* were learned *faster* by the apes. Human children tended to use somewhat slavish imitation, while the chimps were quicker to modify technique to achieve certain goals. This supports the argument that imitation serves a social purpose. It also suggests that the new skill might not be in itself, in the short run, more adaptive for the individual; and, the finding may in fact clarify Deacon's point. A more accurate way of saying this might be: as we became more social, social skills, including imitation, became increasingly important—relative to operant learning—for survival in the group, and indeed for the survival *of* the group. The evolving brain then enhanced imitative skills relative to, or possibly at the expense of, operant-associative learning skills. Thus, as human cultures developed, we might expect that *imitation of rituals*, in themselves not beneficial to the individual, would be supported because they enhance the group's purposes, and its communal identity.

Infant Observation

At this point we have taken an evolutionary approach up to the development of the human infant. This brings us to the science of infant observation, wherein the ontogeny of identification may be observed. That body of information is too vast for this paper, and I will only point to some findings that will most likely be relevant to a more complete description of the process.

The phenomena of imitation in humans have been intensely studied by the recent generation of infant observers, including Stern, Beebe and Lachman, Jaffe and others. One impressive phenomenon is the interaction between mother and infant under the concept of attunement. These researchers have described in detail the kinds of imitative and reactive, contingent interactions that go on all day in the life of an infant. There are imitations particularly of rhythms, of expressions, of sounds in a process of turn-taking that seems a prototype for later conversation and empathic intercourse. This is one of several aspects of human infancy that seems not to be shared with other mammals. One quality of it is its multi-modality, so that a rhythm may be manifested by a rattle in the baby and hand-clapping or body movements in the mother. The process seems to include practice in integrating multiple sensory modes as well as internalizing aspects of the dyadic process.

However, as we learn more about the early infancy experience from the infant observation researchers, we have to deal with a kind of phenomenon different from simple imitation. With Stern's attunement experience there is a trading back and forth of different sensory-modal expressions, which seem to set up an integrated inter-modal experience, leading to results that would seem to be internalization at a very fundamental level. It seems that the infant is being introduced to human experience itself, to the rudiments of taking in the world in a complex multi-modal way, apparently different from the upbringing of other primates. This occurs in a creature that develops into a complex social, symbolic, linguistic being orders of magnitude beyond the pongids.

This interactive biofeedback process must be the first form of internalization in the baby's life. It is an exchange of signs, whose "meanings" develop in the very process of exchanging them. Several workers have described the result of these interactions as a kind of internalization. Bowlby used the term "Internal working models"—mental entities representing the dyad as an internal set of expectations and procedures. Stern used a similar concept, the "RIG" or "representation of interactions that have been generalized."

The Effects of the Genes

Now let's look to an account from the point of view the science of genetics and the inter-generational transfer of traits and behavior patterns. There is considerable research showing the immense influence of the genes. Biological science seems to go through phases wherein the gene becomes all-important. Fonagy (2002) points out that the pendulum has recently swung far in this direction. One argument from this perspective is that one reason children appear to internalize and identify with parents is that they share similar genes. In this way of thinking, the fact that an abused child grows up to be an abusing parent indicates mostly that that child inherited major traits genetically from the parent. There are also many studies of twins that show uncanny similarities in adult twins who were raised apart in very different circumstances. Does this mean that all this discussion of identification is currently irrelevant, since this mechanism might account for only a tiny, possibly insignificant, portion of what is passed down from the parents?

It does complicate the picture, since twins raised apart also do have differences. The picture may be partly clarified if we see that certain genetic configurations seem to have effects on the identification process itself. As Kandel (1999) has argued, experience can alter gene expression. For example, a recent New Zealand study (Caspi, 2002) showed that in a prospectively observed group, followed from childhood to adulthood, one genetic configuration predicted greater similarity in parents and offspring. A sub-group of the children carried a gene coding for a monoamine oxidase that was a variant from the rest (MAOA). Of the whole group, some of the children were seriously physically abused by their parents. Either the nature theory or the nurture theory could predict that those children would become violent abusers. However, it turned out that those with the MAOA variant who were abused were more likely to become abusers, while those who did not have it were not more likely to show that behavior. And those with the variant gene who grew up in non-violent homes were *not* more prone to violence. Here is a complex interaction between gene and environment that seems to influence the tendency to identify. In other words, it may be that some people identify with certain traits more than others, depending on genetic make-up.

Neurobiology and Mirror Neurons

Let us now turn to see what we can learn from another science about internalization, the fertile field of neurobiology. A new viewpoint on imitative learning and some other types of motor learning, including language, makes use of the recently described phenomenon of *mirror neurons*. [2] The work of Rizzolatti and others has demonstrated this entity in monkeys (Rizzolatti, et al., 1996; Gallese & Goldman, 1998). A monkey, in their experiment, wears an array of micro-electrodes that record the activation of individual neurons in the cortex. When the monkey picks up a morsel of food and puts it in its mouth, a characteristic read-out appears, one aspect of which is a recognizable neuronal activity in the pre-motor cortex. The pre-motor cortex has been known for years to be where co-coordinated actions are generated, in contrast to the motor cortex, which controls individual muscle contractions. Therefore, this finding was no surprise. However, it was discovered almost accidentally in one experiment, that when the resting, motionless monkey *sees* an experimenter do the same thing, namely pick up a food morsel and put it in his or her mouth, the *same* cortical read-out occurs in the monkey. In other words, in the experience of viewing a motor event of another, there seems to be a virtual pre-motor-cortical event in the viewer. The same cells fire that would fire had the observer performed the same action.

The phenomenon of the mirror neuron may be less surprising than it at first appears. After all we have to have some way to recognize actions just as we need to recognize objects. When we recognize an object we use our primary sensory cortex to form an iconic representation of the sense datum. For instance, when one sees a square, there is first a square outlined in activated neurons on the retina, and then again there is a retinotopic, square-shaped activation in the visual cortex. Eventually a complex neuronal pattern is recognized as an object, say a hammer or a squirrel, by way of the temporal cortex. But how do we recognize an *action*? There are cells in the visual cortex that represent motion. However, the representation of an action, such as putting food in your mouth, is much more than motion. It is a temporal sequence, with objects, actors and purposes. Thus, the activity of the mirror neurons is part of the process of *perception*. The only way we can recognize an action is to play it out in the brain. This takes us back to Piaget for whom the sensori-motor realm is the basis of perception and representation (Piaget & Inhelder, 1971). It also reminds us of the work by Pulvermuller (1999) that suggests that the neurological activation required to produce a verb, an *action* word, like "walk" or "climb," in language, includes the pre-motor cortex. In other words, a concept of a motor act needs to include a pre-motor activation.[3] So, in order to perceive an action, and in order to symbolize or speak of an action, we draw in the frontal, motor part of the brain. An *action* is a holistic or integrated concept of a piece of behavior; this may be at the same level of complexity as the concept of an *object*.

In pursuit of the argument that an *action* is an important biological concept, these researchers have noted that for mirror neurons to fire during the perception of an action, it must be a recognized action with a beginning and ending, and possibly with a purpose. As with an object it may be that, for this kind of recognition, it must have been seen before. In the experimental situation with the monkey, if the other simply lifts and lowers a hand with no apparent purpose, the neuronal mirror reaction will not occur. Similarly, when the person picks up a nut with a pair of pliers for the first time, that too will not be recognized. After several such events, the monkey will have a mirror neuron response to the action with the pliers.

Recent research has fleshed out the mirroring function in dramatic and useful ways. After much work on the macaque motor neuron mirroring, it became natural to ask if other phenomena are mirrored in a similar way. A number of researchers into the cognitive and neural science of social behavior have been teasing out some of the details. Carr et al. (2003), in a detailed paper on the subject, described a "minimal architecture for imitation." This includes areas in the temporal, parietal and frontal lobes; it is a kind of circuit that "codes" for three components: the perception of another's action, the motor specification for the action to be imitated, and the goal of that action.

Another large issue that is biologically closely related to identification is *empathy*. Recently emerging from this research is the finding that the appreciation of *affects* functions in a similar way. Imaging studies show that certain areas are stimulated and activated when one perceives the affect of another. In simply observing another's emotional state, areas are activated, the same areas that light up when one has that emotion oneself.[4] (Carr et al., 2003; Decety & Chaminade, 2003; Leslie et al., 2004).

What is striking is that perception has more to it than iconic representation. Perception is "being there." Especially with interpersonal perception and recognition, one does not simply perceive, one *becomes*. In this model the visible actions and expressions of the other seem to some extent *invasive* and *controlling*. One replicates or simulates the external world internally, and only in this way can one understand.

The Perception-Action Model

In the psychological theory of the past century there have been several theories of perception. There is no room to review these theories. But it should be noted that the findings described above tend to support a *perception-action model*. In an extensive review article presenting a theory of empathy, Preston and De Waal (2002) describe the model. "According to the perception-action hypothesis, perception of a behavior in another automatically activates one's own representations of the behavior, and output from this shared representation automatically proceeds to motor areas of the brain where responses are prepared and executed." An early version of this theory was proposed by Theodore Lipps, who applied it to perception of both action and emotion. The theory was pushed aside during the days of behaviorism and cognitivism, but now seems to be gaining respectability derived from some of the recent findings described above. In turn, the model encourages the thinking of interpersonal theorists. The dramatic import lets us focus on the permeability of individuals. What I perceive makes automatic and involuntary changes in my brain, in which I simulate what I am perceiving. The most dramatic form of simulation occurs when I experience the affect of the other, because of automatic mirroring of the other's expressions. This model is particularly apt for any transfer of qualities from one to another. Such transfers occur in emotional contagion, empathy, identification, and imitation.

Summary and Some Possibilities

In our brief look at other sciences, what have we gleaned? From the *cognitive psychologists* we have a differentiated view of memory and its subtypes. We can see where identification might fit into this. This may give us a perspective on identification as memory. In the future there may be new information about brain structures that are centrally involved in this function.

From the *animal researchers* we have evidence of evolutionary precursors to identification, particularly the emergence of imitation as a skill in higher primates, leading to its pre-eminent role in *Homo sapiens,* possibly contributing both to identification and to the evolution of human culture.

The *infant observers* have pursued imitation, along with the interactions of mirroring, attunement and attachment phenomena, all of which seem to contribute to identification. They have also, along with some of the primatologists, developed the notion of theory of mind, and its stages of development. Fonagy, Target, Gergely, and others have envisioned a staged scheme in children, similar and more detailed than Tomasello's (Fonagy et al., 2002; Gergely & Watson, 1999).

Recently the *neurobiologists* have discovered the mirror neuron, which has contributed to a revolution in our thinking about perception and the virtual recreation of the external world in the brain. In addition, the mirror neuron may play an as yet unclear role in the evolution of the capacity to imitate, and therefore in the capacity to identify.

At this point it is too early to put these various scientific inputs together into a coherent theory. I hope that the project of this paper, bringing these strands together in one train of thought, might in time lead to new models, and to hypotheses as to their possible integration in a future theory.

Identification occurs as the self takes on characteristics of the other, by way of emulation or imitation. True imitation involves an accurate motor or thought program that copies the other. Mirror neurons may be involved since they are probably involved in the perception and understanding of the other's behavior. They may have evolved as a brain mechanism for the recognition of actions, in a complex sense including the goals and intention of the actor. This could have been a building block towards intentionality, identification and theory of mind.

The novel phenomenon in human primates is the sense of the dyad and the relationship within it. This is a precursor to the appreciation of the other as an intentional and representational mental agent. During the same period of evolution, Homo sapiens became the *symbolic species* (Deacon, 1997; Olds, 2000, 2002). This meant that this whole process involving imitation and the passing down of culture, seen in primitive form in the pongids, exploded in complexity when new levels of semiotic capacity including language became possible. Also, during the same evolutionary era, there developed human consciousness as we know it. It is difficult to separate individual entities from this phalanx of human co-evolved capacities, which includes imitation, iden-tification, causality, language, sociality, and consciousness.

Identification then is the result of a group of functions operating in a complex system. In the process of phylogeny these functions have co-evolved in dynamic relationships with each other. In the individual's ontogeny the same is true; the genetic base and constitutional givens, the behavioral learning environment, the personalities of the parents, chance events, the tendency to imitate, all collaborate in a not quite predictable way.[5]

The evolution of the human function of identification seems to have required 1) several kinds of learning, particularly the procedural; 2) mirror neurons contributing possibly both to the capacity to imitate, but also to understand another's actions and develop a theory of mind; and 3) the ability and the drive to imitate, in humans providing capacities to develop a theory of mind, to identify, and to transmit culture. Among the primates, as the period of infantile plasticity increased in length, the opportunities increased for the ontogeny of identification, through imitation and attunement. In parallel with the capacities for imitation and attunement, grew the ego capacities allowing for the development of mentalism and the understanding of the other as a causal, intentional and representational being. It is not clear yet how theory of mind and identification emerged together. They may require each other. One may need both the capacity to imitate and the capacity to understand the mind of the other, in order to identify with the other. Research into psychopathology, particularly that of autism may shed light on this question. It seems likely that imitation, attunement, and theory of mind, co-evolved with identification, but how they interacted in this process is still far from understood.

Some Implications for Psychoanalysis

What does all this do for the psychoanalyst? Our discipline has limned out the concept of identification, independently of neighboring disciplines, finding it useful in understanding child and adult development, as well as the changes that take place in clinical psychoanalysis. In our developmental theories we have found identification a very useful concept. Most of this essay has tried to trace out some of the components of an identification process that leads to the maturation of the individual. In our theorizing, and in our thinking about the development of individual patients, it seems useful to understand the ways in which traits, patterns and behaviors are passed through the generations.

In our clinical theory, we have long held that the analysand identifies with the analyzing function, and adopts certain new behaviors having to do with thinking rather than acting, introspecting rather than externalizing, questioning what is said, looking for associations and symbolic meanings, becoming more aware of subjective feelings, and seeking evidence of transference, and even of the analyst's counter-transference. Imitation and conditioning would seem both to play a part. When the patient shows instances of introspection and self-reflection there is, often a rewarding word or other encouraging sound from behind the couch. Papers have been written about the operant control in the analytic situation (Schwartz, 1988). But even for the patient to adopt these behaviors there must be the *ability to imitate* the analyst. It is frequently noted that patient and therapist in a vis a vis situation often find themselves in mirroring postures. With some patients this occurs more often than in others; one could speculate that this would be evidence of a more intense, positive or intimate relationship. But one could also imagine that this mirroring could be defensive. I am not aware that this has been researched. On the couch the vis a vis is mostly absent, giving much less opportunity for visually mediated imitation. In fact, there we might expect to see more operant conditioning (responding to reward) compared with imitation. However, there are more abstract kinds of imitation, largely of thinking processes, problem-solving habits, and even theoretical biases. There is the lore that patients eventually justify their analyst's theory, and even that they produce dreams most relevant to that theory.

Another common form of internalization in the analytic situation is the introjection of the analyst so that there are inner dialogues between patient and analyst. In these the analyst may be offering advice, criticism, support, or argument. The analyst may appear in imagination as an approving or disapproving presence. There is a growing and promising research thrust into the nature of patients' representations of their therapists (Orlinsky & Geller, 1993; Orlinsky et al., 1993). In this work a number of questionnaires have been developed to elaborate the ways in which patients bring their therapists to mind between sessions, during therapy, and during the months and years after therapy. They have differentiated types of patterns, such as "supportive guiding representations" and "conflict containing representations," and correlated these with certain kinds of affect during sessions and with certain kinds of therapeutic relationship. Descriptively this research says more about *introjection* than *identification*. It may be that this phenomenon of representation is a part of the process of identification with the analyst. There is suggestive data that there may be correlations between these representations and therapeutic outcome.[6]

These issues relating to the internalization of the analyst have been important as well as troubling to analysts because of the concern about *suggestion*. There has been a general conviction that suggestion is bad, and that it undermines the claims for efficacy made by analysts. Freud differentiated analysis from hypnosis on the basis of the non-directive non-suggestive nature of analytic process. At the same time analysts have looked with favor on the idea that identification takes place in analysis. Is that not a form of influence or even suggestion? One reason for the avoidance of suggestion as part of technique is that the power differential that is inherent in the authoritative relationship in the directive form of psychotherapy, *enacts* a certain kind of transference and renders it unanalyzable. If that is the case then how do we handle the issue of identification? We say it is the accepting of the analytic method on the part of the patient in identification with the analyst. It means the patient has to enact the role of analyst, by assuming a kind of neutrality to the extent that he can step back from himself and allow parts of himself to negotiate with each other at a psychic bargaining table. This must be particularly complex and important with respect to the training analysis, in which there is both the above-mentioned identification with the process for one's own treatment, but also the identification with the analyst as mentor and professional model.

Some critics of the analytic method see the use of the couch by analysts as a deprivation that weakens the process. Those who feel that therapy is a "communication between right brains" (Schore, 1994) know that much of that communication is through visual, non-verbal cues and expressions. Why then give up one of our major assets? Our discussion of imitation and mirroring may provide one suggestion. We have discussed that there is a tremendous pull to involuntarily respond to the actions and the affect states of the other, to actually *have them*, and to some extent *become* the other. It is similar to the above-mentioned phenomenon of adopting similar postures.

The control or influence of the other by one's own expressions is powerful and goes both ways in the dyad. The intuition of Freud, who felt he did not like being observed all day by his patients, turns out to have been prescient; he was not really doing it just for his own convenience. The interactive and mutual control by non-verbal expression may indeed interfere with free association and with the flowering of the transference. But of course, transference interacts in extremely complex ways with identification. In becoming the patient who is identifying with the analyst, the transference must change; and as the transference changes so may the identification. And this in both meanings of the term: both in the sense in which the patient believes he is like the analyst, and also in the sense in which he changes himself to resemble the analyst. This phenomenon must be very important in the match between a patient and a particular analyst. The analyst has the same experience in reverse, with identifications interacting with transference and counter-transference.

For psychoanalytic theory, the mirror-neuron information may also shed light on the somewhat controversial concept of projective identification. One problem with this concept, in which the intense feelings of one person are "projected into" the other, is that there is a kind of metaphoric, almost mystical, "beaming" or forceful transmission of the affect into the other person. The mirror neuron phenomenon may allow for a more parsimonious explanation, namely that all emotions may be communicated via verbal and non-verbal means: and, when they are perceived by the other person, that person has at least a signal form of the emotion. In intense situations such as those in which the concept of projective identification is invoked—most commonly a highly charged but possibly disavowed situation in psychotherapy—the heightened sense of anxiety, or fear, or anger in the therapist, leads to some blurring of ego boundaries, and to the therapist's ownership and possibly enactment of the feeling that is being involuntarily and possibly unconsciously mirrored. Although this is quite speculative, it suggests that the contagion of the affect may derive from the therapist's transient loss of ego boundary in such an interaction.

In Review

1   Psychoanalysis has developed a complex idea of the self, both as a representation and as an agent or ego-like entity. This self develops in an environment of others, particularly parents, whose influence seems to occur at least partly through internalization processes.

2   In this paper I have focused on the process of identification, looking at mostly the unconscious, implicit aspects derived from animal models. This process is a part of the process leading to the formation of the self.

3   Of the forms of memory in current thinking, procedural memory bears some resemblance to our concept of identification. As we have seen there

are a number of different processes that contribute to procedural memory, including instruction, practice, behavioral conditioning and imitation. And, all of these interact in complex ways with gene expression.

4   In the evolution of human mental functions, we see here an example of a newly evolved capacity having multiple results as this capacity becomes integrated with others. It is conceivable that the mirror neuron may have been a precursor that joined with other precursors to produce the capacity for imitation. Imitation then may have contributed to the passing down of complex ritual and culture, for the process of identification, and for the learning of language.

5   The implications of this for the theory of analytic technique may be profound, and could help in our understanding of elements of the method, such as frequency, abstinence, and the use of the couch, as well as theoretical issues having to do with intersubjectivity and the one-versus-two-person model.

6   What I have described represents some aspects of mental function that could help build a model of identification congenial to both psychoanalysis and the cognitive sciences. By beginning with the analytic concept and tracing its history and possible biological roots, we may learn much about the concept and ground it in the world of the sciences.

Notes

1   Previously published in the *Journal of the American Psychoanalytic Association* (2006), Vol. 54: 17–46.
2   This discovery has had a big impact in neuro-biology circles. V. S. Ramachandran has declared, "I predict that mirror neurons will do for psychology what DNA did for biology: they will provide a unifying framework and help explain a host of mental abilities that have hitherto remained mysterious and inaccessible to experiments" (Ramachandran, 2000, p. 5).
3   Why does this activation not lead to the same action in the observer? There must be some inhibition of action that may well be learned and that has not yet been opened to research. In patients with echopraxia, it is possible that this inhibitory function has not been learned, or has been lost because of organic brain damage.
4   The theory has grown that deficits in these mirroring functions are an important part of the autistic syndrome, in which the mirroring system does not function, rendering the person unable to understand or empathize with the other (Williams et al., 2001).
5   This is an example of complex system development, in which so many phenomena are evolving at the same time that although causality is maintained, predictability is not. Attempts to understand such complexity have been made by dynamic systems theorists, some of whom have written for a psychoanalytic audience (Galatzer-Levy, 1985, 2002, 2003; Harris, 2004; Palombo, 1999; Piers, 2015; Pincus et al., 2003).
6   In similar work on supervision, Geller and Schaffer (1988) found a positive correlation between a benign supervisory alliance and the tendency to evoke the supervisor in dealing with therapeutic crises.

References

Byrne, R. W. & Russon, A. E. (1998) Learning by Imitation: A hierarchical approach. *Behavioral and Brain Sciences*, 21: 667–721.

Carr, L., Iacoboni, M., Dubeau, M., Mazziotta, J., & Lenzi, G. L. (2003) Neural mechanisms of empathy in humans: A relay from neural systems for imitation to limbic areas. *Proceedings of the National Academy of Sciences*. 100: 5497–5502.

Caspi et al. (2002) Role of Genotype in the Cycle of Violence in Maltreated Children. *Science*, 297: 851–854.

Clyman, R. B. (1991) The procedural organization of emotions: a contribution from cognitive science to the psychoanalytic theory of therapeutic action. *Journal of the American Psychoanalytic Association*, 39 (suppl.): 349–382.

Coates, S. W. & Moore, S. (1997) The Complexity of Early Trauma; Representation and Transformation. *Psychoanalytic Inquiry*, 17: 286–311.

Damasio, A. (1999) *The Feeling of What Happens*. New York: Harcourt Brace.

Deacon, T. (1997) *The Symbolic Species: The Co-evolution of Language and the Brain*. New York: W.W. Norton.

De Waal, F. (2001) *The Ape and the Sushi Master: Cultural Reflections of a Primatologist*. New York: Basic Books.

Decety, J. & Chaminade, T. (2003) Neural correlates of feeling sympathy. *Neuropsychologia*, 41: 127–138.

Emch, M. (1944) On "the need to know" as Related to Identification and Acting Out. *International Journal of Psychoanalysis*, 25: 13–19.

Etchegoyen, R. (1985) Identification and its Vicissitudes. *International Journal of Psychoanalysis*, 66: 3–18.

Fonagy, P., Gergely, G., Jurist, L., & Target, M. (2002) *Affect Regulation, Mentalization, and the Development of the Self*. New York: Other Press.

Gallese, V. & Goldman, A. (1998) Mirror neurons and the simulation theory of mind-reading. *Trends in Cognitive Sciences*, 12: 493–501).

Geller, J. D., Cooley, R. S., & Hartley, D. (1981) Images of the Psychotherapist: A theoretical and methodological perspective. *Imagination, Cognition and Personality*, 1:123–146.

Geller, J. D. & Schaffer (1981) Internalization in the supervisory relationship: Paper presented to the annual meeting of the society for Psychotherapy Research, Santa Fe, NM.

Gergely, G. & Watson, J. (1999) The social biofeedback model of parental affect mirroring. *International Journal of Psychoanalysis*, 77: 1181–1212.

Harris, A. (2004) *Gender as a Soft Assembly*. Hillsdale, NJ: Analytic Press.

Iacoboni, M. (forthcoming) Understanding others: Imitation, language, empathy. In S. Hurley & N. Chater (Eds), *Perspectives on Imitation: From Cognitive Neuroscience to Social Science*. MIT Press, Cambridge.

Jaffe, J. (2001) *Monographs Society for Research in Child Development*.

Kandel, E. R. (1999) Biology and the Future of Psychoanalysis: a New Intellectual Framework for Psychiatry Revisited. *American Journal of Psychiatry*, 156: 505–524.

Leslie, K. R., Johnson-Frey, S. H., & Grafton, S. T. (2004) Functional imaging of face and hand imitation: towards a motor theory of empathy. *NeuroImage*, 21: 601–607.

Loewald, H. W. (1973) On Internalization. *International Journal of Psychoanalysis*, 54: 9–17.

Meissner, W. W. (1981) *Internalization in Psychoanalysis*. New York: International Universities Press.

Meissner, W. W. (1976) A note on internalization as Process. *Psychoanalytic Quarterly*, 45: 374–393.

Milrod, D. (1982) The Wished-For Self Image. *Psychoanalytic Study of the Child*, 37: 95–120.

Meltzoff, A. N. (1990) Foundations for developing a concept of self: the role of imitation in relating self to other and the value of social mirroring, social modeling, and self practice in infancy. In D. Cicchetti & M. Beeghly (Eds), *The Self in Transition: Infancy to childhood*. Chicago, IL: University of Chicago Press.

Olds, D. (2000) A Semiotic Model of Mind. *Journal of the American Psychoanalytic Association*, 48: 497–529.

Olds, D. (2002) JAPA NetCast: A Semiotic Model of Mind, with discussions: www.psychoanalysis.net/JAPA_Psa-NETCAST.

Orlinsky, D. E. & Geller, J. D. (1993) Patients' Representations of their therapists and therapy: new Measures. In N. Miller, L. Luborsky, J. B. Barber, & J. P. Docherty (Eds), *Psychodynamic Treatment Research: A handbook for clinical practice*. New York: Basic Books. pp. 423–466.

Orlinsky, D. E.; Geller, J. D., & Tarragona, M. (1993) Patients' representations of psychotherapy: A new focus for psychotherapy research. *Journal of Consulting & Clinical Psychology*, 61: 596–610.

Pally, R. (2000) *The Mind-Brain Relationship*. London: Karnac.

Palombo, S. R. (1999) *The Emergent Ego: Complexity and Co-evolution in the Psychoanalytic Process*. Madison, CT: International University Press.

Piers, C. (2015) A Review of Psychoanalytic Complexity: Clinical Attitudes for Therapeutic Change: by William J. Coburn. *Contemporary Psychoanalysis*, 51: 747–755.

Pincus, D, Freeman, R. W., & Modell, A. (2003) *Towards a Neurobiology of Transference*. Paper presented at the Neuroscience, Psychopharmacology and Psychoanalysis Study Group, New York, NY.

Preston, S. D. & De Waal, F. B. M. (2002) Empathy: Its ultimate and proximate bases. *Behavioral and Brain Sciences*, 25: 1–72.

Pulvermüller, F. (1999) Words in the Brain's Language. *Behavioral and Brain Sciences*, 22: 253–336.

Ramachandran V.S. (2000) Mirror neurons and imitation learning as the driving force behind "the great leap forward" in human evolution. *The Edge*, www.edge.org/documents/archive/edge69.html.

Rizzolatti, G & Arbib, M. (1998) Language within our grasp. *Trends in Neurosciences*, 21:188.

Savage-Rumbaugh, S. & Lewin, R. (1994) *Kanzi: the Ape at the Brink of the Human Mind*. New York: Wiley.

Schafer, R. (1968) *Aspects of Internalization*. New York: International Universities Press.

Schafer, R. (1972) Internalization: Process or Fantasy? *Psychoanalytic Study of the Child*, 27: 411–436.

Schore, A. N. (1994). *Affect Regulation and the Origin of the Self: The neurobiology of emotional development*. Hillsdale, NJ: Erlbaum.

Schwartz, A. (1987) Drives, Affects, Behavior and Learning: Approaches to a Psychobiology of Emotion and to an Integration of Psychoanalytic and Neurobiological Thought. *Journal of the American Psychoanalytic Association*, 35: 467–506.

Scoville, W. B. & Milner, B. (1957) Loss of recent memory after bilateral hippocampal lesions. *Journal of Neurology and Neurosurgical Psychiatry*, 20: 11–21.

Shanker, S. G. & King, B. J. (2002) The emergence of a new paradigm in ape language research. *Behavioral and Brain Sciences*, 25: 605–656.

Shevrin, H., Bond, J. A., Brakel, L. A., Hertel, R. K., & Williams, W. L. (1996) *Conscious and Unconscious Processes: Psychodynamic, Cognitive, and Neurophysiological Convergences*. New York: Guilford Press.

Smith, H. (2001) Hearing voices: the fate of the analyst's identifications. *Journal of the American Psychoanalytic Association*, 49: 781–812.

Solms, M. & Kaplan-Solms, K. (2001) *Clinical Studies in Neuro-Psychoanalysis: Introduction to a Depth Neuropsychology*. New York: Other Press.

Solms, M. & Turnbull, O. (2002) *The Brain and the Inner World*. New York: Other Press.

Stern, D. (1984) Affect attunement. In: J. D. Call, E. Galenson, & R. L. Tyson, eds. *Frontiers of Infant Psychiatry*, Vol. 2. New York: Basic Books, pp.3–14.

Stern, D. (1985) *The Interpersonal World of the Infant*. New York: Basic Books.

Thelen, E. & Smith, L. B. (1996) *A Dynamic Systems Approach to the Development of Cognition and Action*. Cambridge, MA: MIT Press.

Tomasello, M. (1999) *The Cultural Origins of Modern Cognition*. Cambridge, MA: Harvard University Press.

Williams, J. H. G., Whiten, A., Suddendorf, T., & Perrett, D. I. (2001) Imitation, mirror neurons and autism. *Neuroscience and Biobehavioral Reviews*, 25: 287–295.

Chapter 13

Interdisciplinary Studies and Our Practice[1]

Introduction

Why should psychoanalysts learn about neighboring disciplines? It is often argued that, although information from neuroscience, neuropsychology, evolutionary psychology, and other fields may be of interest to analysts, it has no real effect on their practice: on the way they listen, the way they react, or the way they treat their patients. A corollary of this position is that there is no reason to include such information in a psychoanalytic curriculum, since it does not help candidates become better analysts. Against this view, two reasons are advanced for the importance of interdisciplinary study. The more general reason is that it grounds psychoanalysis in the broader scientific world, reducing its isolation and inbred parochialism. This can help justify the discipline intellectually, possibly in advance of and independently of supportive research from within the field (e.g., outcome studies). The second reason is that our own minds, and particularly those of the generation now entering training, have been altered by changes in the scientific zeitgeist, and we need to have some grasp of these changes. Finally, six examples of findings from other disciplines are presented that even now may be contributing to thinking about psychoanalytic practice.

The sciences devoted to brain and mind have in recent years made dramatic progress. Many functions of mind have been elucidated and have often been meaningfully related to brain activities. A patchwork of theories has grown up giving us a partial view of how the brain works. Psychoanalysts have faced this deluge of information and responded in various ways. This paper is an attempt to discuss this interchange between psychoanalysis and neighboring sciences.

We are faced with the question: are there any changes in psychoanalytic practice resulting from the new information? It is generally accepted that scientific information has led to changes in psychoanalytic theory building. But it is less certain that it has made much difference in the way we treat our patients. Pulver (2003), discussing the "astonishing clinical irrelevance" of neuroscience, made the argument that our technique is well established and

DOI: 10.4324/9781003399551-14

that neuroscience tells us "nothing we did not already know" (p. 760). And if it does tell us something new about theory, he asserted, it is still irrelevant to practice.[2] Although in the short term this argument may have merit, if we take a longer view, we see that the issue is much more complex.

It may well be that no neuroscience finding is going to suddenly cause a huge shake-up in psychoanalytic practice. One might in fact ask why we should expect such a revolution. Our practice has been developed and honed over a hundred years; it isn't obvious that knowledge of the brain would have a dramatic effect. I think that there are changes and that there will be more, but because our technique is so well established these changes will be modest, especially in the near future. One might also ask how much change our technique could undergo and still be psychoanalysis. That question is a reason for anxiety among analysts dealing with this topic.[3]

What is more important for this discussion is that the accumulation of information from other sciences is already having a profound effect on the way we think about brain and mind. It is changing us and our minds. It is changing the context in which we understand what it is to be a living entity, a mammal, a human being. I think that psychoanalytic practice will evolve slowly and subtly as part of this process.

Reframing the Question

Keeping this in mind, we may see the need to reframe the question concerning the impact of interdisciplinary information on clinical practice. Some analysts will say, in answer to the question, that they cannot think of an instance where interdisciplinary knowledge has led them to practice any differently, treat patients any differently, or even think about their patients any differently. Yet I think most would agree that analytic technique and practice have changed in important ways over the last thirty to forty years. We might rephrase the question this way: There have been important changes in technique in the last half century; is it possible to say what kind of contribution the cognitive sciences have made to this evolution? These changes in clinical theory and practice include a more active and interactive stance toward the patient by the analyst; the shift from a libido-economic model of mind to one based more on information, meaning, and narrative; the development of a "two-person" psychology, according the relational matrix greater prominence; and the increased importance of brain and body in the analytic situation, seen most concretely in the more common use of psychotropic medication as part of the treatment. The short answer to this reframed question may be that the other sciences have contributed to our clinical theory and technique, partly in specific ways we'll discuss below, and partly indirectly, via the impress of changes in the zeitgeist. Even theories we had already espoused take on new meanings because of this change in context and the changes brought about by the new information itself.

Isolation and its Virtues

Over the hundred-year history of psychoanalysis our discipline traveled an increasingly isolated path, divorced from what was happening in the wider scientific world. Although this probably degraded our status as a scientific discipline, it may also have had the effect of preserving some of our central tenets, and allowing us to elaborate our own concepts and theories, particularly those concerning the interiority and agency of the self–a mind in control, a mind in conflict. Had we mingled freely with other disciplines, we might have been buried under the tide of behaviorism and would only now be starting to dig ourselves out. As it happened, we preserved our basic principles, and now it turns out that many of them were valid; as the neuroscientist, Eric Kandel (1999) has pointed out, we had a theory of mind that was the most comprehensive theory available. So, in this most general view, psychoanalysis has preserved some basic principles, and these may ultimately have an effect on the other sciences. In the two-way exchange that now seems to be occurring, we may find some of those principles validated and some losing credibility. We are also finding that some of the phenomena that analysts have alone been working to understand can provide information to other sciences even as they raise questions for those sciences to answer.

Who are our Neighbors?

When we think of our isolation, we must ask what our boundaries are, who our neighbors are. This paper focuses on the nearby biological sciences such as neuroscience, cognitive psychology, primatology, and evolutionary biology. It is part of our lore that Freud aspired to forge connections with such sciences, but the level of knowledge made this impossible until quite recently. Other boundaries were considerably more porous, and the traffic brisk. The earliest insights into oedipal and other family dynamics emerged from Freud's reading of Sophocles and Shakespeare. Freud's thinking was shaped by his deep immersion in philosophy, from the pre-Socratics to the modern era. And of course, psychoanalysis has exerted an influence of its own on literature, history, anthropology, and other social sciences. There has of late been a fruitful back-and-forth between our discipline and a major branch of biologically oriented philosophy, including the works of Cavell, Churchland, Dennett, and Searle, to name a few. Indeed, such interdisciplinary intercourse is the model for the scientific interchange that is now occurring. It is often at the boundaries of disciplines that innovation and creativity emerge, at both theoretical and practical levels. That is why a professional education usually explores the neighboring terrain. It may be impossible to understand the boundaries of one's own discipline until one has seen what is on the other side of it. It is at the borders that differing ideas come into contact to produce new thinking.

Another close neighbor that space considerations prohibit discussing in this paper is the realm of infant and child observation. This vast enterprise has blossomed in recent decades to provide much information of value in our formulations about patients and in our techniques. Even here some have argued that the information is of no importance clinically, the reasoning being similar to that about the other scientific disciplines (Wolff 1996). Yet we often hear notions coming from attachment theory and child development research creeping into our discussions of patients and our techniques of therapy. Another important neighbor that combines developmental and evolutionary perspectives is the research in the components of attachment behavior in infants of other species. (Hofer 2003; Suomi 1995). The end result of the new ecumenism, despite the epistemological difficulties inevitably encountered in trying to integrate disciplines with such different basic concepts and databases, should be that we have firmer standing in the scientific world, positively affecting the way the world views us and improving our morale and self-esteem. These changes will influence how (and how much) we practice psychoanalysis, possibly preserving the discipline from its recently threatened demise. So, one effect may be the influence on whether anyone practices psychoanalysis at all.

Information that Might be Relevant

What sort of data are we talking about? What kind of interdisciplinary information would have any effect on our work? I will present six examples of new knowledge and open for consideration the question, Do they really make a difference? The areas concerned are mirror neurons, procedural memory, cognitive function, affect, trauma, and dynamic systems theories.

Mirror Neurons

My first example is the discovery of mirror neurons, a recently described set of neurons that may be important for imitative learning and other types of motor learning, including language. The work of Rizzolatti, Gallese, and others has demonstrated this entity in monkeys (Rizzolatti et al., 1996; Gallese & Goldman, 1998). A monkey, in their experiment, wears an array of microelectrodes that record the activation of individual neurons in the cortex. When the monkey picks up a morsel of food and puts it in its mouth, a characteristic readout appears from the premotor cortex. This area of the brain has been known for years to be where coordinated actions are generated, in contrast to the motor cortex, which controls individual muscle contractions. This finding was therefore no surprise. However, it was discovered almost accidentally in one experiment that when the resting, motionless monkey sees an experimenter pick up a food morsel and put it in his or her mouth, the same cortical readout occurs in the monkey. In other words, in the experience of viewing a motor event of another, there seems to occur a virtual premotor-cortical event in the viewer. The same cells fire that would fire had the observer performed the same action. have hitherto remained mysterious and inaccessible to experiments.

This finding has caused quite a stir in neuroscience circles. V. S. Ramachandran (2000), an eminent neurobiologist, has declared that "mirror neurons will do for psychology what DNA did for biology: they will provide a unifying framework and help explain a host of mental abilities that have hitherto remained mysterious and inaccessible to experiments" (p. 5).

Why such a fuss? And why should we be interested? For their part, neuroscientists feel that data of this sort reveal something about the biology of higher mental function. From our point of view, they may provide us some insight into interpersonal communication. They reveal an aspect of perception we had not thought of before. To make a bold claim, we might say that this research finding reveals the intense interpenetration of subjective beings who are in personal contact. When you see another person performing an action, you do a virtual performance, or simulation, of that action in your head; that is what it means to perceive an action (Olds, 2006). This lead has been followed by Rizzolatti and his colleagues in Parma, and now some at UC-San Diego (Gallese, Keysers, & Rizzolatti, 2004; Iacoboni, forthcoming). They have also shown that when one perceives another's affect, a similar virtual manifestation occurs in one's brain. It is speculated that one experiences a mild form of the other person's affect; that could help us understand something about empathy.

This gives us another point of view on the phenomena of imitation and identification, and the role of mirroring in development and maturation, and in the psychoanalytic situation. In psychotherapy it is observed that patient and therapist sometimes find themselves in mirroring postures. It is also noted that patients, in a process of identification, take on some of the mannerisms, verbal expressions, and even theories of the therapist. To some this information produces an uncanny feeling that in a dyad each reads the other's mind, unconsciously. But though the reading is unconscious, it influences what happens next–what feelings, associations, and enactments will merge. It may be that we already knew all of this. But these findings tell it to us with more dramatic impact: that every facial and bodily expression will have an effect on the other, and most of it will be unconscious, and it will guide the entire session. With respect to the clinical situation in psychoanalysis, this inter-penetration of selves by nonverbal, largely unconscious means provides arguments both for and against use of the couch. With the couch we give up the intense and mutual interpersonal control arising from the mirroring response. Some have pointed out that the "communication between right brains" is important to therapy, and that to give it up is to lose a major asset (Schore 1994). But in psychoanalysis that may be what we want: a measure of freedom from that control (Olds 2006). This should be a fruitful area of research; it may be difficult or impossible to free-associate while engaged in the kind of interactive mutual control that influences face-to-face interactions.

Procedural Memory

The phenomenon of procedural memory has been known for years, and has recently been seen as important to analysts. The by now well-known report of the case of H.M., who in 1956 underwent surgery resulting in the loss of both hippocampi, in an attempt to treat an intractable seizure disorder, was an early step in the process of distinguishing several different kinds of memory (Scoville & Milner 1957). After the surgery the patient was found to have lost his recent episodic memory (conscious memory for events) but retained his procedural memory (for habits and procedures). This latter mode of memory, usually categorized under the heading of implicit or unconscious memory, can be seen as a way in which repetitive psychological and behavioral schemas are maintained.[3] Procedural memory has captured the attention of analysts, and many see it as a concept that may help us understand what we call the repetition compulsion. It has led to an emphasis on the repetition itself, as opposed to the repressed episodic or the autobiographical memory, which previous theories viewed as the motivation for the repetition. In current practice, many analysts privilege exploration of the transference over recovery of the repressed memory. We encourage the transference to unfold and develop, and allow it to reveal a repetitive structure, which seems to be a basic schema, or set of schemata, governing the patient's life. It is often the case that we can trace this pattern back to childhood and early structural fantasies. The pattern is the way the child responded to family dynamics, and to fantasies related to those dynamics, and perhaps managed a situation that was more or less traumatic. That pattern persists in the patient's later life. In therapy we may observe the pattern in the patient's interactions with others, and in the accompanying fantasies. In analysis we allow the pattern to flourish in the relationship with the analyst. This of course is what we have always done. But I think there has been a change in emphasis. At one time the pursuit of the repressed episodic memory was more central to our work. Now it seems that we emphasize the pattern of behavior and fantasy more, and use the childhood memories, especially those relevant to the pattern, as ways to understand the pattern itself. We have been influenced by what come to be seen as the unreliability of long-term memory and the idea that historical truth is unreachable, that what counts is narrative truth–namely, the underlying set of narratives and fantasies that organize the patient's life.

Fonagy (1999) has emphasized the importance of the effect of psychotherapy on a patient's procedural schemas. In his view, this is the crucial factor bringing about change via analytic therapy, a factor more important than the interpretation and reconstruction of repressed episodic memories.

You may or may not agree with him, but it would seem that your opinion on that matter would have an effect on your clinical practice. The debate between Fonagy (1999) and Blum (2003), and the internet discussion that followed, shows that this change in emphasis, stimulated in part by the discovery of several different types of memory—particularly procedural memory—could definitely make a difference in analytic technique.

We have here mainly a question of emphasis, privileging the patterns of interaction evolved in procedural memory over the recovery of repressed memory. And this interest in patterns seems to accommodate a parallel emphasis on the importance of the dyad in the development of the individual, and the emergence in the analytic dyad of transference and countertransference schemas. The focus on the interacting analytic couple has provided fertile ground for relational and intersubjective models of the analytic encounter. As the analytic relationship evolves there may be more attention to the here and now, which reveals the schemas encoded in procedural memory–another important change in clinical practice.

Cognitive Processes and Capacities

Another significant alteration in technique has emerged as a result of our increasing understanding of cognitive processes and ego functions. The idea of "conflict-free" psychological functions or ego capacities received attention via the adaptational point of view. This directed our attention to the fact that we cannot assume that every patient has the same cognitive equipment. Within the normal range of patients there are variations in such capacities as reality testing, ego boundaries, language abilities, and long- and short-term memory that lead to unique understanding of experience and unique interaction with a given analyst. Increasingly, however, we also see patients not in the normal range, people whose lives have been bedeviled by impairments in these cognitive capacities. With many of these a classical conflict model, in which the understanding would involve a fear of success or oedipal victory, say, may have to give way to the idea that failure is due to cognitive impairment. Analysis may be appropriate for some such patients, but there will be much more need for attention to, and sometimes direct help in countering, reality distortions and organizational difficulties.

Psychoanalysts (as so often, first on the scene) encountered these problems before the cognitive scientists. Hartmann and others wrote extensively about the conflict-free sphere and developed a detailed understanding of cognitive deficits. Only more recently have neural scientists described some of the underpinnings of such deficits. The most dramatic example is the case, described in detail by Damasio (1995), of Phineas Gage, the railroad worker who lost a large portion of his prefrontal cortex in an accident, and whose life deteriorated from then on because of a sociopathic syndrome based on flaws in social judgment.

Kafka (1984), Bellak (1997), and Marcus (2004) have enumerated ego capacities such as boundary definition, reality testing, attention, and integration. Brain studies done by neuroscientists reveal more and more specifically the brain functions impaired in these discrete deficits. Such patients are increasingly treated in analysis. Consequently, the analyst's awareness of the nature of these deficits as they derive from brain pathology, and as they fit into the personal psychodynamics of the individual, is becoming more important. In fact, the recognition of cognitive deficits has produced new techniques and even new resistances. Patients whose academic failure or feeling of incompetence is recognized as a variant of Attention Deficit Disorder may be quite relieved, taking comfort in the idea that their difficulties are caused not by "bad personality" but by a neural deficit. In such cases, the treatment may have to take account of how the patient uses the diagnosis as a defense, or as a cover for other conflicts and inhibitions.[4]

Affect Systems and Disorders

A crucial change in both theory and technique has been forced by research into affect systems and the treatment of affect disorders. Cognitive scientists entered the game late, having spent much of the last century studying various forms of cognition and memory. Psychiatrists, however, were working on the clinical front, finding that medications can have direct and dramatic effects on disorders such as depression and mania. More recently, "affective neuroscientists" such as Panksepp (1994, 1998) and LeDoux (1996) have done important work integrating the cognitive and affective systems.

The implications for psychoanalysis have been profound. In recent decades analysts have been faced with the fact that psychotropic drugs can have major effects on patients, in many cases enhancing the effects of the psychotherapies. Analysts have made the adjustment, and many now accept that change in a brain function—in this case affect and affect regulation mechanisms—alters the dynamic formulations we can make and the kinds of interpretations we might venture. Here again, the phenomenon mentioned above, a success phobia previously interpreted as oedipal in origin, may turn out to have an affective aspect. In this situation the patient's capacity improves dramatically when medication produces a shift in mood, with a consequent alteration in self-esteem, self-confidence, assertiveness, and adventurousness. With a patient thus improved, we might in hindsight decide that the oedipal competition with a parent was less important than we thought; or, alternatively, that it was very important, and that the improvement in mood made the patient less inhibited in the competitive situation; or that improved mental functioning allowed the patient to use the treatment more productively in analyzing the conflict.

Trauma

Another major contribution to clinical practice has come from research into the effects of trauma. Freud's trajectory from seeing the source of pathology in early real trauma, to viewing much of pathology as the result of imagined trauma, is now to some extent being reversed, the spotlight again turning to the actuality of traumatic losses and sexual or violent assaults that have lasting psychic effects based on biological change.

Regarding defects in memory arising from trauma, it is understood that some distortions are the result not simply of repression mobilized to avoid painful recollection. Research suggests that the hippocampus, mentioned above as the organ important in remembering events in one's life, may be chemically disrupted by the flood of stress hormones during a traumatic event. This makes a difference clinically when one is trying to evaluate possible false memories, and also in the degree to which one tries to undo "repression" in patients suffering the aftereffects of trauma. Today we appreciate the difference between a defensive alteration or distortion of memory in a neurotically conflicted person, whose brain is functioning within normal limits, and the omissions and misconstructions arising from a brain with trauma-induced interferences of memory storage and retrieval.

As with the other areas of new information that I have discussed, this one too adds to clinical complexity. It is not clear when an issue crosses from conflict between psychic structures, or between motivations, to trauma that produces functional brain distortion. In all cases there will be interactions between the trauma, its psychic reconstruction, and the desire to repress or dissociate memories. Busch (2005) discusses conflicts that arise from the patient's need to avoid trauma-induced feelings. There are also significant differences in degree with respect to kinds of trauma. Terrorizing experiences such as being held hostage, being tortured, or witnessing the murder of loved ones seem qualitatively different from the traumas within emotionally abusive families, yet we may not be able to predict the degree of brain damage, of memory distortion, or intrapsychic conflict in an individual. Even more complicating is the issue of identification with aggressors that is often part of the traumatic and posttraumatic experience. When repressed and elaborated in fantasy, such identifications become factors in intra-psychic conflicts. In the more severe traumas, we do not tend to recommend psychoanalysis, but again the boundary is blurred between the severe and the not-too-severe. Neuroimaging tools may help us map the degree of damage to the brain, and this may in turn help us decide on the choice of therapy.

In any given patient there may be a complex combination of the ego deficits discussed in the previous section and their mutual interaction with the results of trauma. Both sets of factors interact also with the affective systems. In the severe personality disorders, there can be synergies among traumatic brain effects, ego deficits, and affective instabilities (Kernberg, 2005; Depue, 2005).

Complex Models of Mind

A more subtle but pervasive influence on our practice may come from what might be called "complexity theories." These theories have emerged from a need in the biological sciences for less mechanistic models with which to explain complicated dynamic processes. Biologists, like psychoanalysts, were finding mechanistic linear models limiting and unsatisfactory in their attempts to describe phenomena that have so many interdependent variables that prediction is virtually impossible. Several theories have been developed by mathematicians responding to the challenge to understand discontinuous, seemingly chaotic phenomena. We have had the General Systems Theory of von Bertalanffy, and after that chaos theory, connectionist or neural network theory, and updated versions of dynamic systems theory. Examples are Palombo's integration of dynamic systems models and psychoanalysis (1999) and Westen and Gabbard's use of connectionist theory in updating the concepts of psychological conflict and transference (2002a, 2002b; see also Olds, 1994; Piers, 2005).

Here I can only sketchily describe these models. Underlying all of them is the fact that in biological systems there are so many variables that the mechanistic predictability afforded by the linear model of physical systems, such as the interaction of billiard balls, must be given up. Although we assume that physical causality holds in biological systems, we cannot claim the possibility of complete predictability. With billiard balls you can re-create the experience of hitting one ball with another to send it into a pocket. You can put the balls back in the same place and hit the first ball at the same angle and be sure of the result. But in a biological system–or even a complex nonbiological system such as the weather–with thousands of variables, you can never perfectly re-create the setup and therefore cannot absolutely predict the outcome. This phenomenon, called "sensitivity to initial conditions," means that you can never completely re-create the scene. You can predict that the rat will push the lever to get a food reward, but only if it is hungry, and not anxious, and not otherwise trained, and not in a different cage and so on and on. Behavioral experiments are designed to reduce the number of variables, but with many biological systems, including human thought and action, we have found that we always run into limits.

Models of complexity may importantly influence our theorizing and, ultimately, our practice.[5] The new thinking has allowed us to understand discontinuities in child development, such that children go through sudden shifts, not completely predictable, in maturation, object relations, and skills. The kind of predictions we used to make, assured that a person from a certain kind of childhood would become socio-pathic, or depressed, or unanalyzable, are made less often today. Also, the epigenetic model, which implies a set blueprint in which developmental stages are timed to go off in a prescribed sequence, has had to be loosened (Galatzer-Levy, 2004). This does not mean that all bets are off; we do indeed make fairly reliable predictions about people, but we are more modest. It means, among other things, that we may be less willing to foreclose our patients' potentials. Complexity models have also opened the way to relational theories emphasizing that one's behavior is often influenced by another, that in a dyad there may be mutual influence, making the behavior of either person less predictable and more interactive. This dyadic interactivity may be explained in part by the mirror neuron phenomenon described above.

Interdisciplinary Knowledge and Psychoanalytic Training

Let me turn briefly to some of the implications of this discussion on how we think about analytic training. Scientific interdisciplinary courses are appearing in analytic institutes, sometimes against resistance. An argument frequently raised is the one that initiated this paper–namely, that these studies have no effect on clinical practice, so why teach them? Behind this argument may lie the conviction that analytic education is training for a craft on the apprenticeship model. The argument taken to its extreme would suggest that all we need to study is what the patient and analyst say and do in the consulting room; we learn how to do this with no need for theory. This argument can be extended to say that no body of theory, even that traditionally taught in our institutes, has much effect on practice; we learn practice from practice, and from supervision. The model is more the training of a technician than the training of a professional student.

Analytic theorists who focus on meaning might agree here with those who are antagonistic to the scientific search for underlying mechanisms. The anchor of their agreement is that the only thing that counts is the patient's behavioral output, including what the patient says and means. Ironically, this puts both of them in the bed of the behaviorist, where I'm not sure they would be comfortable. The behaviorist argument has always been this: we are interested in the behavior, not the interior; we are interested in probabilities and patterns, but only in behavioral and verbal output. It is that output that can to some extent be scientifically studied. Mentalism, or the sense that there is an inner source of agency, an ego, or a central self, is ruled out. Paradoxically, the integration of psychoanalysis and science could allow mentalism to be ruled back in.

This raises the question of how integration with the sciences affects analytic education. I have been involved in developing a course for analytic candidates that attempts to integrate information from other disciplines with psychoanalysis. A point we have recently come to appreciate in teaching the course is that the introduction of information from neighboring sciences enhances learning, rather than confusing students, as we had initially feared. Where there are biological correlates relevant to psychoanalytic theories, they make the theories more comprehensible and credible than before. When we "learned" psychoanalytic theory by the voice of authority, we often found ourselves parroting ideas without really understanding them. An example might be the success phobia mentioned above. It may be appropriate with one patient to apply an oedipal model in understanding the dynamics, but in other instances it might be confusing and distorting to use that model alone; issues of trauma, affect, and cognitive capacity may help produce an explanatory picture more helpful to both analyst and patient.

It seems clear that good, testable theories are easier to understand than outmoded or unsubstantiated theories we must twist and turn to relate to clinical experience. We get a bonus from our interdisciplinary studies: theory is more understandable and satisfying.[6]

What About Theory?

As intimated above, one could question whether any theory has an effect on practice. Certainly, metapsychological theories have been denigrated in recent years. Michels (1999) makes an important point about the function of theories. He reviews Sandler's argument (1983) that analysts use both a conscious "official, standard or public" theory, and a less conscious patchwork of theories derived from the personal, clinical situation. The latter set of theories covers more of the analyst's clinical experience, and guides much of the daily work. These theories may not be well organized, they may contradict each other, but they guide practice, often in our most "intuitive" interventions.

Among the formal theories, Michels identifies bridging theories, which can be traced 1) to the biological theories of Freud's 1895 Project; 2) to the evolutionary concerns of Totem and Taboo and ethologists like Bowlby; and 3) to the ontogenetic interests of the Three Essays and later developmental researchers. These are all interdisciplinary theories of the sort I've been discussing. Michels next mentions psychological theories, which attempt to describe and categorize mental functioning, with less regard to origins and more to phenomenology. Finally come clinical theories, which may be traced to Studies on Hysteria and "Analysis Terminable and Interminable." These deal with the clinical experience with transference, resistance, and working through. It seems clear that the current biological interests are in the tradition of bridging theories. Among the functions of these theories is to provide a scientific grounding for practice, as sources for the understanding by which we generate interpretations, and as theoretical bases for the analyst's role, the way we practice. It is likely that interdisciplinary information is already changing our unconscious, workaday theories, and that only later will they become part of our formal theories. In other words, it seems clear that the culture, including the scientific culture, influences our informal, implicit clinical model. That is what I meant by saying that the interdisciplinary interests are "changing us and our minds." But the change has not yet advanced to the point of modifying our formal theories; this may be one reason many analysts see these interests as irrelevant.

Conclusion

One result of all this interdisciplinary input is that we deal today with a much more complex situation than we at least thought we dealt with in the past. The number of points of view from different fields of inquiry is mind-numbing. Instead of a central dynamic that we can be confident will fit all patients, we have information applicable at several levels and from many different disciplines, as well as patients with all kinds of unique characteristics. There is some danger that such complexity will lead analysts to throw up their hands and give up trying to adapt to this changing scene. It is possible, however, that we will integrate much of this information in our unconscious procedural memories, leading to subtle changes in technique. Once we get the idea about different kinds of memory, or the idea of ego deficit based in organic cerebral dysfunction, it permanently changes the way we think. We will still follow our hunches, our frissons, our counter-transference signals, but they will be richer in information.

When psychoanalysis was the only game in town, everybody got analyzed. The success rate in that situation was doubtful. This may be one factor that led to a general disillusionment with psychoanalysis, as high expectations often lead to disappointment. In recent years, competing treatments have taken away much of the work of analysts. But the work that remained, with a more select group of patients, has probably been blessed with better results. This very likely is due in part to selection processes ensuring that analysis is indeed the most appropriate treatment for today's analysands, and in part to changes in technique, some influenced by new understanding of the brain.

Although I have tried to show specific instances in which findings from other disciplines have contributed to clinical work, these instances are but small steps in the process we are at present undergoing. As I hope is evident from some of my examples, one effect of information from other sciences is to provide fodder for controversies in our field (e.g., the value of the couch, or the Fonagy-Blum debate). The new information will not suddenly revolutionize the way we work. We will use it in our deliberations about clinical theory and technique, and that will contribute to the evolution of our work.

We may now be entering a new phase in this interdisciplinary exchange. The advance of neuroimaging technology and techniques has opened the brain up to increasingly refined exploration. We see more studies showing the two-way street between brain function and mind function. Some of these studies are already elucidating some basic psychoanalytic constructs (e.g., the interaction of conscious and unconscious mental processes), the neuroanatomical impact of trauma, and some effects of psychotherapy on the brain (Gabbard 2000; Beutel, Stern, & Silbersweig, 2003). In the future we may be able to use imaging and other techniques to actually support analytic theories, and at times support one analytic theory over another. In other words, in the future we may see a corralling of analytic theory into a more consistent and less fragmented discipline. Currently we have several quite divergent models calling themselves psychoanalytic; in the future there may be fewer, and they may be more similar.

A possible result of developing a more scientific basis for psychoanalysis may be a firmer foundation for our discipline in the public mind, leading to a greater sense that we are part of a spectrum of effective psychological modalities. The mechanisms of action of behavioral, cognitive, hypnotic, and pharmacological treatments have become known and at least partially elucidated by psychological and neuro-scientific theories. There is no reason that psychoanalytic concepts cannot be studied similarly. Over the years, measures of the efficacy of analytic therapies have been only partially successful, an urgent problem in this time of "evidence-based" treatments. Efficacy studies have proven difficult to do, though in future they may become more possible. In the meantime, an important support for psychoanalysis will be its credibility derived from parallel sciences. Making our concepts supportable and understandable as part of the wider biological and psychological universe will be helpful in presenting it as a rational endeavor. It will become evident that the psychoanalytic approach is different from other forms of therapy, that for certain types of patients it has a clear rationale, and that for them it is the best possible treatment.

Notes

1　Previously published in the *Journal of the American Psychoanalytic Association* (2006b), Vol. 54: 857–876.
2　Other leading analysts have voiced agreement with Pulver's view. Goldberg (2004) has argued that there is in principle no reason to expect information from other sciences to influence our clinical discipline. Sciences have boundaries, and once you cross a border into neuroscience or evolutionary biology, you are in that discipline, not the one you left. Despite its provocative title, Pulver's paper gives a thoughtful consideration of a "congruence model" embracing both psychoanalysis and the cognitive sciences at the level of theory. My area of disagreement concerns the larger picture, which includes the clinical realm.
3　Clyman (1991) introduced the concept of procedural memory as having implications for child development, the phenomenon of transference, and all kinds of repetitive schemas of behavior. Reviews of the different kinds of memory can be found in Pally (2000), Schacter (1996), and Westen and Gabbard (2002a, b,). Rosenblatt (2004) discusses the relationship of procedural memory to working through in analysis.
4　The neurobiology of executive function is a growing and massive undertaking. Damasio, a major contributor, has demonstrated the need for integration of

cognitive and emotional elements in adaptive decision making. His books, The Feeling of What Happens (2002), and Looking for Spinoza (2003), are important works. The topic is addressed in Beer, Shimamura, and Knight (2004), Depue (2005), Kernberg (2005), and Solms and Turnbull (2002).

5 There is a large and growing literature on the importance of systems theories to clinical practice and technique. Introductions to the theoretical models include Galatzer-Levy (2002, 2004), Harris (2004), Piers (2005), Thelen (2005), and Thelen and Smith (1994). Important works relating systems theories to practice include Schlessinger (2003) and Seligman (2005). Two recent journal issues have been thematically focused on this topic: *Psychoanalytic Dialogues* (Vol. 15, No. 2, 2005) and *Psychoanalytic Inquiry* (Vol. 22, No. 5, 2002).

6 Interestingly, Lewin (1965) suggests that theories may originate in attempts to teach. Good theory makes a good pedagogical tool, often providing rich and useful metaphors and analogies to aid in understanding. He says that "teaching and theorizing coincide and that the business of teaching leads to the production of theories" (p. 138).

References

Beer, J. S., Shimamura, A. P., & Knight, R. T. (2004) Frontal lobe contributions to executive control of cognitive and social behavior. In M. S. Gazzaniga (Ed.), *The Cognitive Neurosciences* III. Cambridge, MA: MIT Press.

Bellak, L. (1997) The use of ego function assessment for the study of ADHD in adults. *Psychiatric Annals*, 27:563–571.

Beutel, M. E., Stern, E., & Silbersweig, D. A. (2003) The emerging dialogue between psychoanalysis and neuroscience: Neuroimaging perspectives. *Journal of the American Psychoanalytic Association*, 51: 773–801.

Blum, H. P. (2003) Repression, transference, and reconstruction. *International Journal of Psychoanalysis*, 84:497–503.

Busch, F. (2005) Conflict theory/trauma theory. *Psychoanalytic Quarterly*, 74: 27–45.

Clyman, R.B. (1991) The procedural organization of emotions: a contribution from cognitive science to the psychoanalytic theory of therapeutic action. *Journal of the American Psychoanalytic Association*, 39 (Suppl.): 349–382.

Damasio, A. (1995) *Descartes' Error: Emotion, Reason, and the Human Brain*. New York: Penguin.

Damasio, A. (1999) *The Feeling of What Happens*. New York: Harcourt Brace.

Damasio, A. (2003) *Looking for Spinoza*. New York: Harcourt Brace.

Depue, R.A. (2005) A neurobehavioral dimensional model of personality disturbance. In *Major Theories of Personality Disorders*, ed. J. F. Clarkin & M.F. Lenzenweger. New York: Guilford Press, pp. 391–453.

Fonagy, P. (1999) Memory and therapeutic action. *International Journal of Psychoanalysis*, 80: 215–223.

Gabbard, G. O. (2000) A neurobiologically informed perspective on psychotherapy. *British Journal of Psychiatry*, 177: 117–122.

Galatzer-Levy, R. M. (2002) Emergence. *Psychoanalytic Inquiry*, 22: 708–727.

Galatzer-Levy, R. M. (2004) Chaotic possibilities: Toward a new model of development. *International Journal of Psychoanalysis*, 85: 419–441.

Gallese, V. & Goldman, A. (1998) Mirror neurons and the simulation theory of mind-reading. *Trends in Cognitive Sciences*, 2: 493–501.

Gallese, V., Keysers, C., & Rizzolatti, G. (2004) A unifying view of the basis of social cognition. *Trends in Cognitive Sciences*, 8: 396–403.

Goldberg, A. (2004) Delineating a discipline. Panel discussion at the 2004 Winter Meeting of the American Psychoanalytic Association, New York, January.

Harris, A. (2004) *Gender as a Soft Assembly.* Hillsdale, NJ: Analytic Press.

Hofer, M. A. (2003) The emerging neurobiology of attachment: How parents shape their infant's brain and behavior. In, S. Coates, J. Rosenthal, & D. Schechter (Eds), *September 11: Trauma and the Human Bond.* Hillsdale, NJ: Analytic Press, pp. 191–209.

Iacoboni, M. (forthcoming) Understanding others: Imitation, language, empathy. In S. Hurley & N. Chater (Eds), *Perspectives on Imitation: From Cognitive Neuroscience to Social Science.* Cambridge, MA: MIT Press.

Kafka, E. (1984) Cognitive difficulties in psychoanalysis. *Psychoanalytic Quarterly*, 53: 533–550.

Kandel, E. R. (1999) Biology and the future of psychoanalysis: A new intellectual framework for psychiatry revisited. *American Journal of Psychiatry*, 156: 505–524.

Kernberg, O. (2005) Unconscious conflict in the light of contemporary psychoanalytic findings. *Psychoanalytic Quarterly*, 74: 65–81.

LeDoux, J. (1996) *The Emotional Brain.* New York: Simon & Schuster.

Lewin, B. (1965) Teaching and the beginnings of theory. *International Journal of Psychoanalysis*, 46: 137–139.

Marcus, E. R. (2004) *Psychosis and Near Psychosis.* Madison, CT: International Universities Press.

Michels, R. (1999) Psychoanalysts' theories. In P. Fonagy, A. M. Cooper, & R. Wallerstein (Eds), *Psychoanalysis on the Move: The Work of Joseph Sandler.* New York: Routledge, pp. 187–200.

Olds, D. D. (1994) Connectionism and psychoanalysis. *Journal of the American Psychoanalytic Association*, 42: 581–611.

Olds, D. D. (2006) Identification: Psychoanalytic and biological perspectives. *Journal of the American Psychoanalytic Association*, 54: 17–46.

Pally, R. (2000) *The Mind-Brain Relationship.* London: Karnac Books.

Palombo, S. R. (1999) *The Emergent Ego: Complexity and Coevolution in the Psychoanalytic Process.* Madison, CT: International Universities Press.

Panksepp, J. (1994) The basics of basic emotion. In , P. Ekman & R. J. Davidson (Eds), *The Nature of Emotion: Fundamental Questions.* New York: Oxford University Press, pp. 20–24.

Panksepp, J. (1998) *Affective Neuroscience.* New York: Oxford University Press.

Piers, C. (2005) The mind's multiplicity and continuity. *Psychoanalytic Dialogues*, 15: 229–254.

Pulver, S. (2003) On the astonishing clinical irrelevance of neuroscience. *Journal of the American Psychoanalytic Association*, 51: 755–772.

Ramachandran, V. S. (2000) Mirror neurons and imitation learning as the driving force behind "the great leap forward" in human evolution. *The Edge*, www.edge.org/documents/archive/edge69.html.

Rizzolatti, G. & Arbib, M. (1998) Language within our grasp. *Trends in Neurosciences*, 21: 188–194.

Rizzolatti, G., Faddiga, L., Gallese, V., & Fogassi, L. (1996) Premotor cortex and the recognition of motor actions. *Cognition & Brain Research*, 3: 131–141.

Rosenblatt, A. (2004) Insight, working through, and practice: The role of procedural knowledge. *Journal of the American Psychoanalytic Association*, 52: 189–207.

Sandler, J. (1983) Reflections on some relations between psychoanalytic concepts and psychoanalytic practice. *International Journal of Psychoanalysis*, 64: 35–45.

Schacter, D. L. (1996) *Searching for Memory: The Brain, the Mind, and the Past*. New York: Basic Books.

Schlessinger, H. (2003) *The Texture of Treatment*. Hillsdale, NJ: Analytic Press.

Schore, A. N. (1994) *Affect Regulation and the Origin of the Self: The Neurobiology of Emotional Development*. Hillsdale, NJ: Erlbaum.

Scoville, W. B. & Milner, B. (1957) Loss of recent memory after bilateral hippocampal lesions. *Journal of Neurology, Neurosurgery & Psychiatry*, 20: 11–21.

Seligman, S. (2005) Systems theories as a meta-framework for psychoanalysis. *Psychoanalytic Dialogues*, 15: 285–319.

Solms, M. & Turnbull, O. (2002) *The Brain and the Inner World*. New York: Other Press.

Suomi, S. J. (1995) Attachment theory in non-human primates. In S. Goldberg, R. Muir, & J. Kerr (Eds), *Attachment Theory: Social, Developmental, and Clinical Perspectives*. Hillsdale, NJ: Analytic Press.

Thelen, E. (2005) Dynamic systems theory and the complexity of change. *Psychoanalytic. Dialogues*, 15: 255–283.

Thelen, E. & Smith, L. B. (1994) *A Dynamic Systems Approach to the Development of Perception and Action*. Cambridge: MIT Press.

Westen, D. & Gabbard, G. (2002a) Developments in cognitive neuroscience: I. Conflict, compromise, and connectionism. *Journal of the American Psychoanalytic Association*, 50: 53–98.

Westen, D. & Gabbard, G. (2002b) Developments in cognitive neuroscience: II. Implications for theories of transference. *Journal of the American Psychoanalytic Association*, 50: 99–134.

Wolff, P. H. (1996) The irrelevance of infant observations for psychoanalysis. *Journal of the American Psychoanalytic Association*, 44: 369–392.

Chapter 14

Leap Carefully from Brain to Mind; But It Can Be Done

Commentary on Jeanine Vivona's Paper: Leaping from Brain to Mind: A Critique of Mirror Neuron Explanations of Countertransference[1]

In this elegant and scholarly paper, Jeanine Vivona draws our attention to a possibly overhasty embrace by analysts of the mirror neuron phenomenon. The advent of Rizzolatti's discovery of mirror neurons has created quite a stir in many areas of psychology, neuroscience, social psychology, and psychoanalysis. V. S. Ramachandran, a leading neuro-scientist, has declared this to be a major finding, in league with the discovery of DNA. Psychoanalysts have jumped on the bandwagon, hoping that the mirror neuron would give crucial insights into psychological phenomena such as empathy, imitation learning, identification, transference, and countertransference. There has then been the inevitable backlash, from several quarters. These would include those who want to slow down the bandwagon to make sure all the claims about mirror neurons have some empirical basis, those who feel that even if there are mirror neurons they are of no consequence for psychoanalysts, and those who oppose the whole neuroscience game as something both useless and even threatening to psychoanalysis.

As part of this backlash, I would mention Sidney Pulver's plenary address (2003) at our Winter Meeting a few years ago, and more recently a much-discussed paper in the International Journal by Rachel Blass and Zvi Carmeli (2007). In the end Pulver took aim more at what he considered the clinical irrelevance of neuroscience to analysts—in other words, his view that none of this neuroscience information affects the way we practice. He allowed that it has probably made some difference to analytic theory. His address was one reason I wrote my paper on interdisciplinary studies and analytic practice (Olds, 2006). I wanted to explore whether indeed interdisciplinary science might have some influence on our clinical work.

The Blass and Carmeli paper takes a more extreme view and sees the whole neuroscience effort as bad for us analysts. They make three main points, which are the current staples of neuropsychoanalysis bashing. These are:

> 1) neuropsychoanalysis is irrelevant to psychoanalysis; 2) it is non-analytic, since it deals only with the physical brain and not with meaning,

DOI: 10.4324/9781003399551-15

and meaning is what analysis is about; 3) it is dangerous to psycho-analysis, in that it leads us down the wrong path, a path where only the biological is real, and the meaning-making in psychoanalysis is ignored, thus misdirecting and impoverishing psychoanalysis.

These papers, among others, form part of the context surrounding Vivona's paper. Her target is a narrower one, more specifically a questioning of the enthusiasm for mirror neurons in explaining psychoanalytic phenomena such as transference and empathy. As I understand her view, it too is a tripartite one. In her opinion the mirror neuron theory, as directed at the issues rele-vant to psychoanalysis, is based on three assumptions, all erroneous: that there is correspondence between brain activity and mental activity; that similarity of brain activity across individuals indicates a similar or shared psychological experience in the individuals; and that this sharing is effected by a direct, automatic biological mechanism that is unmediated by cognition, language, or any other conscious or unconscious mental process.

We can be grateful to Vivona for offering these cautions, and also pointing to where the rather indistinct boundaries now may be placed between the empirically demonstrated and the conjectural or hypothetical ideas about the implications of mirror neurons. I'll briefly give my reaction to these three points, with which I have some sympathy and agreement, and about which I make some points in amplification.

The Correspondence Assumption

As to the correspondence between brain and mental activity, this may mean that brain events cause, or are necessary, for mental events to occur. Even Blass and Carmeli allow that this is the case. In fact, this assumption is probably at the heart of all the sciences that study the brain. And a great deal of science has succeeded in the presence of the assumption. So, in itself, it should not condemn the explanatory uses of mirror neurons. The alternative to correspondence would seem to be a dualism of the Cartesian sort, where mind is somehow independent of brain. A milder alternative is advanced by those who agree that you need a brain to have a mind, but that the two levels are logically distinct, so that you can't talk meaningfully across the boundary. To try to do so is to commit a category error. In the dualist view, brain has many functions, and some of them have to do with conscious thoughts and language. But we talk about thoughts, wishes, intentions, and feelings differently than we do parts of the brain. We seem to arrive here at a kind of Kantian antinomy whereby the arguments for dualism and for monism are both incontrovertible, and the question cannot be resolved, or is resolved almost as a matter of personal preference.

But Vivona's argument has a temporal dimension, namely, the idea that we cannot at present characterize the correspondence in a definitive and detailed way. Indeed, her argument that our measuring techniques are not precise, and are open to disagreement as to their interpretation, is correct.

Her argument can be extended by reference to other papers on this subject. The earliest work on correspondence was that of the anatomists who made "clinico-pathological" connections at autopsy—for instance, Broca and the speech center. More recently, researchers working with animals, including primates, have used microelectrodes measuring the activation of individual neurons. Here the results can be quite focused and specific. This was the method used in the first mirror neuron discoveries. The findings were persuasive in making the case that these particular neurons fired both when action was initiated, and when another's action was observed. But even here we see a problem with correspondence. It is clear from these data that if the only information you had was the readout from the electrodes, you would not know if the monkey was acting or observing action. And further work showed that the mirror neurons are distributed and are present in several parts of the brain. Later research has worked with human subjects, with whom electrode research is not possible, and has turned to imaging studies. Here we have the problem of very poor resolution; someone has compared these efforts to "studying the motions of a water molecule by observing ocean currents." Current imaging technology measures differential blood oxygen levels, and measurements tend to be of groups of thousands of cells.

With respect to the bandwagon effect encouraged by neuroimaging technology, there is another intriguing finding, by McCabe and Castel (2008), who did experiments comparing the believability of certain ways of presenting research data. Their work showed that findings presented in prose description alone, those presented using bar graphs, and those presented using fMRI pictures of the brain met different levels of acceptance by readers as to their scientific validity. Not surprisingly, the reports with imaging data were significantly more likely to be accepted as scientifically valid. Many neuroimagers themselves feel the need to counter this persuasiveness with frequent caveats and statements of caution in interpreting imaging presentations. For instance, Freed (2008) provides a good discussion of the perils of both condemning and idealizing the work of neuroimagers.

Then there is the problem of whether, when brain events are reliably correlated with subjective introspective reports, a causal connection has been established. Many would argue the negative: the brain event that we measured, seductively but inaccurately, cannot be said to cause the mind event (see Poldrack, 2008).

These points make clear that it is still risky to draw conclusions about the brain-mind connection from the sorts of measuring devices we have available. But the fact that measurements are inaccurate does not imply there is no correspondence between brain and mind. Now if correspondence means something like temporal correlation, that is an easy argument to make. But it is harder at this point to say that there is a causal correspondence, although most monists would accept that this will turn out to be true. Here I think we are dealing with basic assumptions, or belief systems, and these systems involve a fundamental view of reality. The monistic view has the problem that it conflicts with our subjective experience, which is normally dualistic. And dualism has the problem that it requires two different kinds of matter or substance. A compromise that many neuroscientists are comfortable with is so-called dual-aspect monism. In this view there is only one kind of matter. But for humans there are two aspects from which to view the brain; one is the "objective view," which may use measuring devices, microscopes, and radiological techniques, and a "subjective view," provided by introspection, in which we use certain brain mechanisms to register mental processes in consciousness. I think that if you are going to scientifically study the brain, dual-aspect monism is an attractive model to use (Solms & Turnbull, 2002). This model leaves open the possibility of correspondence.

The Shared Experience Assumption

As for the shared experience idea, it has problems similar to those of the correspondence theory. Folk psychology asserts that we do share experience with others; that's why we feel we can empathize, understand another's behavior, even to some extent predict that behavior. It could be that this is an illusion, as some believe that free will is an illusion. But the illusion makes sense of the world and leads to a stable social experience. It may be that mirror neurons play a part in this potential sharing. Now, Vivona is right that it has not been demonstrated that when there is activity in a discrete area of the brain, we can predict that the subject is having a certain mental experience; and, we cannot say that activation of that same area in another person's brain will produce the same experience in the other person. This is largely the effect of the lack of precision in our current technology. But it may, even with future technology, be a result of some indeterminacy in the complex system of the brain, so that there are ultimate limits to predictability between neuron populations and subjective experiences.

The Directness Assumption

Third, the directness concept goes to the heart of the paper's objection to mirror neurons. It takes issue with how we empathize, how we apprehend another's feelings or intentions. Gallese, Eagle, and Migone (2007) have spelled out this discussion as one between two theories of the way we represent things. These have been called theory-theory and simulation theory.

When I perceive an object or an action or emotion, theory-theory would hold that I figure out from various cues what it is I am seeing, in a rapid process of assembling sense data, matching the assemblage with an inner template, and "recognizing" the perceived entity. According to the theory-theory view, "our understanding of another's mind is based on explicit and implicit theories of how minds function and that account for people's behavior in terms of inferences regarding their beliefs, desires, and intentions" (Gallese, Eagle, & Migone 2007, p. 164). In other words, we put the details of perception together, and match it up with images from past experience, and then recognize the object or phenomenon.

By contrast, simulation theory, or Gallese's "embodied simulation" model, says that one immediately and unconsciously makes a kind of copy in one's brain that is similar to the object. The major difference is that the mirror system is engaged unconsciously and automatically, and initiates a bodily, partial imitation of the phenomenon.

I believe Vivona would be considered a theory theorist and possibly a linguistically oriented theory theorist, in that she would consider language to be always playing an important part in any human cognition. She makes a very important point when she mentions possible alternative models in perception theory. One is that of Csibra (2004), who takes an opposite stance—clearly a theory theory—holding that we decide what the action or the emotion is by inference, mostly from the context and the entity perceived. Once the inference is made, the brain generates the faint activation that mirrors the other's affect. The procedure is the reverse of the mirror neuron simulation theory. This difference in theories is quite important and may be the most fundamental disagreement in the evolution and possible acceptance of mirror neuron theory. It will take further research to resolve the differences here.

In several of her arguments Vivona points out that only a few experiments have been done with respect to a phenomenon, or that none have been done in humans, implying that we cannot infer that humans manifest the same phenomena. This could be true, but it is not necessarily an absolute or useful argument. We infer across species about many things, and the inferences are usually accurate. Until we have done a definitive electrode study in the human premotor cortex, we could say we don't know for sure. But I don't think we should give up and wait until that experiment is done. Neuroscience carries many promissory notes of this kind, where we generate hypotheses based on such inferences or assumptions and move ahead, usually listening to see if there is an unexpected result that would lead us to a rethinking.

There is one part of Vivona's argument about the Directness Assumption that I can't quite agree with. She says that it emphasizes a direct nonverbal biological mechanism of understanding, and neglects the operation of verbal and cognitive processes. It is true that in the process of apprehending another's emotional state, the simulation model proposes a direct replay of the other's emotion; but as with the perception of purposeful action, the replay is at the signal level and does not necessarily evoke an action or a full-blown emotion. If the model turns out to be right, that simulation will be an early step in the complex process of empathy, or of "understanding" what the other person is feeling. That process will involve several areas of the brain, the autonomic system, and possibly language, until one is conscious of one's perception of the other's affect. A speculative analogy might be made to Joseph LeDoux's model of fear induction (1996). He suggests that there are two circuits that mediate a fear response. LeDoux has presented a by now well-known example about the sight of a stick that could be a snake. The perceptual mechanism has a short circuit through the amygdala to the reflex action centers, and then a longer circuit, which includes cortical areas and possibly the language areas. For affect recognition, the mirror neuron activity (simulation) may be something like the short circuit, which is usually followed by cortical elaboration (theory).

Vivona offers us a useful challenge to be careful when we jump categories, when we import from other sciences. This may go double for our attempts not only to understand what we do clinically with patients, but also to decide how, or whether, to use such scientific data to modify our techniques. Therapists change their techniques for many reasons. Some have to do with the perceived needs of certain patients, some to do with influence by teachers and by the changing zeitgeist, some to do with countertransference, and there are many more. Using what we learn from other sciences is another one, and it can be risky. As Vivona points out, much of our science is still in its infancy, and the findings keep changing. An example might be this. The mirror neuron model indicates that we powerfully influence our interlocutors by nonconscious mirroring mechanisms, although as we see above there is some debate about this. That could influence whether one uses the couch or not. But there are two views on that. You might want to face the patient because of this treasure trove of nonverbal transfer of affect, intention, and mutual mind-reading; or you might see that as distracting—that is, if you feel that it would interfere with free association, and you value free association. It could very well be that at this point a decision based on mirror neurons would be premature. But I would say that simply contemplating this question leads to a richer understanding of how free association might work, and how it might change under various conditions surrounding the analytic dyad. There are many similar questions that will allow analysts to be jointly engaged with other sciences. It almost doesn't matter what the answers turn out to be; the conversation is what counts.

Note

1 Previously published in the *Journal of the American Psychoanalytic Association*, 57: 551–558.

References

Blass, R. B. & Carmeli, Z. (2007) The case against neuropsychoanalysis: On fallacies underlying psychoanalysis' latest scientific trend and its negative impact on psychoanalytic discourse. *International Journal of Psychoanalysis*, 88: 19–40.

Csibra, G. (2004) Mirror neurons and action observation: Is simulation involved? *Interdisciplines.* www.interdisciplines.org/mirror/papers/4.

Freed, P. (2008) Can words become numbers? Sources of blur in the quantification of brain and mind: Commentary on "Functional neuroimaging-can it contribute to our understanding of processes of change?" *Neuropsychoanalysis,* 10: 17–23.

Gallese, V., Eagle, M. N., & Migone, P. (2007) Intentional attunement: Mirror neurons and the neural underpinnings of interpersonal relations. *Journal of the American Psychoanalytic Association,* 55: 131–176.

Ledoux, J. (1996) *The Emotional Brain.* New York: Simon & Schuster.

McCabe, D. P. & Castel, A. D. (2008) Seeing is believing: The effect of brain images on judgments of scientific reasoning. *Cognition,* 107: 343–352.

Olds, D. D. (2006) Interdisciplinary studies and our practice. *Journal of the American Psychoanalytic Association,* 54: 857–876.

Poldrack, R. A. (2008) Can cognitive processes be inferred from neuroimaging data? *Trends in Cognitive Sciences,* 10: 59–63.

Pulver, S. (2003) The astonishing clinical irrelevance of neuroscience. *Journal of the American Psychoanalytic Association,* 51: 755–772.

Solms, M. & Turnbull, O. (2002) *The Brain and the Inner World,* New York: Other Press.

Chapter 15

What if Freud Hadn't? Commentary on Arnold Modell's paper

Psychoanalysis, Neuroscience, and the Unconscious Self

Dr. Modell's paper is an enjoyable and helpful review of some of the important integrative work he has done in bringing other scientific and theoretical approaches to psychoanalysts, most important being the ideas of Gerald Edelman and Walter Freeman. I would like to comment on the author's view on 1) Freud's turning from his Project to a more psychological model; and 2) The unconscious as the biological source of meaning[1].

The first discussion arises from Modell's statement that Freud's turning away from attention to the brain, and abandonment of the efforts of the Project, was an unfortunate choice on his part, one which delayed the neuroscientific understanding of psychoanalysis. At the manifest level, that may have some truth, but there are other aspects to that history that we might think about. One is that it may have been a necessary choice at the time. It is commonly accepted that the neuroscience of the time was nowhere near ready to tackle the understanding of brain and mind. This is despite the work of Pribram and Gill (1976), whose classic monograph shows some of Freud's ideas in his neuro-psychological works to be quite prescient and in tune with current views of brain function. However, one might wonder what would have happened had Freud stuck with the Project, and his paper on Aphasia (Solms & Saling, 1986; Greenberg, 1997), which are deemed the cornerstones of his neuroscientific work?

We could fantasize that he would have not erected the *psychological* model that we know as psychoanalysis, but would have continued with a reductionist model eventually merging with the psychology that came to appear to be the most scientific approach, namely behaviorism. In this fantasy the psychoanalytic psychology would not have been invented, and the behavioral model would have been the only model available in the scientific realm. Instead of that, Freud developed the psychological model as a semi-scientific model, which continued separately and in parallel with behavioral science. Freud's model grew, and it was able to intellectually frame psychological events, underpinned by theories that later might not hold up, but for almost a century could create a meaningful comprehensive system, a model that

DOI: 10.4324/9781003399551-16

some consider the most comprehensive model available in the twentieth century.

To maintain a model with unsound and inconsistent foundations, scientific rigor, and demand for empirical validation could not be required. If they had been required, the discipline might have died in infancy. The model had to be maintained using a quasi-religious paradigm, and an institution on the model of a monastic order. Support would come from authorities—mostly Freud and other leaders in the field, from precedent, and from the experience of clinicians and their supervisors.

In a currently prevalent, somewhat negative view, this was a holding operation, awaiting the technology that would be able to study the brain at molecular, cellular and neuroanatomic levels. Using this psychological model psychoanalysts were free to observe, record and explain behavior in satisfying ways, many of which were useful clinically and accepted as helpful to patients. However, we may take a more positive perspective, such as that of the honoree of this journal issue, (Kandel, 2012) who makes a very important point:

> "(Freud) realized that before human behavior could be linked to brain science, a coherent, dynamic psychology of mind had to be developed... In developing this view, Freud was employing a strategy that had been applied repeatedly in science, one based on the belief that insights into causes are most likely to emerge if a subject has been systematically observed and described."
>
> (pp. 58–59)

Thus, rather than being a retreat to an inferior model because of a lack of neuroscientific knowledge, it was a necessary leap into a creative, descriptive framework that would contain the vast phenomenological detail for a future science to interpret.

In this historical fantasy in which Freud pursues the nascent neuroscientific approach, he and his colleagues would have made many premature connections and devised many incomplete theories. In the academic realm, behaviorism would have been dominant, would have progressed to uncover much of scientific merit, and would have evolved into the cognitive model. It would eventually arrive at the point of needing to explain higher-level mental functions. In this scenario, there would be no psychoanalysis on the parallel track with its rich lode of information about the complexities of the human mind. A psychoanalytic or mentalistic kind of model would have to be invented, using the behavioral and cognitive data at hand. It is interesting to speculate if this would have been a more productive route to have taken.

To pursue a second idea in Modell's paper, we might think about his view of the unconscious as our information processor, which essentially turns its inputs into meanings—at a different level—in which they can become conscious *as meanings*. Following Libet, who showed that, in a person making a choice, the brain event precedes the conscious event by a fraction of a second, he sees consciousness as a read-out phenomenon. "Consciousness is only an observational faculty, and in itself does not cause anything." Here I would demur. It seems to be a slip into dualism, which most of us foreswear, but which we find it difficult to avoid. In this version it is implied that the conscious experience is an end-state, the end of the neurological line, which has no further effect. That would be like saying something similar about perception, which is the end of the line—from the sense organ, through the thalamus, to the sensory cortex and the executive cortex, having no further causal effect. Knowing what we do about reflex arcs, operant conditioning and the like, this would be an absurd conclusion. A perception does cause other brain phenomena leading to actions, feeling and thoughts.

Consciousness, as an end process, is also a feedback event. It feeds back into the system and is part of the process leading to the next conscious experience. Indeed its major purpose may be this feedback, the subjective aspect being an affective jolt that indicates salience—"this is important." In Panksepp's (1998) model of three levels of mental process, the primary includes the basic affects, which provide the value aspect that influences the secondary and tertiary processes of the more evolved mental functions. Affect is basic to conscious experience, which is inherently subjective. In this model the affective basis for consciousness is present in all mammals, and probably other creatures as well.

A dual aspect monism approach (Solms & Turnbull, 2002, 2011) would hold that a conscious experience can be seen from the biological aspect involving the activation of certain brain circuits—possibly revealed by way of brain imaging—and also the subjective aspect, viewed by way of introspection. In this mode of thinking what do we do with *meaning?* Meaning is a catch-all word that seems to carry dualism all the way to an end game and provides no solution. As Modell points out meaning is a brain process on a different level in a hierarchy of biological structures, functioning at the level of symbolism both verbal and non-verbal. There are several ways to talk about this. One popular way is to say that meaning *emerges* from brain processes, a novel product, not quite predictable from knowledge of the brain. Another is to use a semiotic model and say that meanings are *signs* of brain processes, or entities that stand for such processes that communicate to the self, and to others, what is going on in the brain. Such a hierarchical model is an important aspect of Modell's work and is an important part of his contribution to the integrative thinking about mind and brain.

Note

1 Previously published in the *Psychoanalytic Review*, Vol. 99, No. 4: 485–489.

References

Greenberg, V. D. (1997) *Freud and his Aphasia Book: Language and the Sources of Psychoanalysis.* Cornell University Press.

Kandel, E. R. (2012) *The Age of Insight: The Quest to Understand the Unconscious in Art, Mind, and Brain, from Vienna 1900 to the Present.* New York: Random House.

Panksepp J. (1998) *Affective Neuroscience.* New York, Oxford.

Pribram, K. H. & Gill, M. M. (1976) *Freud's "Project" Re-assessed.* New York: Basic Books.

Solms, M. & Saling, M. (1986) On psychoanalysis and neuroscience: Freud's attitude to the localizationist tradition. *The International Journal of Psychoanalysis*, 67: 397–416.

Solms, M. & Turnbull, O. (2002) *The Brain and the Inner World.* New York: Other Press.

Solms, M. & Turnbull, O. (2011) What is Neuropsychoanalysis? *Neuropsychoanalysis*, 13 (2): 133–145.

Chapter 16

Thinking about Curriculum

An Interdisciplinary Perspective

Introduction

This paper discusses the role that curriculum development can play in preparing future psychoanalysts to participate in an on-going dialogue with colleagues in neighboring disciplines. Curriculum design can be used to encourage the development of an interdisciplinary perspective that can serve as an organizing framework to help candidates think about psychoanalytic knowledge in the context of what is known about the functioning of the mind and brain in other disciplines. It is possible to teach these complex matters in a way that students can find accessible and useful. We present exemplars taken from the curriculum designed and taught at the Columbia Center. We also present some of the problems we have faced and the lessons we have learned[1].

The rapid growth of knowledge in the biological sciences offers the possibility of a fruitful dialogue between those primarily interested in how the mind functions and those primarily interested in how the brain functions. Phenomena in the domain of psychoanalysis are beginning to interest colleagues in neighboring scientific disciplines, and phenomena in the domains of these disciplines are beginning to interest psychoanalysts. There are areas of mutual interest, the study of development, defense, representation, memory, motivation and affect for example, that may eventually allow for the development of bridging concepts and theories cast in a language that can help relate or correlate phenomena from these different domains. Kandel (1999) describes the emerging biology of mental processes as a new foundation for psychoanalysis; but for this new foundation to be useful, psychoanalysts need to pose the question that Kandel raises, "How does the biologically delineated unconscious relate to Freud's unconscious?" This of course harkens back to the questions Freud tried to answer for himself in the Project (1950 [1985]). Asking such questions again requires collaboration with neighboring sciences.

DOI: 10.4324/9781003399551-17

As Freud pointed out in *The Future of an Illusion*: "No, our science is no illusion. But an illusion it would be to suppose that what science cannot give us we can get elsewhere."

The focus of this paper will be the role psychoanalytic institutes can play in preparing future psychoanalysts to participate in an on-going dialogue with other scientific disciplines. We will begin by describing an interdisciplinary perspective and what this perspective is designed to achieve for our candidates and for our field. We will then describe a course for fourth year candidates at the Columbia Center for Psychoanalytic Training and Research, *Psychoanalytic Concepts: An Interdisciplinary Perspective*. This course has evolved over twenty-five years as we have grappled with the possibilities and problems involved in teaching information from neighboring sciences.

An Interdisciplinary Perspective

If candidates are to think critically and creatively about psychoanalytic knowledge and to help us end our intellectual isolation as a field, they must be able to understand and to evaluate psychoanalytic knowledge in the context of the knowledge in other disciplines. An interdisciplinary perspective helps candidates see the possibility of thinking across disciplinary boundaries, grounds psychoanalytic knowledge in the larger scientific culture and community of ideas, and so opens the way for dialogue with other fields. However, a meaningful dialogue with scholars and researchers in neighboring disciplines will only be possible if candidates begin to develop an acquaintance with language and concepts of others so that we can help these colleagues understand ours. Even if we do not yet know if or how the thinking and research in other fields can be relevant for psychoanalytic theorizing and technique, candidates benefit from an opportunity to consider this possibility. Our focus is on the cognitive and affective neurosciences and developmental studies. Institutes may be able to use our experience to fit their own faculty, trainees and educational interests. An interdisciplinary perspective can be focused on scientific developments in gender and sexuality, race and other aspects of the social-political environment as well.

As an example, let's return for a moment to the beginnings of our discipline, the collaboration between Freud and Breuer on the treatment of symptoms of hysteria. The diverging interests of Freud and Breuer regarding the origin and nature of hysterical phenomena can be thought about as containing the roots of two traditions. Freud's interest in the functioning of psychological defense, conflict, and fantasy led him to hypothesize the centrality of a dynamically determined unconscious in mental life and in symptom formation. Breuer's interest in states of mind, states of arousal or excitation of the nervous system and splits of consciousness or dissociation led him to emphasize state phenomena that are descriptively unconscious.

Freud and Breuer eventually broke off their collaboration. Freud, after his abandonment of his seduction hypothesis, left the trauma model behind, and with it his interest in states of mind. Repression became the cornerstone of psychoanalysis. However, today the widening scope of our treatment includes patients with trauma. Trauma is accompanied by hyperarousal, psychic numbing and dissociation, and these states can become traits (Perry et al., 1996). How are we to conceptualize the nature and functioning of residues and memories of trauma in relation to fantasy and conflict? What are the forms of remembering and the defenses against remembering trauma, as these are manifest in the analytic process? Do memories of trauma function differently from other memories because they are laid down during times when the brain is functioning differently? And if they do, what are the implications for our technique?

Evolution of the Course

The long term aim of our interdisciplinary curriculum is to bring the psychoanalytic discipline into as cogent a relationship as is possible with disciplines that study the functioning and development of the brain, particularly regarding unconscious processes, dreams, memory and affect. A more immediate aim is to offer candidates an opportunity to expand their appreciation of the potential for understanding the biological underpinnings of psychoanalytic theory and technique. We hope that this enriched theoretical foundation will encourage the creativity that will allow psychoanalytic theory to develop within the larger culture of science and in the community of ideas. Psychoanalysis has a vast body of clinical data and theory developed over the past century, indeed several bodies of theory, which relate in different ways to the brain-mind theories that are emerging. Our scientific colleagues can benefit from our unique data as we can from theirs.

In what follows we will describe innovations in the interdisciplinary curriculum at the Columbia University Center for Psychoanalytic Training and Research at a stage of its on going development. It may help the reader to take in the presentation if we describe very briefly the evolution of the curriculum.

The course began as a four-session course within the fourth year theory course, Advanced Psychoanalytic Concepts. This was in 1988 and at that time, the models of interest to psychoanalysts were from semiotics, information theory, neural networks and connectionism. From this tentative beginning, the course evolved into the course of twenty-two sessions that we will describe. Faculty development has been crucial in developing the course. Each faculty member had to gain some expertise and become somewhat specialized in an area of interest in these neighboring disciplines. Then we had to learn how to teach what we had learned in a meaningful way. This latter has been more difficult, and we continue to struggle to find ways to help candidates appreciate the clinical relevance of this new information when the bridges to psychoanalysis are still sparse.

At first, we organized the course around basic concepts in the cognitive sciences: representation, memory, consciousness, cognition and affect, for example. The candidates found this organization too distant from their psychoanalytic work. In response to this feedback, we decided to organize the course around basic psychoanalytic concepts. Topic headings included: The Body, The Ego and Modes of Representation; Transference and the Compulsion to Repeat; Trauma and Memory; Drive, Motivation and Affect; and Internalization, for example. We devoted two to four classes to each topic. In the first class, we explored the historical and current use of the concepts by psychoanalysts. In the next class or classes, we introduced information from other disciplines and, where possible, attempted to illustrate the usefulness of this information in relation to clinical cases. We found that the candidates needed to be able to think about the new concepts in immediate relation to clinical material for these concepts to be meaningful to them.

We expected that the course would change as the candidates' needs changed, as the faculty developed, and as the information and knowledge in our neighboring disciplines changed. After the first years, the Curriculum Committee asked us to include a more definite ego psychological perspective when it was thought that our candidates needed more depth in this perspective. We added a topic, Introduction to Modern Ego Psychology and a sequence of classes that compared the trauma model, the deficit model and the conflict model. Later, as candidates became interested in inter-subjectivity and attachment theory, we added Modes of Relating that included the classes: Attachment; Emergence of the Infant from the Dyad; and Intersubjectivity. As non-linear models emerged, we added Complex Systems Models to our topics. More recently the course has taken Embodiment as an integrating thread. Evolution and change in response to candidate feedback and changing training priorities is essential to this curriculum design.

Given the fact that the course has evolved over the years, we have chosen in this paper to present an iteration of the course that we think will be most useful to institutes that are considering an interdisciplinary curriculum for their candidates. We will describe the topics that the authors have taught in some detail. Thus, this paper is based on our experience organizing the course, and its continuing evolution over its first twenty-five years. Over the past five years, we have continued to teach some classes in the course, but the leadership of the course has appropriately passed from our hands, and the direction moved towards a relational orientation and a more intentional focus on theories of embodiment. We think this is a positive change and, to some extent, an attempt to provide a continuing theoretical underpinning to the changes occurring in the general psychoanalytic theory. The reading list in the Appendix represents an amalgam of the early structure of the course.

What We Have Learned

Teaching Methods

Our most challenging problem has been to find ways to answer the two questions most asked by our candidates. "Why do we need to know this? What difference does this make in what we do?" Our ways of answering have evolved since the course began and we have discovered that we must continually look for new ways to reach candidates. This is a delicate matter because our answers must reflect the fact that adequate bridging concepts do not yet exist. It is crucial that premature bridging not be encouraged as we try to interest candidates in the potential for bridging as our knowledge advances. With each year's class, we assess the degree of interest and skepticism and redirect our approach accordingly. We find that about half the candidates are more or less interested and the other half are not, with some inclined to reject what we hope to offer them. We have found that the rationale for the course must be presented at the beginning. We begin with the question, why do we need to know this? In the first class, we hope to show candidates that their thinking and clinical actions have already been affected by new clinical realities brought about largely by the nature of the patients they take into analysis. These new clinical realities—analyzing patients who are being medicated for depression and anxiety disorders, patients with PTSD and OCD, patients with attention and learning disorders—have already raised questions for them at the boundary between psychoanalysis and the biological sciences.

Teaching cannot be by the traditional method—read a paper and open a discussion with the hope that candidates will carry the discussion. Teaching must be actively guided and illustrated with clinical process or vignettes whenever possible. We have found two methods particularly effective. The first is a lecture conducted in a seminar style that is rich with information that calls for discussion. Questions can be posed to suggest the potential for clinical relevance. For example, when presenting the findings about the mirror neuron phenomenon we might discuss the implications for our use of the couch. The second method is to present a clinical case using clinical vignettes that include clinical process and present new information and concepts in relation to the clinical presentation. For instance, the class comparing the concepts of schema and unconscious fantasy is taught in this way. A case thought to demonstrate the influence of schema on the transference as well as the influence of unconscious fantasy in transference fantasies and dreams is presented for consideration. In this method, teaching points are drawn from the case presentation itself. The lecture format is only used to introduce the concepts.

As the course developed, we learned to teach more actively using the readings as a backdrop and as enrichment for those who chose to read.

Interactive discussion and guided learning with reference to clinical material worked best.

Organization of the Course

The course is organized around topic areas of two to four classes. Different teachers teach these topic areas. Consequently, providing an integrated skeleton for the course as a whole and coordinating the teaching of each topic with the others has been a challenge. Candidates have told us that they experience the course as discontinuous and bumpy. The effort to coordinate teaching has been addressed by a junior teacher serving as coordinator for at least half of the course or ideally for the whole course. We have found the coordinator to be essential to the smooth functioning of the course. The coordinator is able to harken back to information from earlier classes, and other teachers, to help integrate earlier topics with the current material. The benefit for the coordinator is that they learn a great deal, and in a number of cases have developed an interest in some particular topic, which they can use to prepare a class to teach in subsequent years.

Curriculum Exemplars

Before the course begins, we provide a four-session introduction discussing the epistemological problems associated with our discipline. Before embarking on an exploration of the possibilities for new knowledge across disciplinary boundaries, it is important for candidates to have an understanding that epistemological considerations present difficult and sometimes insurmountable problems. This preceding segment, entitled A Critical Evaluation of Psychoanalytic Knowledge, is designed to familiarize candidates with an epistemological perspective that gives them the tools to appreciate these problems.

We want candidates to understand the epistemological questions that confront our field. What is a psychoanalytic fact? Is our goal to understand and/or explain phenomena? Are we interested in causes? What do we consider evidence that would confirm or disconfirm our ideas? How are we to tell if one idea is better than another?

As an introduction to the interdisciplinary curriculum, we ask, what do you consider the proper relationship between neuroscience and psychoanalysis? Is the relationship between the mind and the brain relevant for psychoanalysis? If yes, or possibly yes, what are the problems that we face when we attempt to import and integrate information from outside the psychoanalytic situation?

In the year we are presenting, we wanted to highlight Kandel's critical question for psychoanalysis, mentioned above, "How does the biologically determined unconscious relate to Freud's dynamic unconscious?" As an illustration of the epistemological problems that Kandel's question poses, we decided to contrast the views of Peter Fonagy (1999) and Harold Blum (2003) on memory and therapeutic action. Blum's views rely on processes of a dynamic unconscious, while Fonagy's rely on non-conscious processes in a descriptive sense. The role of repression is central in their debate as it is in the exploration of the relationship between the dynamic unconscious and the biologically determined unconscious.

Blum argues that repressed early memories in the form of unconscious fantasies are expressed in the transference. These transference fantasies are compromise formations and so are not literal representations of early experience. A defensive element is inherent in the constellation. For Blum, the aim of psychoanalytic treatment is the analysis and working through of intrapsychic conflict and residues of trauma as these are manifest in the transference. As this occurs, memory can be revised.

Fonagy's model holds that early experience is encoded in parts of the brain different from those responsible for autobiographical memory. Early experiences with significant others are encoded in the form of mental models of self-other relationships. He envisions these models as constellations of non-conscious procedures that create expectancies in relationships with others. These expectancies are expressed in the transference in the way an analysand is with us, and in the way they experience being with us. These constellations do not exist in words or images. They are essentially nonverbal. According to Fonagy, the aim of a psychoanalytic treatment is to modify these mental models which can be modified in the context of the relationship with the analyst. The emphasis is on the process of being with the analyst rather than on the interpretation of unconscious fantasy. Consequently, psychoanalysis allows the active construction of new ways of experiencing with the analyst.

Fonagy and Blum offer alternative hypotheses about the nature of early memory and the nature of the transference. Repression is central to Blum's hypothesis. The activation of non-conscious mental models is central to Fonagy's hypothesis. We ask the candidates what problems they think Fonagy's hypothesis raises for a psychoanalytic perspective. We discuss the nature of the evidence cited by Blum and Fonagy. Blum cites clinical evidence—that emerging from the analysis of the transference—which brings to light long repressed childhood memories. Fonagy cites evidence from the cognitive and neurosciences, which reveal unconscious emotional processes that were never visualized or spoken about. We try to clarify the problems that arise when we use evidence from different methodological traditions.

Our candidates are aware that non-conscious processes are thought to be involved in the therapeutic action of psychoanalysis by some analysts. Consequently, some members of the class say that these hypotheses can be thought about together, even if we don't yet know how this works. Daniel Stern, who was for some time on our faculty, thought that non-conscious schemas of being with another shaped the formation of unconscious fantasy.

Such an idea opens the way for the possible collaboration between different types of memory encoding in the shaping of fantasy and transference.

Introduction to the Course: Interdisciplinary Studies and Our Practice

In 2006, we began introducing the course with a paper written to answer the question most asked by candidates: Why do we need to study this topic? (Olds, 2006). The paper discusses six topics that seemed most likely to have already had an effect on psychoanalytic thinking, so that they would be somewhat familiar to candidates: mirror neuron discoveries; memory research; cognitive processes and capacities; affect systems and disorders; trauma; and complex models of mind.

Mirror Neurons

The mirror neuron phenomenon, discovered by the Italian neuroscientists Rizzolatti and Gallese and colleagues in 1996, revealed the possibility that in order to perceive the actions of another person, and even to perceive another's affect, we simulate this movement or this affect in our own minds, using a complex brain system that includes the pre-motor cortex. Thus, we partially enact what we are seeing and therefore experience a signal aspect of it. This implies that when facing another person we are willy-nilly captivated in some way by the other's affect, this being a crucial aspect of all social interaction.

We invite candidates to think about how this observation might bear on the therapeutic encounter and the use of the couch. Candidates typically mention that the couch robs us of much information, since we are not vis-à-vis. Some argue that this is the purpose of the couch—to free us from the unconscious capture by the other, allowing both analyst and analysand to freely associate. Others think about the implications for processes like projective identification or internalization. All seem eager to think about aspects of the frame in new ways. We return to the mirror neuron concept later in the course in classes discussing inter-subjectivity, identification and, projective identification.

Modes of Memory

We move on to our thinking about memory. The concept of memory has been relatively undifferentiated in psychoanalytic thinking. The concept of procedural memory has emerged as part of the research into different types of memory, probably beginning with an observation in the case of HM, a patient. HM was treated for intractable epilepsy by the bilateral surgical removal of his hippocampus. After the surgery, he was found to have lost all recent memory for events but had not lost his previously learned skills in playing games or in social interaction. The memory for skills was seen as different from memory for recent events or episodic memory and was called procedural memory.

The important debate between Blum and Fonagy presented in the classes on a critical evaluation of psychoanalytic knowledge focused on just this issue, the role of memory and the nature of therapeutic change. Procedural or implicit memory has now become part of psychoanalytic discourse on therapeutic process and change. In 2006 the concept of memory systems based in different brain processes was new to candidates. However, their familiarity with the then emerging understanding of the role of facilitating enactments in the analytic process served as a conceptual bridge for them. We return to a consideration of the functioning of different kinds of memory in the classes on trauma and memories of trauma.

Cognitive Capacities

We turn next to differences in the cognitive and perceptual capacities in our analysands. People with variants of ADHD, learning disabilities, strabismus in childhood, or brain trauma, may have brains that function somewhat differently. When people with developmental challenges with stimulation, various learning demands and perceptional differences are taken into analysis they pose a challenge for analytic technique. Analytic technique modified to take their differences into account can be very effective. Important in this, however, is that the analyst understands the nature of these differences and their potential impact on fantasy and conflict as well as on cognitive function. We find that candidates have struggled with how to work with such analysands, and so are intrigued with thinking about ways to work with them within an analytic frame.

We have two classes devoted to the study of clinical material from an analysis of such a patient.

Affect and Affect Disorders

Probably the most dramatic intrusion into psychoanalytic practice results from research on affects and affect disorders. This research has led to an explosion in the use of psychopharmacological agents in all forms of psychotherapy. Most candidates have analysands who take medication. In many cases, the analysis could not take place without it. Candidates are concerned with how to think about how we can work with psychic reality when internal biological reality is being manipulated.

We can also note that the analytic profession has changed such that it is no longer the sole domain of medically trained analysts. Analysts now in training are more frequently from the disciplines of clinical psychology or social work. These differences in background knowledge present challenges for an institute's curriculum. For some candidates knowledge in the biological realm may need more attention than before. However, we now need also to be aware that while the medically trained candidates may be more prepared in biology and neurology, other candidates may have stronger training in the social sciences and the phenomenology of mental activity. We could now say that medically trained candidates need intensive training in psychoanalytic theory and social science and that the majority of current students need more in the realm of brain science, especially since that science is forging ahead rapidly. We feel that this greater diversity in our profession makes the kind of course herein described even more crucial.

Working with Trauma

In our brief survey of very complicated topics, we move on to begin a discussion about how we might think about working with trauma in the light of new information from trauma research. Analysts have been concerned with how to conceptualize memories of trauma and their function in the analytic process. Research on memory of trauma has shown that severe trauma leads to stress hormone flooding that has biological effects on the brain. The hippocampus, which plays an important role in autobiographical memory, can be inhibited in memory formation by stress hormones. If the trauma is prolonged, hippocampal cells can be destroyed. This means that we might consider that memories are absent not only due to repression, but they may not have been laid down at all. In that case, the memory is not recoverable. This raises a new technical question. How are we to handle the issue analytically? It is possible that our technique will not be aimed at the lifting of repression, but rather will be aimed at providing a narrative for an experience that is remembered in nonverbal fragments. We are left with a question: how do these nonverbal fragments influence fantasy and behavior? Candidates find this question interesting and perplexing. Here we have a biological underpinning of the Blum/Fonagy debate mentioned above. The unrepressed unconscious may also be relevant to the disruption from later life traumas, which overwhelm the hippocampus and its memory capacity. This can lead to important discussions about the technique of early encouragement to retell the trauma story, which some feel re-traumatizes the patient. It may be that the shutting down of the hippocampus has a protective function, and that the careful and slow bringing the memory into verbal consciousness, has a later curative function.

Complex Systems Models

Lastly, we introduce complex systems theories, a philosophically important addition to our thinking and theorizing. Complex systems theories focus on the complexity inherent in biological systems and some non-biological ones such as the weather and climate change. These theories present the view that phenomena in nature are caused, but that the more complex ones are not necessarily predictable. The important point for thinkers about human behavior is that predictability cannot be assumed. Our more linear causal theories might suggest more predictability than is warranted.

As may now be apparent, the Olds paper and its discussion form a kind of table of contents for the course, since in later classes these issues are explored more deeply in both their brain-science and clinical aspects. Topics not included in this list as described above, including attachment theory and modes of consciousness and unconsciousness, were added in later years.

We will now give more detailed accounts of classes that are or have been taught by the authors so that the educational intent and class process can be described. We try to give an impression of what we are trying to do, and to some extent how the students respond, and what kind of dialogue ensues.

The Body, The Ego, and Modes of Representation

For some years, following the introductory material just described, we began the interdisciplinary approach by exploring modes of representation, viewing this perspective as helpful when considering psychoanalysis in relationship to the neighboring sciences. Analysts have been more and more interested in exploring the unrepressed, the unthought, and the non-conscious aspects of mind. The ideas of Blum and Fonagy presented earlier are an example of analysts coming to grips with a focus on new modes of remembering, thinking and internalizing experience. Sensation, perception, object awareness, fantasy, memory, affect, and consciousness all involve modes of representation of different kinds. We discuss and compare modes of representation that are drawn from body experience and that contribute to schema formation, and fantasy.

Psychoanalytic Concepts

We begin the class with a quote from Freud. "If we consider mental life from a biological point of view...an instinct appears to us as a concept on the frontier between the mental and the somatic, as the psychical representative of the stimuli originating within the organism and reaching the mind, as a measure of the demand made upon the mind for work" [Instincts and Their Vicissitudes, 1915]. Freud's words allow us to begin on familiar ground. Freud is describing the transformation of somatic energy into psychic energy. He envisions instinct as a bridging concept between body and mind. "An instinct can never become the object of consciousness-only the idea that represents the instinct can" [The Unconscious, 1915]. We then explore Freud's concepts of fantasy and dreams. The motive force for the formation of fantasy, whether conscious or unconscious, and dreams, is a wish. A wish for Freud is a biologically determined unconscious state of urgency that activates memory traces of earlier experiences of satisfaction, and so makes a demand on the mind for representation, and on the organism for action in order to satisfy an instinctual need. The fantasy or the dream represents the disguised fulfillment of the wish in consciousness. Representation is a concept from the cognitive and neurosciences. However, Freud described fantasy as the mental representative of the drive. We hope to place this concept in a psychoanalytic frame of reference for the candidates using Freud's early study of "means of representation" in dreams. In describing the dream-work, Freud said, "The dream-thoughts and the dream-content are presented to us like two versions of the same subject-matter in two different languages. Or more properly, the dream-content seems like a transcript of the dream-thought in another mode of expression, whose characters and syntactic laws it is our business to discover by comparing the original and the translation." [Interpretation of Dreams, 1900] Freud envisioned the manifest dream as a pictorial script that was related to the dream-thoughts that had been transformed by processes that constituted the dream-work—condensation and displacement, for example. He illustrated these ideas in his specimen dream, The Dream of Irma's Injection.

We use Erik Erikson's analysis of the Irma Dream as a basis for the discussion. In his paper, Erikson (1954) extended Freud's understanding of the influence of heredity, constitution, somatic functioning and the developmental unfolding of sexuality on mental representation to include context and culture. Like Freud, Erikson was interested in the form of things, the shape and configuration of the dream as well as the content. We want the candidates to appreciate that there are modes of representation formed in intimate connection with our perceptual, sensory, affective and interpersonal experience. Erikson highlights the dimensions of the manifest dream in these terms. He thought that the ego manifests its unique nature in the style of its representations. These could be studied in the manifest dream itself.

We next consider another of Freud's concepts that we think bears on mental representation, the concept of presentation. Freud described two forms, a thing presentation and a word presentation. A presentation is a cathexis of a memory trace derived from sense perceptions. A presentation is a process for Freud, a process that has its origin in memories of body experience. Candidates are often thinking in terms of mental *content,* and we want to help them begin to think about mental *processes* that constitute the mind.

With this preparation, we can now ask, what is a mental representation? Mental representation is the transformation in the mental sphere of biological drives, body states, perceptions, affects, memories and the patterns and configurations determined by the functioning of the brain and the internalization of experience. Representation is thus a phenomenon whereby one thing can *stand for* another. As Freud told us, the instinct can only be known by the idea that represents it. The idea stands for the activity of the instinct. We now think that there are other forms beyond ideas, pre-conceptual schemas and mental models, for example. Drive, affect, perception and memory are the ingredients for a variety of modes of representations of mental processes: images, gestures, words, schema, fantasy and dreams. We want to interest the candidates in what determines and shapes these processes at the levels of brain and mind. We want the candidates to appreciate that a fantasy or a dream or a schema is the result of a representational process or chain of neural and mental events.

Unconscious Fantasy and Schema

In this class, we explore the ways in which our psychoanalytic concept of unconscious fantasy can be related to or differs from the concept of schema (Rees, 2012). The discussion is based on process material from the analysis of a man whose mother was depressed and so neglectful in his early years of life. Aspects of the transference seemed best described by the schema of being with such a mother. Other aspects were better described as the enactment of unconscious fantasies.

Schema is a concept from the developmental and cognitive neurosciences. Schema, in the sense we are using this concept, is an organization of mental processes that takes on the character of a structure that then shapes subjective experience. This is a description that could also describe unconscious fantasy. The projection of body experience to the realm of meaning recalls Freud's understanding of the impact of the somatic functions on the structuring of the sexual drive and fantasy. We compare and contrast Daniel Stern's (1985, 1995) ideas about the representation of subjective experience in the infant with the psychoanalytic concept of unconscious fantasy.

We begin with the notion of schema because this is much less familiar to candidates. A schema embodies patterns of experience. It is not a template but a malleable dynamic structure that organizes mental representations pre-conceptually. Disparate experiences are connected, "yoked together" in Stern's terms. He tells us that the infant has the capacity to transfer perceptual experience from one sensory modality to another. He calls this trans modal perception. Stern's *schema of being with another* brings together the realms of affect, sensation, perception, action and intentionality. A schematic structure thus operates as a gestalt or a unified meaningful whole that can structure perceptions and images and organize mental representations. These structures influence expectations of others and of the world, as do unconscious fantasies.

As an example of such a network of schemas, we ask the candidates to imagine the experience of nursing as Stern describes this. Stern envisions the subjective experience of feeding as like a series of musical phrases. The infant experiences hunger, hears and feels the approach of the mother, feels the movement to the breast, experiences the smell, sights, sounds and feel of the mother/breast, feels milk in the mouth and the sense of satiation then rest. This experience exists in time and has what Stern refers to as a shape in time. To help clarify this, we ask the candidates to remember Freud's description of the situation of satisfaction. The situation of satisfaction includes all the perceptual aspects of sight, smell, touch, sounds, movements, feelings and rhythms associated with the breast, the mother, sucking and the relief of tension or hunger. In his *Project for a Scientific Psychology* (1950, [1895]), Freud envisioned the neuronal underpinnings for a wish as facilitation among complexes of perceptual neurons that associated a state of urgency with the memory of satisfaction. When this network of neurons was activated, a state of hunger could be represented consciously as a hallucination of the situation of satisfaction. Later, a frustrated wish could find representation as a fantasy. Freud hypothesized the formation of wishes embedded in wishful fantasies: while Stern hypothesizes the formation of schemas that are later refigured in fantasy. We ask the candidates to tell us how they think these concepts differ with respect to our theories of unconscious motivation. Although Stern includes the infant's perception of intentionality in the other, this is probably very different from the infant's perception of the other's unconscious motivation and fantasy life. Stern does not discuss the issue of innate motivational factors other than affect and hedonics.

Stern does not see schema as functioning in the same way as fantasy. He sees schema of early experience as something like a building block as fantasy develops. This then leaves room for the refiguring of schema in response to unconscious motivation. However, Stern thinks that the experiences of the "real child" that have been encoded in schema must be given weight in our understanding of the experience and the fantasies of the adult.

We move on to the Kleinian concept of unconscious phantasy as this is presented in Susan Isaacs' paper, The Nature and Function of Phantasy (1952). We chose to include the Kleinian concept because it connects to and makes it necessary to ask developmental questions about the nature of mental representation in the earliest years of life. The Kleinians consider unconscious phantasy the primary content of unconscious mental life and the direct representative of the instinctual drives. Perception, affect, sensation, impulses and psychological defenses are experienced as unconscious phantasies from the beginning of life. There has been controversy about the possibility of unconscious phantasy so early in life. Here it is interesting to wonder with the candidates whether Stern's concept of pre-conceptual schema might be helpful in understanding the nature and functioning of unconscious phantasies and their development.

Trauma and Memory

Neurobiological research and theorizing about memory systems with particular focus on autobiographical memory, emotional memory and memories of emotions and more than a century of trauma research offer an opportunity for us to think again about leaving Freud's early work on trauma behind. We can ask questions now with more expectation that, with the help of other disciplines, we can achieve greater understanding over time. We pose for the candidates the questions raised in the introduction. How are we to conceptualize the nature and functioning of residues and memories of trauma in relation to fantasy and conflict? What are the forms of remembering and the defenses against remembering trauma, as these are manifest in the analytic process? Do memories of trauma function differently than other memories because they are laid down during times when the brain is functioning differently? And if they do, what are the implications for our technique?

Clinical observations from two analysands following the 9/11 terrorist attack in New York City provide the clinical basis for an exploration of the relationship between trauma in adulthood and residues of trauma from earlier in life (Rees, 2002). The focus is on the experience of the terrorist attack as it apparently affected memory and defense in the therapeutic process.

K and H each had conscious memories and fantasies about trauma in childhood but without the expected feelings. Attempts to help them gain access to these feelings were repeatedly met with an unusual tenacity of resistance. However, in the weeks following the terrorist attack, K and H gained access to feelings associated with childhood trauma or more precisely that they associated with childhood trauma. Defenses against an awareness of these feelings in the transference diminished so that the transference was more alive. This new emotional intensity lasted about three months and then gradually subsided. Even after an awareness of these emotions receded, conscious memories of childhood trauma remained altered. An emotional dimension seemed to have been added. K and H felt that a missing piece of themselves had been restored. An emotional context for familiar memories and fantasies seemed to deepen their self-understanding. As time went on, these narrative memories were sometimes remembered with feeling. More usually, they were remembered in close association with the *memory* of the feeling.

We ask the candidates how they understand what happened in the analytic process after September 11? Two hypotheses emerged in the discussion. The first is that the current trauma awakened emotional memories from the past because the current trauma involved sensory and affective elements that resembled the past trauma. The second is that states of mind in the present recruited memories of trauma from the past as in the way that anxiety recruits content. We remind the candidates that Freud and Breuer studied the influence of affect and states of mind on the remembering and forgetting of trauma. Breuer was particularly interested in the affect of fright and the effects of hyper excitability of the nervous system. Freud was interested in psychological defenses against stimuli that overwhelmed the mind leading to splits in consciousness and defenses triggered by anxiety in the face of wishes that were intolerable when conscious. The focus on states of mind led to an investigation of dissociation. The focus on conflict, fantasy and meaning led to an investigation of the functioning of repression. We ask the candidates to think about how these two kinds of defenses might shape the analytic process, and how they might contribute to understanding the nature of resistances to remembering when they operate together.

In order to ground the discussion in research, we turn to the work of Joseph Le Doux (1996), a neuroscientist interested in the brain mechanisms underlying emotion and memory, particularly anxiety and fear. We are interested in his work on the memory system associated with the amygdala, a group of neurons at the tip of the temporal lobe. The amygdala is thought to mediate the emotional experience of fear and to preserve information that promotes survival and safety in the form of implicit emotional memories. Le Doux differentiates emotional memories from memories of emotions. Emotional memories are of bodily responses and emotional arousal. Memories of emotions are explicit memories of events in narrative form. The hippocampus is thought to mediate these memories. In an emotional situation, these separate memory systems operate in parallel, but they function differently and are dissociable one from another. These systems are also anatomically and developmentally distinct. The amygdala represents features of things and fragments of experience. The hippocampus represents objects and events. The hippocampal system provides narrative and autobiographical context; the amygdala provides emotional coloring and body states. These two systems have different triggers for remembering and different mechanisms for not remembering.

The concept of triggers for emotional memories leads into a discussion of the nature of memories of trauma. Memories of trauma tend to be experienced as fragments of sensory components, images, sensations, feelings without narrative at first (Van der Kolk & Fisler, 1995). Recall is triggered by exposure to sensory or affective stimuli that match sensory or affective elements associated with the trauma. The affect, *terror* for example, seems to be a critical cue. Meaningless stimuli become cues that signal potentially dangerous situations on the basis of past experience with similar situations. One example for many New Yorkers is the clear blue sky and the bright sunny day on September 11.

Le Doux points out that the two memory systems can be represented together in working memory. This finding offers a way of understanding what K and H experienced after the terrorist attack. We raise the possibility that the terror experienced on September 11 served as a trigger for memories of trauma from earlier in life for K and H. The affects in the present and/or the remembered affect from the past could then be held in working memory along with the narrative memories of the earlier trauma. A new memory would be formed in the present that had emotional coloring. This new memory faded with time but the memory of the feelings in this new memory persisted as part of the narrative.

These clinical observations allow us to hypothesize about the interaction of psychological forms of defense and two kinds of dissociation. First, the emotional memories mediated by the amygdala have no access to consciousness. They are dissociated from consciousness as a result of their brain circuitry. Second, it is in the nature of trauma to overwhelm thought and cognitive processing. Trauma is experienced without words and without categories for narrative at first. Technically, we need to provide words, and form narratives, for these fragments of bodily experience. Psychological defenses presuppose that the experience has been available to consciousness but has been dynamically removed from awareness. Technically, we are on more familiar ground as we attempt to analyze the fantasies and conflicts that motivated the defenses. It is important for candidates to appreciate that when trauma is involved, the tenacity of the apparent resistance may be inherent in the nature of memories of trauma as well as motivated by fears of re-traumatization based in a memory of the mind having been actually overwhelmed.

Our clinical experience with memories of trauma offers us an opportunity to observe the interaction of phenomena based in the descriptive unconscious and the dynamic unconscious. As we learn more, we can differentiate our technique to more effectively address the way the mind is functioning.

Internalization

Internalization is a concept that lends itself to an interdisciplinary exploration. We hope to interest candidates in the diverse processes that contribute to the phenomenon. The psychoanalytic construct of internalization has included the concepts of *incorporation*—a primitive fantasy of ingestion, taking the other inside one's own body; *introjection*—a sense of taking in the other as a virtual object, as a conscious advisor or critic, an internalized parent and; *identification*—a change of the self to resemble the other—often related to ego and superego development. The construct of internalization now may include phenomena and processes from the neural, genetic and, epigenetic domains. Consequently, processes and phenomena that are conscious, dynamically unconscious and non-conscious may contribute to our current understanding of this psychoanalytic concept. For example, imitation, modeling of self on other is largely a conscious process as is learning, while intrapsychic processes such as identification and introjection are dynamically unconscious, and neural. Genetic and epigenetic processes are descriptively unconscious or non-conscious. Brief examples using these threads serve to expand the candidates' appreciation of the concept of internalization and as an example of integrating biological knowledge and psychoanalytic phenomena and concepts (Olds, 2006a).

We begin our discussion with an evolutionary perspective. We think it is important that candidates think about human capacities in an evolutionary context because this will help them understand the development of these capacities and their functioning in possible relationship to psychoanalytic theory. Over the span of the history of our species, internalization has been part of the development of our mental capacities and our culture. If we look to what is known in primates, we can find evidence for imitation and possibly for identification. In primates, the process of "aping" is actually primitive, but it does lead to modest examples of culture. A chimp raised by humans was photographed sitting on a boulder paging through a book, as if reading. Another, when asked to sort his own photo with photos of other chimps or with people, placed his photo with the people. Humans have taken on imitation in a big way, and it is one of the prime movers of the capacity for the development of culture. Babies can be seen to imitate shortly after birth. Imitation is so important that it may excede obvious behavioral rewards; for example painful religious rituals, which are non-rewarding except for the reward of social approval and bonding.

Humans are more inclined to imitate than primates, and in some cases this may put them at a disadvantage in relation to apes. An experiment by Tomasello (1999) compared chimpanzees and human two-year-olds in regard to learning. Both groups were given a rake and the opportunity to use it to rake in candy rewards. One group was shown how to do it the wrong way with the rake teeth side down, and the other was shown the right way, teeth side up. Human children tried to imitate the instructor and so do it the wrong way for much longer than chimps. Chimps quickly tried different methods and succeeded faster—and got much more candy—than the children.

In the analytic situation, there may be imitation of the analyst in various ways, these having little to do with behavioral rewards, and more to do with fantasies about approval from the analyst, or approval from others if one becomes more like the analyst, and therefore part of the analytic culture. There is much to be learned about the role of imitation in bonding and in cultural evolution.

Another evolutionary link at the neuronal level is the mirror neuron phenomenon, mentioned earlier. This may be one mechanism underlying imitation, as well as perception and interpretation of behavior and affect in both primates and humans. The idea that we perceive and may simulate what we perceive in our minds is somewhat surprising and thought provoking for our understanding of the analytic process. As one sits with a patient, one can imagine how this works, not like a camera sending light patterns to passive film or data disk, but a much more interactive, motoric, responsiveness, which includes all the perceptual properties and relevant emotions as well. This may be an aspect of embodied listening and responsiveness. When the neuroscience research is explored, our views of the interpersonal field become much more exciting, dramatic and complex than we could ever have thought. For example, how does this form of internal imitation or simulation influence identification or fantasies of incorporation or the capacity for empathy and understanding?

We move from an evolutionary and neuronal context to the level of genes and gene expression. It is becoming apparent that experience can alter gene expression. For example, a New Zealand study (Caspi, 2002) showed that in a prospectively observed group followed from childhood through adulthood, one genetic configuration predicted greater similarity in parents and offspring. A sub-group of children carried a gene coding for a variant form of the monoamine oxidase (MAO), which was named MAOA. Of the group, some parents had seriously physically abused their children. Either the nature theory or the nurture theory could predict that these children would become violent abusers. However, it turned out that those children with the MAOA variant who were abused were more likely to become abusers, while those children who had the normal MAO were not more likely to become abusers. Also, those with the MAOA variant raised in non-violent homes were *not* more likely to become abusers. Here is a complex interaction between gene and environment that may influence the tendency to identify. This raises the interesting question; does genetic make-up influence processes of identification and if so how? However, this brings us back to our earlier discussion of dynamic systems and unpredictability. Here we see that the outcome with the abused child with a MAOA variant must be considered in terms of *probability*, and we ought to include gene variance. When the outcome includes a healthy adult we now tend to attribute this to "resilience."

Our educational goal for this class is that candidates have an opportunity to envision the complexity that may underlie our fundamental concepts. The new information about imitation, mirror neurons and gene expression gives us a glimpse of how complex these processes can be. This complexity can be intimidating. When all we could do was interpret aspects of the Oedipus complex, our job was simpler. Now we have to deal with several levels of causation. We must now ask, how do we understand the interaction of these levels as they may influence our concepts and our technique? This is a difficult issue and it requires a number of class discussions for candidates to sort through and be more comfortable with the complexity involved.

Reductionism and its Discontents

We may be approaching the time in the history of our discipline that Freud anticipated, when we are able to rethink our theoretical foundations in light of a growing body of knowledge from interdisciplinary science. This new knowledge offers our candidates flexibility and creativity in thinking about their clinical work and in making contributions to the evolution of our profession.

One of the things we discuss to varying degrees in different classes is the issue of reductionism. Candidates are concerned about this possibility. Some consider psychoanalysis a special field where dualism must be maintained if we are to maintain complexity. There has recently been a heated debate between Mark Solms and Rachel Blass (Blass & Carmelli, 2007; Sandberg, 2016; Yovell et al., 2015) that in recent years we have presented to candidates to help them think about whether an interdisciplinary perspective is – according to Blass – irrelevant and dangerous to psychoanalysis. This is certainly an issue to confront.

We offer conceptual tools that we hope will aid their thinking. One is the philosophical concept of *dual aspect monism*. In this model, the mind and brain can be viewed from two different *aspects* (Solms & Turnbull, 2002). One aspect includes viewing the brain and mind from an external perspective using all the techniques at our command: observation; fMRI and PET imaging; electroencephalogram (EEG) studies; for example. The second aspect views the brain's function and the mind from within using introspection and self-reflective awareness. For now, we don't understand how these two perspectives relate to one another so we use a heuristic that may provide a bridge. The heuristic that we use is the semiotic "standing for" relationship in which meanings are forms of representation that stand for neuronal forms of representation (Olds, 2000). We hope this more complex model will help avoid slipping into a simplistic monism.

These ways of framing the problem of reductionism are not intended to minimize the problem or the concern but rather to allow the candidates to hold their concerns in mind while considering how neural and mental phenomena might be thought about together.

Among the candidates we teach there are some who have a resistance to scientific understanding about psychoanalysis. However, more and more often there are candidates who are already quite knowledgeable about the brain sciences. This difference allows for vigorous discussion among the candidates. In this context, we find it helpful to discuss again the different epistemological stances about the nature of our discipline, the scientific and the hermeneutic. We hope to show candidates that these stances can complement one another.

Change and Future Evolution

This kind of course is different from the usual in the demands that it makes on faculty to keep up with developments in neighboring disciplines. The main thing we can predict is that the course must change as it tries to integrate the constant input from scientific neighbors. At the same time, psychoanalysis will change as it develops from one generation of psychoanalysts to another. In other words, each generation of beginning candidates, is facing a landscape, shaped by different brain knowledge and evolving models of analytic theory. Our hope is that a proactive interdisciplinary perspective can foster the best possible dialogue and integration with our scientific neighbors.

Why teach this? Let us return to that question. Why do we even ask it? If we are to end our isolation as a discipline, psychoanalytic knowledge must be consistent with knowledge of the mind and brain in neighboring disciplines, and dialogue with colleagues in these disciplines must be established. However, in the current climate of training and practice, we ask this because many candidates undertake the additional training in psychoanalysis hoping to enrich their skills in doing psychoanalytic psychotherapy. In this context, the emerging knowledge from, for example, child developmental studies, and from the study of the descriptively unconscious processes like procedural memory, offers the analyst/psychotherapist a multidimensional framework in which to think about theory and to differentiate technique. How might this interdisciplinary knowledge help improve concepts, theory and technique? Some possibilities include the following:

1   The analyst who has this multi-layered knowledge can use it to augment the training and supervision that teaches analytic method. New sources of possible causation and influences on the patient's current thought, feeling and behavior can be considered. The interdisciplinary information adds new kinds of information and a more complex picture of mental functioning, which can allow for innovation in technique within an analytic frame, refinement of analytic concepts, and the evolution of analytic theory.

2   This wealth of detail helps avoid some absurd conclusions such as that everything boils down to the Oedipal, that affect disorder is irrelevant, or misconceptions about the nature of memory. We do not want to follow leads that are incompatible with what we know about biology.

3   The possibility that psychoanalytic understanding will be replaced by or interfered with by biological understanding should be looked at carefully. When such a replacement seems to be occurring, this could be an opportunity for bringing analytical and biological learning together in a way that enhances each. In the future, we may use the dual aspect perspective to broaden our thinking and our research possibilities so that we do not compromise the essence of the psychoanalytic point of view.

4   If analysts have good current knowledge of how the brain/mind operates, they may be more comfortable doing their work, thus reducing the sometimes excessive tension in the analytic hour, which may indeed arise from errors of understanding and emphasis, i.e. inappropriately emphasizing Oedipal issues over depression, or failing to understand the immediate and long-term effects of childhood trauma.

Conclusion

In this chapter, we have described one iteration of a fourth-year theory course at the Columbia Psychoanalytic Center, whose goal is to provide candidates with information from neighboring sciences that is relevant or potentially relevant for psychoanalysis. This interdisciplinary perspective can allow analytic candidates to consider a biological underpinning to their knowledge of psychoanalytic theory and technique. The hope is that, in a way similar to that in other graduate programs, our candidates, as educated professionals, will learn more than a technique. A theoretical background that includes and is coherent with information and ideas in neighboring sciences enriches one's knowledge and understanding allowing for greater depth and possibly creativity in the field. Our larger aim is to give candidates an opportunity to bring psychoanalysis as a discipline into a cogent relationship with an evolving understanding of the brain and its functioning, with particular interest in unconscious processes. We hope that an interdisciplinary perspective will encourage a dialogue with other disciplines that will allow psychoanalytic theory to make sense in the larger culture of science.

Note

1 Previously published by David Olds and Ellen Rees in the *Journal of the American Psychoanalytic Association* (2018), 66: 1089–1120.

References

Blass, R. B. & Carmelli, Z. (2007) The case against neuropsychoanalysis. On fallacies underlying psychoanalysis' latest scientific trend and its negative impact on psychoanalytic discourse. *The International Journal of Psychoanalysis*, 88 (1): 19–40.

Blum, H. (2003) Psychoanalytic controversies, repression, transference and reconstruction. *International Journal of Psychoanalysis*, 84: 497–513.

Caspi, A. et al. (2002) Role of genotype in the cycle of violence in maltreated children. *Science*, 297: 851–854.

Damasio, A. (2018) *The Strange Order of Things: Life Feeling and the Making of Cultures*. New York: Pantheon.

Erikson, E. (1954) The dream specimen of psychoanalysis. *Journal of the American Psychoanalytic Association*, 2:16–52.

Freud, S. (1950 [1985]) The project for a scientific psychology. *Standard Edition* 1: pp. 283–397.

Freud, S. (1893–95) Studies on hysteria. *Standard Edition* 2: pp. 3–305.

Freud, S. (1900) The interpretation of dreams. *Standard Edition* 4 and 5

Freud, S. (1913) Totem and taboo. *Standard Edition* 13: pp. 1–161.

Freud, S. (1915) The unconscious. *Standard Edition* 14: pp. 161–215.

Freud, S. (1915) Instincts and their vicissitudes. *Standard Edition* 14: pp. 117–140.

Freud, S. (1927) Future of an illusion. *Standard Edition* 21: pp. 56.

Fonagy, P. (1999) Guest Editorial, Memory and therapeutic action. *International Journal of Psychoanalysis*, 80: 215–223.

Isaacs, S. (1952) The nature and function of fantasy. *Developments in Psychoanalysis*. London: Hogarth Press.

Kandel, E. (1999) Biology and the future of psychoanalysis. *American Journal of Psychiatry*, 156: 505–524.

Le Doux, J. (1996) *The Emotional Brain*. New York: Simon & Schuster.

Olds, D. D. (2000) A semiotic model of mind. *Journal of the American Psychoanalytic Association*, 48: 497–529.

Olds, D. D. (2006a) Identification: psychoanalytic and biological perspectives. *Journal of the American Psychoanalytic Association*, 54: 17–46.

Olds, D. D. (2006b) Interdisciplinary studies and our practice. *Journal of the American Psychoanalytic Association*, 54: 857–876.

Perry, B. D., Pollard, R. A., Blakley, T. L. , Baker, W. L., & Vigilante, D. (1996) Childhood trauma, the neurobiology of adaptation and use-dependent development of the brain: How states become traits. *Infant Mental Health Journal*, 16: 271–291.

Rees, E. (2002) *Some clinical observations after September 11: awakening the past September 11: Trauma and Human Bonds*. Hillsdale, NJ: Analytic Press.

Rees, E. (2012). Unconscious fantasy and schema: A comparison of concepts. In *From the Couch to the Lab: Trends in Psychodynamic Neuroscience*. Oxford: Oxford University Press.

Rizzolatti, G., Gallese, V. et al. (1996) Premotor cortex and the recognition of motor actions. *Cognitive Brain Research*, 3 (2): 131–141.

Sandberg, L. S. (2016) The argument for (and against) neuropsychoanalysis. *The International Journal of Psychoanalysis*, 97 (4): 1149–1150.

Solms, M. & Turnbull, O. (2002) *The Brain and the Inner World: An Introduction to the Neuroscience of Subjective Experience*. London: Karnac.

Stern, D. (1985) *The Interpersonal World of the Infant*. New York: Basic Books.

Stern, D. (1995) The nature and formation of the infant's representations. In *The Motherhood Constellation*. New York: Basic Books.

Tomasselo, M. (1999) *The Cultural Origins of Modern Cognition*. Cambridge, MA: Harvard University Press.

Van der Kolk, B. A. & Fisler, R. (1995) Dissociation and the fragmentary nature of traumatic memories: Overview and exploratory study. *J. Traumatic Stress*, 8:505–525.

Yovell, Y., Solms, M., & Fotopoulou, A. (2015) The case for neuropsychoanalysis: Why a dialogue with neuroscience is necessary but not sufficient for psychoanalysis. *The International Journal of Psychoanalysis*, 96: 1515–1553.

Index